AMYLOIDOSIS – AN INSIGHT TO DISEASE OF SYSTEMS AND NOVEL THERAPIES

Edited by **Işil Adadan Güvenç**

Amyloidosis – An Insight to Disease of Systems and Novel Therapies
Edited by Işil Adadan Güvenç

Published by InTech

Janeza Trdine 9, 51000 Rijeka, Croatia

Publishing Process Manager Petra Zobic

Technical Editor Teodora Smiljanic

Cover Designer InTech Design Team

Additional hard copies can be obtained from orders@intechopen.com

Amyloidosis – An Insight to Disease of Systems and Novel Therapies,
Edited by Işil Adadan Güvenç
p. cm.
ISBN 978-953-307-795-6

For EU product safety concerns:
IN TECH d.o.o., Prolaz Marije Krucifikse Kozulić 3, 51000 Rijeka, Croatia,
info@intechopen.com or visit our website at intechopen.com.

Meet the editor

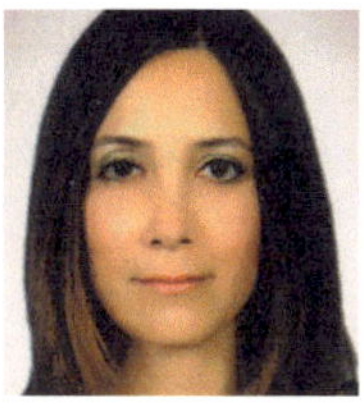

Dr. Işıl Adadan Güvenç was born in 1976, in İzmir, Turkey. After graduating from American Collegiate Institute in İzmir, she received her medical degree at Hacettepe University, Faculty of Medicine in 2000. Then she specialized in Otorhinolaryngology-Head and Neck Surgery at İzmir Atatürk Research and Training Hospital. Today she works in Zübeyde Hanım Research and Training Hospital, related to Başkent University in İzmir as a specialist. She has 12 published articles in respectable international journals and three articles in national journals. She is married to an architect and has a 9 month-old son, named Kaan.

Contents

Preface

Amyloidosis is a benign, slowly progressive condition characterized by the presence of extracellular fibrillar proteins in various organs and tissues. It has systemic or localized forms. Systemic amyloidosis can involve multiple organs, and shortens life expectancy, whereas localized amyloidosis usually has a benign course.

Both systemic and localized amyloidosis have been a point of interest for many researchers and there have been a growing number of case reports in the literature for the last decade. The aim of this book is to help the reader become familiar with the presentation, diagnosis and treatment modalities of systemic and localized amyloidosis.

The first and second sections focus on systemic and localized amyloidosis. Each chapter discusses a specific organ or system and is based on review of the literature in English language. The last section consists of three chapters in which novel therapies of amyloidosis are introduced.

I would like to thank all of the authors who have contributed to this book and I believe that this book will provide useful information to physicians and other health professionals practicing in various medical fields.

Işıl ADADAN GÜVENÇ, MD
Department of Otorhinolarygology
Head and Neck Surgery
Başkent University
Zübeyde Hanım Research and Training Hospital
İzmir,
Turkey

Part 1

Systemic Amyloidosis

1

Clinical Presentation of Amyloid A Amyloidosis

Nurşen Düzgün
Ankara University; Faculty of Medicine
Department of Rheumatology
Turkey

1. Introduction

Amyloid is an eosinophilic substance which appears "apple-green birefringence" in Congo red stained tissue sections under polarized light. This standard histological analysis is supported with immunochemistry technic using specific antibodies directed against most of the common human amyloid proteins, and also amyloid proteins can be identified with characteristic fibrillar appearance by electron microscopy (1).

Amyloidosis is a name given to a heterogenous group diseases. It is caused by the extracellular amyloid deposition as insolubl fibrillar aggregates that destroy normal tissue architecture and interfere normal function of tissues and organs. The biochemical nature of the precursor protein forming the amyloid fibrils differs in the different clinical conditions such as chronic inflammatory infectious or non-infectious diseases, malignancies, hereditary diseases and other less common disorders. Identification of the type of amyloidosis is important to assess clinical management, prognosis and treatment. Amyloid fibril protein nomenclature "2010 recommendations of the nomenclature commitee of the International Society of Amyloidosis" was reported and 27 human fibril proteins were described. In current nomenclature, a prefix "A" shows amyloid, followed by an abbreviation orginated from the name of the precursor protein (for example, AL addresses amyloid derived from immunglobulin light chain, AH shows amyloid derived from immunglobulin heavy chain, AA indicates amyloid derived from serum amyloid A (SAA) protein, $Aß_2M$ shows amyloid orginated from $ß_2$ microglobulin, ATTR describes amyloid derived from transthretin, and others). The amyloidoses can be classified according to localized or systemic deposits along with its biochemical nature (2).

Localised amyloid depositions usually lead to mechanical interference and generally are considered to be benign. Alzheimer's disease is the only form of localized amyloid fibril deposition which often leads to serious disorder.

Systemic amyloid forms include mainly immunoglobulin light chain (AL) amyloidosis, secondary, reactive (AA amyloidosis), hereditary familial form (for example, ATTR amyloidosis) and dialysis-related ($A\beta_2M$) amyloidosis (3,4). AA, AL and ATTR amyloidosis involve more than 90% of systemic amyloidosis (5).

AL amyloidosis is the most common form of systemic amyloidosis in western world. The ratio AL/AA amyloidosis appears 2/1 in the Netherlands (6). A retrospective study from

France suggests a 3/1 AL/AA ratio (7). These ratios should be supported by prospective studies in the world. AL amyloidosis is caused by clonal plasma cells that produce misfolded light chains, associated with B cell lymphoproliferative diseases such as multiple myeloma, and rarely malignant lymphoma and macroglonulinemia. Cardiac involvement is main clinical characteristic of AL amyloidosis (8). Demonstration of a monoclonal immunoglobulin (Ig) protein in the blood, in urine, or in clonal plasma cells in the bone marrow is an important finding for the diagnosis.

AA amyloidosis is the second most common type of amyloidosis worldwide. Acquired and hereditary diseases can cause to AA amyloidosis, including chronic inflammatory diseases, such as rheumatoid arthritis (RA), inflammatory bowel disease (IBD), familial Mediterranean fever (FMF) or other periodic fever syndromes, bronchiectasis, tuberculosis, chronic osteomyelitis and rarely malignancies. The prevalence rates of AA amyloidosis in these disorders show the wide variations due in part to geographic differences, possibly genetic factors, and also according to the methods of the resarch performed by the native biopsies or postmortem studies. The underlying inflammatory disease is usually longstanding and characterized with persistent inflammation. Renal involvement is the major cause of morbidity and mortality in AA amyloidosis (9).

Hereditary amyloidosis occurs by deposition of genetically variant proteins and it is associated with mutations in the genes such as transthyretin, apolipoprotein AI, apolipoprotein AII, apolipoprotein AIV, lysozyme, fibrinogen A, gelsolin, cystatin C. The transthyretin amyloidosis is the most common form of hereditary amyloidosis, and consists in two varieties; as "senil" and hereditary. Clinic characteristics are polyneuropathy and cardiac involvement, and renal involvement may be clinically silent (10).

This review includes the following issues: (1) epidemiology and incidence of the underlying diseases related AA amyloidosis, (2) the clinical manifestations of the involved tissues/organs, and (3) diagnostic approach and treatment strategy in AA amyloidosis.

In AA amyloidosis (secondary, reactive), amyloid fibril proteins are composed of fragments of serum amyloid A (SAA) protein, a major acute-phase reactant protein, an apolipoprotein. Its serum concentration increases 100 to 1000-fold under inflammatory signals, predominantly interleukin (IL)-I β, tumor necrosis factor (TNF)-α and IL-6. In chronic inflammatory diseases, persistent or intermittent elevated SAA concentrations are the basic factor promoting amyloidosis (9). Increased SAA levels were showed to be correlate to disease course in patients with amyloidosis. Also the increased amyloid load and deteriorated organ function were demonstrated to be associated with persistently high SAA concentration (>50m/L) (11). However, amyloidosis does not develop in every patient with chronic active inflammatory diseases, only a subset of patients with persistently increased SAA levels may develop AA amyloidosis. Several forms of SAA have been identified in human plasma, SAA1 seems a predominate factor in the formation AA deposits. The genetic factors may increase the risk of amyloidosis, but it is not fully clear. The main suspects focus on the genes of the SAA1 protein, however there are differences related to ethnicity (12-14). The frequency of the SAA1.3 allele is about 40% for Japanese, it is lower in whites (15). It was reported that the SAA1.3 allele is a risk factor for the association of AA amyloidosis and alsoa poor prognostic factor in survival for Japanese patients with RA (16).

Environment can affect onset of amyloidosis in chronic inflammatory disease. Toitou et al. suggested that country of recruitment is an important factor for the development of renal amyloidosis in FMF and authors suggested that the patient's country should be considered (17).

2. Epidemiology and incidence of underlying diseases due to AA Amyloidosis

AA amyloidosis occurs in association with chronic infectious (i.e. tuberculosis, bronchiectasis, osteomyelitis, leprosy) and chronic inflammatory diseases (i.e. RA, JIA, AS, IBD, psoriatic arthritis, Behçet's disease, adult Still's disease), malignancies (i.e.Hodgkin's disease, renal carsinoma, Castleman's tumor) and hereditary periodic fever (i.e. FMF, others). The prevalence rates of AA amyloidosis in these disorders show a wide variation due in part to geographic differences, possibly genetic factors, and also according to the study's material (i.e. biopsy or autopsy) and method (i.e. immunohistochemistry).

AA amyloidosis associated with chronic infections such as tuberculosis and osteomyelitis was common in early 20th century. These cases appear less frequent after the eradication of some infectious diseases and due to advances in the management of diseases. Von Hutten et al. reassesed renal amyloidosis in 233 renal biopsies and demonstrated that chronic non-infectious inflammmatory diseases were more than chronic infectious diseases (73.8%, 24.6% respectively) (18). Similar results were found in the Western countries (19,20). Malignancy related AA amyloidosis is rare causes. Among malignities renal cancer, hepatocellular carcinoma and lymphoma are most frequently implicated in AA amyloidosis. Castleman's disease is one of the most recently recognized causes in case reports (21).

Rheumatoid arthritis is one of non-infectious, inflammatory, longstanding rheumatic disases. It is generally an inflammatory disease in synovial joints, and also affects systemic organs including lungs, heart, kidneys, nervous system. A major factor responsible for the development of AA amyloidosis seems sustained overproduction of SAA under chronic inflammatory conditions. The prevalence of AA amyloidosis in RA is a range from 7% to 26% and it varies due to clinical severity of patients and duration of arthritis (22-24). In a Dutch series, RA was the most frequent cause of AA amyloidosis, followed by recurrent pulmonary infection (11%), Crohn's disease (5%), ankylosing spondylitis (5%), tuberculosis (3%), osteomyelitis (2%), FMF (2%) and Hodgkin's disease (2%) (25). A study from Finland (26) based on Finnish Registry for Kidney Diseases identified 264 patients suffering from amyloidosis associated with RA, AS or JIA over the period 1995-2008, most of cases were RA (n=229), followed JIA (n=20) and AS (n=15). A cohort study of patients with RA showed 16.3% AA fibril depositions in the abdominal fat samples of patients (27).

In general, the development of AA amyloidosis in RA takes a long time, often more than 15 years (28,29). Morigush et al. reported that secondary amiloidosis developed in a shorter period in Japanese RA patients with the γ/γ homozygotes in the SAAI gene (14).

Juvenil idiopathic arthritis is also a cause of AA amyloid which has been observed in systemic (Still disease) and polyarticular forms (30). However, the effective suppression of the disease activity with new immunosuppressive treatment agents (i.e.biologics) in early stages may change prognosis in both RA and JIA.

AA amyloidosis also complicates 4 hereditary diseases with varying frequencies: FMF, the tumor necrosis factor receptor–associated periodic syndrome (TRAPS), Muckle-Wells syndrome (MWS) and hyperimmunoglobulinemia IgD with periodic fever (HIDS) (31).

Familial Mediterranean fever is well recognised among the hereditary periodic fever syndromes, also called as autoinflammatory syndromes. Autoinflammatory diseases are characterised by unprokoved inflammatory episodes without any recognizable pathogens. FMF mainly affects people of Mediterranean origin (Sephardic Jews, Turks, Armenians, Araps). Its prevalance is between 1/500-1/1000 and carrier rate is very high in the Eastern

Mediterranean (32). Its a monogenic autoinflammatory disease associated with mutations in a gene called MEFV (MEditerranean FeVer) (33,34).
There are two phenotypes of FMF as types 1 and 2. Familial Mediterranean fever type 1 is characterised by recurrent short episodes of fever, peritonitis, synovitis, pleuritis, rarely pericarditis or erysipelas-like skin disease, along with increased acute phase reactants. Familial Mediterranean fever type 2 is probably quite rare characterized by amyloidosis as the first clinical manifestation of FMF without classical FMF attacks, but their family members have often characteristic FMF signs (35,36).
The symptoms and severity of FMF vary among affected individuals. During attacks,acute phase reactants such as C-reactive protein, fibrinogen, ceruloplasmin, serum amyloid A are elevated. After attacks, all these abnormal tests usually return to normal values. In %30-63 of patients, inflammation can persist in attack-free periods with elevated acute -phase proteins (37-39). Chronic subclinical inflammation can cause the risk of developing complications such as AA amyloidosis.
In a retrospective analysis of 287 patients with renal amyloidosis from Turkey, FMF appears most frequent among the causes of AA amyloidosis, the etiological distribution was found as follows; FMF 64%, tuberculosis 10%, bronchiectasis and chronic obstructive lung disease 6%, RA 4%, spondyloarthropathy 3%, chronic osteomyelitis 2%, miscellaneous 4%, unknown 7%. Oedema accompanied by proteinuria was the most prominent presenting finding in 88% of the cases. Hepatomegaly in 17%, and splenomegaly in 11% of the patients were found in this study (40). In pediatric FMF series, 29% of 110 cases developed AA amyloidosis (41). In Sephardic Jews, the incidence of FMF related amyloidosis was 37.2 % (42). The frequency of amyloidosis varies among different ethnic groups and also due to regular the use of colchicine which is beneficial in preventing FMF amyloidosis by a reduction in the number and severity of attacks.
The mutations in exon 10, in the region between 680 and 694 and especially M694V homozygosity were demonstrated to be associated with AA amyloidosis (43-45), however the different mutations were also shown (46). M694V homozygosity and/or SAA alpha/alpha genotype, male gender,delay in diagnosis of FMF and the presence of secondary amyloidosis in the family has been suggested to be risk factors for the development of amyloidosis in FMF patients (43-47). The frequency of the main signs and symptoms of FMF were found fever 92.5%, peritonitis 93.7%,arthritis 47.4%, pleurisy 31.2%, amyloidosis 12.9% (44).
TRAPS is a rare autosomal-dominant disorder characterised by recurrent attacks of fever, abdominal pain, rash and periorbital edema. AA amyloidosis is more common among patients with cystein mutations compared to non-cystein ones (48).
MWS is also autosomal dominant disease, characterised by recurrent attacks of urticaria, fever, polyarthralgia. Amyloidosis may develop in later life (49). It was estimated that approximately one-third of patients suffer from amyloidosis and there is familial clustering (50).
Hyperimmunglobulin D syndrome is an autosomal recessively inherited disease manifested by recurrent attacks of fever, arthralgia, abdominal pain, diarrhea, maculopapular rash, and lymphadenopathy lasting 3-7 days. The incidence of amyloidosis in hyper IgD syndrome is remarkably low compared to other periodic fever syndromes.
Secondary amyloidosis in ankylosing spondylitis is less frequent. Sing et al. detected that subclinical amyloid deposits by abdominal subcutaneous fat aspiration in 5 patients (7%) with ankylosing spondylitis (n= 72) with disease duration longer than 5 years (51).

In other chronic rheumatic inflammatory diseases including systemic lupus erythematosus, polymyalgia rheumatica and Behçet's disease, AA amyloidosis has been rarely reported in case reports (52-59).

The development of AA amyloidosis was reported in 28 SLE patients (one of them overlapping with systemic sclerosis) between 1956-2011 (up to March, based on Pubmed). The lack of acute phase response in SLE compared to other inflammatory diseases has contributed to reduce the incidence (52-54). Most of patients presented proteinuria/nephrotic-range proteinuria or nephrotic syndrome or progressive renal insufficiency when the amyloidosis was diagnosed. Renal failure was a major cause of death of these patients. Cardiac presentations with arrthmia and congestive heart failure in SLE related AA amyloidosis is not common. Hepatic, splenic pulmoner, intestinal, adrenal involvement with amyloidosis and mononeuropathy were very rare in SLE patients (54).

Behçet's disease is a multisystem inflammatory disorder with a genetic background, characterised by oral and genital ulcers, uveitis, cutaneous pustular erythematous lesions, arthritis, central nerveous system involvement and/or vascular manifestations such as veneous thrombosis, arteritis and aneurysms. Behçet's disease is more frequent in the regions along the Mediterranean, Middle East and Far East countries. Amyloidosis is a rare complication, its frequency changes between 0.01 and 4.8 % in several clinical series (57). Major risk factors for the development of AA amyloidosis are peripheral or pulmonary arterial involvement and venous thrombosis, and the presence of arthritis has also been implicated as a predictor in Behçet's disease (58-59).

Secondary amyloidosis rarely occurs in long-lasting inflammatory bowel diseases. In the retrospective studies the prevalance is ranging from 0.5% to 3% among patients with Crohn's disease (60,61).

3. Clinical manifestations of AA Amyloidosis

Clinical amyloidosis is defined as the presence of symptoms or signs of visseral involvement by amyloid. General signs such as fatique and weight loss are often. Clinical signs of amyloidosis generate according to its locations, and most of them are not specific. Kidney, liver, spleen, heart, intestinal and respiratory tract are the main involved organs or systems in AA amyloidosis (4,19,20,55,60-66). Adrenal and thyroid glands, testes, skin, synovial membrane and bone marrow are other sites of involvement and less common presentations (67-69). Most of clinical symptoms are caused by distortion of the normal tissue architecture. The patients can present with organ enlargement such as hepatomegaly, splenomegaly, renomegali, enlarged thyroid, rarely hypertophy of lymph nodes by massive amyloid deposition, easy bruising by weakening of the vascular walls (65,70), proteinuria, renal failure and malabsorbtion (4,19,20,61,65). Unexplained kidney, heart, or systemic disease, hepatomegaly and splenomegaly are among suspicious for amyloidosis.

In AA amyloidosis, kidney is the most affected organ (4). The first sign of renal amyloidosis is asemptomatic proteinuria, gradually progressing to nephrotic syndrome and /or renal dysfunction. Amyloidosis is one of the major differential diagnoses of proteinüria. The most common clinical manifestation is peripheral edema due to the development of nephrotic syndrome. Haematuria, renal vein thrombosis and tubuler defects are very rare. Hematuria reflects amyloid deposition anywhere in the genitourinary tract. The blood pressure may often remain normal. It is not clear that development of hypertension in renal amiloidosis whether due to renal involvement or a coincidental finding. Persistent nephrotic syndrome and advanced renal insufficiency and enlarged kidney suggest amyloidosis. Occasionally the kidneys are small and scarred. Rarely, a sudden onset of acute renal failure may occur due to renal vein thrombosis. It is very rare for the presenting symptoms to be those of chronic renal failure. AA amyloidosis usually progresses toward end- stage renal failure which is the main cause of mortality.

Amyloid deposits can occur in the mesangium, glomerular capillary loops, tubulo-interstitium, and vasculature of the kidney. It was showed that the patients having glomerular amyloid deposition are more common and have a poor prognosis than patients having vascular and tubular amyloid deposition in secondary amyloidosis to RA (63).

Once the disease established, prognosis remains poor. Renal failure and low serum albumin levels are the most important predictors for poor prognosis (19). Survival of patients with AA amyloidosis appears greatly improved as compared to past decades. Torregrosa et al. reported in a group of patients a survival of 67% and 53% at 12 and 24 months without dialysis respectively (64). Amyloidosis without therapy usually progresses to end-stage kidney disease. Progression of renal amyloidosis can be delayed or slowed by treatments that reduce the production of amyloidogenic precursor proteins, deposits may also regress.

Hepatic involvement is usually expressed as hepatomegaly and increased in serum alkaline phosphatase levels. However, hepatic amyloidosis may remain asymptomatic for a long time or show only mild liver enzymes abnormalities. In the differantial diagnosis in patients with long-standing inflammatory disease, hepatomegaly and liver function tests abnormalities hepatic amyloidosis should be considered. Some complications such as portal hypertension, jaundice, ascites are rare. Gioeva et al. retrieved all liver biopsies from a series of 588 cases with histologically confirmed amyloidosis and reported that hepatic amyloidosis is most commonly AL amyloid of lambda- and kappa-light chain origin (87%). Hepatic AA amyloidosis was found in a single patient (2%) in this study (71).

The spleen is affected and splenomegaly is seen in early periods, functional hyposplenism and splenic rupture rarely may develop(66).

Gastrointestinal amyloidosis manifestations such as abdominal pain, vomiting, disphagia, diarrhea, malabsorbtion, obstruction, bleeding, perforation may occur in about 20% of patients (65), these symptoms are largely nonspecific. The rectum is a commonly affected site and rectal biopsy is the initial diagnostic tool. The hypoproteinemia may not only be due to proteinuria but also to a decreased rate of protein synthesis as a consequence of hepatic amyloidosis, and also to malabsorption of amino-acids because of amyloid infiltration in intestinal mucosa.

Heart disease in secondary amyloidosis is less common (<10%) than it is in other types of amyloidosis and is the main cause of death. Cardiac involvement has been associated with myopathic syndrome and coronary vascular syndrome. Arrithmias may occur at any time. Cardiac amyloidosis should be suspected in any patient who presents with restrictive cardiomyopathy, prominent signs of right-sided heart failure or left sided heart failure in the absence of ischemia disease. Valvular disease, pericarditis, systemic arterial emboli are rare. The combination of clinical and echocardiographic findings suggest amyloidosis (9).

The involvement of adrenal glands may cause adrenal insufficiency. The involvement of thyroid may lead to hypotyroidsm. Although microscopic amyloid deposition may be demonstrated in thyroid gland, a significant enlargement of thyroid and its dysfunction are not often, goiter as a first evidence of AA amyloidosis is rarely seen and thyroid function tests are usually in normal limits. Enlarged thyroid gland making pressure to the near tissues and leading operation is a rare condition in systemic amyloidosis associated with

inflammatory disease. Bleeding is an important complication in thyroid operation of patients with secondary amyloidosis (66,70).
Pulmonary amyloidosis is uncommon (72) and presents with cough, hemoptysis and dyspne. Amyloid depositions may find in bronchial, mediastinal and alveolar area and interferes with tumor mass.
Skin involvement can present with petechiae, purpura and ecchymoses. Rarely papules, nodules, plaques can be seen.
Arthritis is associated with febril attacks in patients with FMF. The patients with MWS patients have polyarthralgias accompanying urticaria.
Spinal cord lesions and cranial nerve involvement are uncommon. Peripheral neuropathy or carpal tunnel syndrome occasionally may occur during the course of AA amyloidosis.
Uretral and bladder amyloidosis are rare and present with pain and hematuria. Amyloid deposits in the wall of blood vessel may lead to vascular fragility, impaired hemostasis, and bleeding (70). Amyloid fibrils can also accumulate in the bone marrow (68).

4. Diagnostic approach of AA Amyloidosis

The approach of the diagnosis based on clinical mainifestations, clinical examination, biochemical nature of AA amyloidosis for differentiation with respect to other varieties, biochemical tests and genetic analysis. Clinical examination and evaluation of the various signs described above should be sistematically performed. The diagnosis of amyloidosis should be confirmed by biopsy from suspicious tissue (s) such as kidney, intestine, liver, thyroid, skin, bone marrow and endomyocard. If biopsy could not be taken from these tissues or clinical signs are not present, biopsy may be taken from intestinal mucosa (rectal), abdominal subcutaneous fat tissue, labial salivary gland samples. The results of gastrointestinal biopsy are highly corelated with those of renal biopsy but the results of abdominal fat samples are not (73).
Abdominal fat aspiration biopsy is easy to perform and repeatable. However, fat aspiration biopsy is less sensitive than kidney and rectal biopsy. Labial salivary gland biopsy is now replaced the old gingiva biopsy. Endomyocardial biopsy can be needed in cardiac involvement. The aim is to detect amyloid early and to type it correctly.
Congo red stain is the gold standard for amyloid detection. The amyloid type must be identified based on amyloid protein within the deposits by immunohistochemistry or immunoelectronmicroscopy and Western blotting. AA amyloidosis can also be diagnosed using serum amyloid P component scintigraphy (74).

5. Treatment strategy of AA Amyloidosis

The main therapeutic target of the chronic inflammatory diseases is to suppress the inflammatory activity of the underlying disease and to prevent the development of AA amyloidoisis. The concentration or production of SAA is reduced by the treatment of underlying chronic inflammatory rheumatic diseases including anti -inflammatory drugs, immunosuppressants or biologics. Treatment with corticosteroids and immunosuppressive drugs in mainly RA and JIA have proved the suppression of the underlying inflammatory process (26). It is suggested that immunosuppressants can improve prognosis of patient with AA amyloidosis (75). Each patient requires systematically evaluation to determine their optimal treatment. Earlier and powerfull treatments of underlying diseases should be aimed.

Colchicine is the most effective drug for prevention of acute inflammatory attacks and development of amyloidosis in most patients with FMF. Early treatment of amyloidosis is associated with much better prognosis and survival, but even reverse established deposits. Colchicine dose of 1.5-2 mg daily is necessary for prevention of the progression of amyloidosis (76). It was shown that colchicine can reduce proteinuria in patients with renal amyloidosis of FMF by case series (77,78).

Epradisate (anti-amyloid compounds) for treating with AA amyloidosis which leads a significant delay in the progression to dialysis or end-satge renal disease (79,80).

In recent years, new biological therapies were approved for the treatment, especially in patients with RA, JIA, spondyloarthropathy, who is unresponsive to conventional treatment.

Several isolated cases and small series have demonstrated a marked clinical improvement and complete or partial resolution of AA amyloid deposits in patients with RA,JIA, herditary periodic fever syndromes under these agents (81-90).

Anti-cytokine biologicals including TNF-alpha antagonists (infliximab, etanercept, adalimumab) (81-84) and a humanised IL-6 R antibodies (tocilizumab) suppresse strongly SAA production by liver and also inflammatory process (85-87). These biologics have been reported to be highly effective in patients with AA amyloidosis secondary to RA and JIA. IL-I receptor antagonist (anakinra) showed a persisted effect in patients with familial cold autoinflammatory syndrome (88-89).

The trial of rituximab (anti-CD 20 monoclonal antibody) was reported the effficacy for a few patients with AA amyloidosis secondary to RA (91).

A new class of antiamyloid agents, currently in clinical trials, also appear to be amyloid type for AA and ATTR (92).

6. References

[1] Howie AJ, Brewer DB, Howell D, Jones AP. Physical basis of colors seen in Congo red-stained amyloid in polarized light. Lab Invest. 2008;88:232–42.

[2] Amyloid fibril protein nomenclature: 2010 recommendations of the nomenclature commitee of the International Society of Amyloidosis. Amyloid 2010;17:101-4.

[3] Picken MM. New insights into systemic amyloidosis: the importance of diagnosis of specific type. Curr Opin Nephrol Hypertens 2007:16:196-203.

[4] Dember LM. Amyloidosis -associated kidney disease. J Am Soc Nephrol 2006; 17: 3458-3471.

[5] Magy-Bertrand N, Dupond JL, Mauny F, Dupond AS, Duchene F, Gil H et al. Incidence of amyloidosis over 3 years: the AMYPRO study. Clin Exp Rheumatol 2008; 26: 1074-1078.

[6] Hazenberg BP, van Rijswijk MH. Where has secondary amyloid gone. Ann Rheum Dis 2000; 59:577-579.

[7] Cazalets C, Cador B, Mauduit N, Decaux O, Ramee MP, Le Pogamp P et al. Epidemiologic description of amyloidosis at the University Hospital of Rennes from 1995-1999. Rev Med Interne 2003; 24: 424-433.

[8] Merlini G, Seldin DC, Gertz MA. Amyloidosis: Pathogenesis and New Therapeutic Options. J Clin Oncol 2010 Apr 11 [Epub ahead of print]

[9] Lachmann HJ, Goodman HJ, Gilbertson JA, Gallimore JR, Sabin CA, Gillmore JD, et al.Natural history and outcome in systemic AA amyloidosis. New Engl Med 2007; 356: 2361-2371.
[10] Rapezzi C, Quarta CC, Riva L,Longhi S,Galleli I, Cilberti P et al. Transthyretin-related amyloidoses and the heart: a clinical overview. Nat Rev Cardiol 2010;7:398-408.
[11] Gillmore JD, Lovat LB, Persey MR, Pepys MB, Hawkins PN. Amyloid load and clinical outcome in AA amyloidosis in relation to circulating concentration of serum amyloid A protein. Lancet 2001;358: 24–29.
[12] Baba S, Masago SA, Takahashi T, Kasama T, Sugimura H, Tsugane S, et al. A novel allelic variant of serum amyloid A, SAAI γ: genomic evidence, evolution,frequency and implication as a risk factor for reactive systemic AA-amyloidosis. Hum Mol Genet 1995;4:1083-1087.
[13] Gershoni-Baruch R, Brik R, Zacks N, Shinawi M, Lidar M, Livneh A, The contribution of genotypes at the MEFV and SAA1 loci to amyloidosis and disease severity in patients with Familial Mediterranean fever. Arthritis Rheum 2003; 48; 1149–1155.
[14] Moriguchi M, Terai C, Koseki Y, Uesato M, Nakajima A, Inada S, et al. Influence of genotypes at SAA1 and SAA2 loci on the development and the length of latent period of secondary AA-amyloidosis in patients with rheumatoid arthritis. Hum. Genet 1999;105: 360–366.
[15] Yamada T, Okuda Y, Takasugi K, Wang L, Marks D, Benson MD et al. An allele of serum amyloid A1 associated with amyloidosis in both Japanese and Caucasians: Amyloid 2003; 10: 7-11.
[16] Nakamura T. Clinical strategies for amyloid A amyloidosis secondary to rheumatoid arthritis. Mod Rheumatol 2008; 18: 109-118.
[17] Touitou I, Sarkisian T, Medlej-Hashim M, Tunca M, Livneh A, Cattan D, et al. Country as the primary risk factor for renal amyloidosis in familial Mediterranean fever. Arthritis Rheum 2007; 56:1706–1712.
[18] Von Hutten H, Mihatsch M, Lobeck H, Rudolph B, Eriksson M, Röcken C. Prevalance and origin of amyloid in kidney biopsies. Am J Surg Pathol 2009;33:1198-1205.
[19] Joss N, McLaughlin K, Simpson K, Boulton-Jones JM.Presentation ,survival and prognostic markers in AA amyloidosis . QJ Med 2000;93:535-542
[20] Bergesio F, Ciciani AM, Santostefano M, Brugnano R.M, Angagaro M, Palldini G, et al. Immunopathology Group, Italian Society of Nephrology Renal involvement in systemic amyloidosis -an Italian retrospective study on epidemiological and clinical data at diagnosis. Nephrol Dial Transplant 2007;22:1608-1618.
[21] Lachmann HJ, Gilbertson JA.Gilmore JD. Unicentric Castleman's disease complicated bay systemic AA amyloidosis: a curable disease.QJM 2002;95: 211-218.
[22] Wakhlu A, Krisnani N, Hissatia P, Aggarwal A, Misra R. Prevalence of secondary amyloidosis in Asian north Indian patients with rheumatoid arthritis. J Rheumatol. 2003;30:948–51.
[23] El Mansoury TM, Hazenberg BP, El Badawy SA, Ahmed AH, Bijzet J, Limburg PC, et al. Screeningfor amyloid in subcutaneous fat tissue of Egyptian patients with rheumatoid arthritis: clinical and laboratory characteristics. Ann Rheum Dis. 2002;61:42–47.

[24] Kobayashi H, Tada S, Fuchigami T, Okuda Y, Takasugi K, Miyamoto T, et al. Secondary amyloidosis in patients with rheumatoid arthritis: diagnostic and prognostic value of gastroduodenal biopsy. Br J Rheumatol. 1996;35:44–49.

[25] Hazenberg BP, van Rijswijk MH., Clinical and therapeutic aspects of AA amyloidosis, Bailliere's Clin Rheumatol. 1994;8:661–690.

[26] Immonen K, Finne P, Grönhagen-Riska C, Petterson T, Kautiainen H, et al. A marked decline in the incidence of renal replacement therapy for amyloidosis associated with inflammatory rheumatic diseases-data from nationwide registries in Finland.Amyloid 2011; 18(1):25-8. 25-8

[27] Gomez-Casonava E et al. Secondary amyloidosis in rheumatoid arthritis: a 9 year experience with abdominal fat aspiration. XVII the Congress of Rheumatology, Barcelona Spain July 1993.

[28] Özdemir AI, Wright JR, Calkins E. Influence of rheumatoid arthritis on amyloidosis of ageing. New Eng J Med 1971;285: 534-538.

[29] Nakai H, Ozaki S, Kano S, et al. Clinical characteristics and genetic background of secondary amyloidosis associated with rheumatoid arthritis in Japanese. Ryumachi (Rheumatism) 1996;36: 25-33 (Abstract in English)

[30] Beşbaş N, Saatci U, Bakkaloğlu A, Ozen S. Amyloidosis of juvenile chronic arthritis in Turkish children. Scand J Rheumatol 1992; 21: 257-259.

[31] Drenth, J. P. and J. W. van der Meer. Hereditary periodic fever. N Engl J Med 2001. 345:1748–1757

[32] Ozen S, Karaaslan Y, Özdemir O, Saatçi U, Bakkaloğlu A, Koroglu E, Tezcan S Prevalance of juvenil chronic arthritis and familial Mediterranean fever in Turkey. J Rheumatol 1998; 25: 2445-2449.

[33] Ancient missense mutations in a new member of the RoRet gene familia likely to cause familial Mediterranean fever. The International FMA Consortium. Cell 1997 22;90: 797-807

[34] A candidate gene for familial Mediterranean fever French FMF Consortium. Nature Gene 1997;17:25-31

[35] Livneh A, Langevitz P, Shinar Y, Zaks N, Kastner DL, Pras M et al. Amyloid 1999;6:1-6.

[36] Kutlay S, Yılmaz E, Koytak ES, Tulunay O O, Keven K, Ozcan M, Ertürk S. A case of familial Mediterranean fever with amyloidosis as the first manifestation. Am J Kidney 2001; 38(6):E34.

[37] Lidar M, Livneh A. Familial Mediterranean fever: clinical,molecular and manegement advancements. Neth J Med 2007;65: 318-324.

[38] Lachman HJ, Şengül B, Yavuzşen TU et al. Clinical and subclinical inflammation in patients with familial Mediterranean fever and heterozygous carries of MEFV mutations. Rheumatology 2006; 45:746-750.

[39] Korkmaz C, Özdoğan H, Kasapçapur Ö, Yazıcı H. Acute phase response in familial Mediterranean fever. Ann Rheum Dis 2002;61:79-81.

[40] Tuglular, F. Yalcinkaya, S. Paydas, A. Oner, C. Utas and S. Bozfakioglu et al., A retrospective analysis for aetiology and clinical findings of 287 secondary amyloidosis cases in Turkey Nephrol Dial Transplant 2002; 17 : 2003–2005.

[41] Yalçınkaya F, Tümer N, Tekin M, Akar N, Akçakuş M.. Familial Mediterranean fever in Turkish children (analysis of 110 cases) In Familial Mediterranean Fever Sohar E,

Gafni J, Pras M (eds) Freund Publishing Hause London and Telaviv, 1997 pp: 157-61

[42] Pras MM, Gafni J, Jacob ET, Cabili S, Zemer D, Sohar E. Recent advances in familial Mediterranean fever. Adv Nephrol 1984;13:261-70.

[43] Akar N, Hasipek M, Akar E, Ekim M, Yalçınkaya F, Cakar N. Serum amyloiod A and tumor necrosis factor- alpha alleles in Turkish familial Mediterranean fever with and without amyloidosis. Amiloid 2003;10:12-16.

[44] Tunca M, Akar S, Onen F, Ozdogan H, Kasapcopur O, Yalcınkaya F, Tutar E, Ozen S, Topaloglu R, Yılmaz E, Arici N, Bakkaloglu A, Besbas N, Akpolat T, Dinc A, Erken E; Turkish FMF study group, Familial Mediterranean fever in Turkey. Results of a nation wide multicenter study. Medicine 2005; 84:1-11.

[45] Ben-Chetrit E, Backenroth R. Amyloidosis induced end stage renal disease in patients with familial Mediterranean fever is highly associated with point mutations in the MEFV gene. Ann Rheum Dis 2001; 60:146-9.

[46] Yalcınkaya F, Topaloğlu R, Yılmaz E, Emre S, Erken E.; on behalf of the Turkish Family Study Clin Exp Rheumatol 2002; 20 (Suppl 26), S90 (abstract).

[47] Saatci U, Ozen S, Ozdemir S, Bakkaloglu A, Besbas N, Topaloglu R, Arslan S (1997) FMF in children: report of a large series and discussions of the risk and prognostic factors of amyloidosis. Eur J Pediatr 1997; 156:619–23.

[48] Aksentijevich I,Galon J, Soares M, Mansfield E, Hull K, Oh HH et al. The Tumor necrosis factor receptor-associated periodic syndrome:new mutations in TNFRIA, ancestral orgins, genotype-phenotype studies and evidence for further genetic heterogeneity of periodic fevers. Am J Hum Genet 2001; 69:301-14.

[49] Hoffmann HM, Mueller JL, Broide DH, Wanderer AA, Kolodner RD. Mutation of a new gene encoding a putative pyrin like protein causes familial cold autoinflammatory syndrome and Muckle Wells syndrome. Nat Genet 2001;29:301–5

[50] Muckle TJ. The 'Muckle–Wells' syndrome. Br J Dermatol 1979 100:87–92.

[51] Sing G,Kumari N, Aggrawal A, Krisnani N, Misra R. Prevalance of subclinical amyloidosis in ankylosing spondylitis J Rheumatol 2007 ;34: 371-3

[52] Düzgün N, Tokgöz G, Ölmez Ü, Aydıntuğ O, Sonel B, Sak S. Systemic amyloidosis and sacroiliitis in a patient with systemic lupus erythematosus. Rheumatol Int 1999;18:153-55.

[53] Düzgün N. AA Amyloidosis and systemic lupus erythematosus: Literature review.Expert Review Clin Immunol 2007;16:201-8.

[54] Aktaş YB, Düzgün N, Mete T, Yazıcıoğlu L, Saykı M, Ensari A, Ertürk S. AA amyloidosis associated with systemic lupus erythematosus: impact on clinical course and outcome. Rheumatol Int 2008;28: 367-70.

[55] Javaid MM, Karnalathan M, Kon SP. Rapid development of renal failure secondary to AA type amyloidois in a patient with polymyalgia rheumatica. J Ren Care 2010: 36: 199-202.

[56] Akpolat T, Dilek M, Aksu K, Keser K, Toprak Ö, Cirit M et al. Renal Behçet's disease: An Update. Semin Arthritis Rheum 2008; 38: 241-48.

[57] Yurdakul S, Tüzüner N,Yurdakul I, Hamuryudan V, Yazıcı H. Amyloidosis in Behçet's syndrome. Arthritis Rheum 1990;33:1586-1589.

[58] Melikoğlu M, Altıparmak M, Fresko I, Tunç R Yurdakul S, Hamuryudan V. A reappraisal of amyloidosis in Behçet's syndrome. Rheumatology (Oxford) 2001 40; 212-15.
[59] Stankovic K, Grateau G. Amylose AA Nephrol Ther 2008; 4: 281–287.
[60] Serra I, Oller B, Manosa M, Naves JE, Zabana Y, Cabre E, et al. Systemic amyloidosis in inflammatory bowel disease: retrospective study. J Crohns Colitis 2010 4(3): 269-74.
[61] Miyoka M, Matsui T, Hisabe T,Yano Y, Hirai F Takaki Y et al. Clinical and endoscopic features of amyloidosis secondary to Crohn's disease : diagnostic value of duaodenal observation and biopsy. Dig Endosc 2011; 23(2): 157-65.
[62] Uda H, Yokota A, Kobayashi K, Miyake T, Fushimu H, Maeda A, Saiki O. Two distinc clinical courses of renal involvement in rheumatoid patients with AA amyloidosis J Rheumatol 2006; 33:1482-1487.
[63] Torregrosa E, Hernandez-Jaras J, Calvo C, Ríus A, García-Pérez H, Maduell F, et al. Secondary amyloidosis (AA) and renal disease. Nefrologia 2003;23: 321-326.
[64] Ebert EC, Nagar M. Gastrointestinal manifestations of amyloidosis. Am J Gastroent 2008; 103;776-787.
[65] Renzulli P, Schoepfer A, Mueller E, Condias D. Atravmatic splenic rupture in amyloidosis. Amiloid 2009; 16; 47-53.
[66] Düzgün N, Morris Y, Yıldız HI, Öztürk S, Küpana Ayva Ş, et al. Amyloid goiter in juvenil onset rheumatoid arthritis (Letter to the Editor). Scan J Rheumatol 2003;32 (4):254-255.
[67] Srivastava A, Baxi M, Yadav S, Agarwal A, Gupta RK, Misra SK, Mithal A. Juvenil rheumatoid arthritis with amyloid goiter: report of a case with review of the literature. Endocr Pathol 2001;12(4): 437-441.
[68] Sungur C, Sungur A, Ruacan S, Arık N, Yasavul U, Turgan C, Çağlar S. Diagnostic value of bone marrow biopsy in patients with renal diseases secondary familial Mediterranean fever. Kidney Int 1993;44: 834-836.
[69] Sueker C, Hetzel GR, Grabensee B, Stockschlaeder M, Scharf RE. Amyloidosis and bleeding pathophysiology,diagnosis and therapy Am J Kidney 2006;47:947-955.
[70] Giova Z, Kieninger B, Röken C. Amyloidosis in liver biopsies. Pathologe 2009; 30: 240-245.
[71] Lachmann HJ, Hawkins PN. Amyloidosis and the lung. Chron Respir Dis 2006; 3:203-214.
[72] Kuroda T, Tanabe N, Sakatsume M, Nozawa S, Mitsuka T, Ishikawa H et al. Comparison of gastroduodenal,renal and abdominal fat biopsies for diagnosing amyloidosis in rheumatoid arthritis. Clin Rheumatol 2002 ; 21(2): 123-128.
[73] Hawkins PN, Pepys MB. Imaging amyloidosis with radiolabeled SAP. Eur J Nucl Med 1995;22:595-59
[74] Chevrel G, Jenvrin C, McGregor B, Miossec P. Renal type AA amyloidosis associated with rheumatoid arthritis: a cohort study showing improved survival on treatment with pulse cyclo- phosphamide. Rheumatology 2001;40:821-825.
[75] Zemer D, Pras M, Sohar E. Colchicine in the prevention and treatment of the amyloidosis of familial Mediterranean fever. N Eng J Med 1986;314:1001-1005.
[76] Öner A, Erdoğan O, Demircin G. Efficacy of colchicine therapy in amyloid nephropathy of familial Mediterranean fever. Pediatr Nephrol 2003;18:521-526.

[77] Livneh A, Zemer D, Langevitz P. Colchicine treatment of AA amyloidosis of familial Mediterranean fever.An analysis of factors affecting outcome. Arthritis Rheum 1994;37:1804-1811.
[78] Dember LM, Hawkins PN, Hanzenberg BPC, Gorevic PD, Merlini GM, Butrimiene I, et al. Eprodisate for the treatment of renal disease in AA amyloidosis. N Eng J Med 2007;356:2349- 2360.
[79] Gorevic PD, Hawkins PN, Skinner M, Nasonov EL, Butrimiene I, Benson MD, et al. Treatment with eprodisate results in a significant delay in the progression to dialysis /end stage renal disease in amyloid A amyloidosis patients: analysis including retrieved follow-up data. Arthritis Rheum 2007; 56 (Suppl): 520.
[80] Gottenberg JE, Merle-Vincent F, Bentaberry F, Allonore Y, Berenbaum F, Fautrel B et al and for the Club Rheumatism and Inflammation. Anti-tumor necrosis factor alpha therapy in fifteen patients with AA amyloidosis secondary to inflammatory arthritides: a follow up report of tolerability and efficacy. Arthritis Rheum 2003; 48: 2019-2024.
[81] Fernandez-Nebro A, Olive A, Castro MC, Varela AH, Riera E, Irigoven MV et al. Long-term TNF- alpha blockade in patients with amyloid A amyloidosis complicating rheumatic diseases. Am J Med 2010;123(5): 454-61.
[82] Nakamura T, Higashi S, Tomoda K, Tsukano M, Shono M. Etanercept can induce resolution of renal deteriotion in patients with amyloid A amyloidosis secondary to rheumatoid arthritis. Clin Rheumatol 2010;29 (12);1395-401.
[83] Metyas S, Arkfield DG, Forrester DM, Ehresmann GR. Infliximab treatment of familial Medditeranean fever and its effect on secondary AA amyloidosis. J Clin Rheumatol 2004; 10(3):134-137.
[84] Maini RN, Taylor PC, Szechinski J, Pavelka K, Broll J, Balint G et al. Double-blind randomised controlled clinical trial of the interleukin-6 receptor antagonist, tocilizumab, in European patients with rheumatoid arthritis who had an incomplete response to methotrexate. Arthritis Rheum 2006; 54:2817-2829.
[85] Sato H, Sakai T, Sugaya T, Otaki Y, Aoki K, Ishii K et al. Tocilizumab dramatically ameliorated life threatening diarrhea due to secondary amyloidosis associated with rheumatoid arthritis. Clin Rheumatol 2009;28:1113-1116.
[86] Okuda Y,Takasugi K. Successful use of a humanized anti-interleukin -6 receptor antibody, tocilizumab, to treat amyloid A amyloidosis complicating juvenile idiopathic arthritis. Arthritis Rheum 2006;54: 2997-3000.
[87] Leslie KS, Lachmann HJ, Bruning E, et al. Phenotype, genotype and sustained response to anakinra in 22 patients with autoinflammatory diseases associated with CIAS-1/NALP3 mutations. Arch Dermatol 2006; 142: 1591-1597.
[88] Thornton BD, Hoffman HM, Bhat A, et al. Successfull treatment of renal amyloidosis due to familial cold auto inflammatory syndrome using an interleukin 1 receptor antagonist. Am J Kidney Dis 2007; 49: 477-481.
[89] Sacre K, Brihaye B, Lidove O, Papo T, Pocidalo MA, Cuisset L, Dode C. Dramatic improvement following interleukin 1 beta blockade in tumor necrosis factor receptor -1 –associated syndrome (TRAPS) resistant to anti-TNF-alpha therapy. J Rheumatol 2008; 35(2):357-358.

[90] Narvaez J, Hernandez MV, Ruiz JM, Vaquero CG, Juanola X, Nollaa JM. Rituximab therapy for AA-Amyloidosis secondary to rheumatoid arthritis. Joint Bone Spine 2011;78: 101-103.
[91] Dember, LM. Modern treatment of amyloidosis: unresolved questions. J Am Soc Nephrol 2009;20 3:469–472

2

An Overview of the Amyloidosis in Children with Rheumatic Disease

Betül Sözeri, Nida Dincel and Sevgi Mir
Ege University Faculty of Medicine, Department of Pediatrics
Bornova, Izmir
Turkey

1. Introduction

Amyloidosis is a disease resulting from extra cellular accumulation of insoluble proteins in different organs and blood vessels. The term systemic amyloidosis is used to define applied to a variety of disease entities with a wide morphological and clinical spectrum (1). All amyloid proteins have biophysically comparable features (congo red binding, green color in polarized light, fibrillar appearance on electron microscopy) (2). Depending on the organ involvement type and amount, amyloid may cause progressive and life threatening organ dysfunction (3). There are numerous distractive types of amyloid fibrils are now known (4-7). The main protein types leading to amyloidosis are shown in Table 1.

In children, the most common form of amyloidosis is reactive AA amyloidosis due to hereditary periodic fever (HPF) syndromes. The genetics causes of these syndromes derive from defects of the innate immunity and have been well defined at the clinical and genetically level are. Familial Mediterranean Fever (FMF), Hyperimmunoglobulinaemia D and periodic fever syndrome (HIDS), tumor necrosis factor (TNF) receptor-associated periodic syndrome (TRAPS) and the cryopyrin-associated periodic syndrome (CAPS), which encompasses Muckle- Wells syndrome (MWS), familial cold autoinflammatory syndrome (FCAS), and chronic infantile neurological cutaneous and articular syndrome (CINCA).

Juvenile idiopathic arthritis (JIA) is one of the more common chronic diseases of childhood, with a prevalence of approximately 1 per 1,000 (8). The most dramatic systemic inflammation is seen in patients with systemic JIA. This disorder is somewhat different from the other forms of JIA. A role for T cell and antigen –specific responses and many of the manifestations seem to be caused by the overproduction of IL-6 (figure 1). The prevalence of secondary amyloidosis in JIA varies between 1% and 10% (9-11). Risk for amyloidosis in systemic JIA patients is associated with a long-lasting inflammation (12). Although its frequency is dramatically decreasing, probably in relation with a more active DMARD treatment policy (13) Cantarini et al (14) suggest that MEFV may represent a triggering factor for the development of inflammatory state in systemic JIA, that may be an autoinflammatory disorder in itself rather than a subtype of JIA. Amyloid A precursor, serum amyloid A (SAA), is a major acute phase reactant, therefore being raised in chronic inflammatory diseases (15,16).

Amyloid protein	Precursor protein
AA	Serum amyloid A protein
AL	Monoclonal Ig light chains
AH	Monoclonal Ig light chains
Aβ2M	β2-microglobulin
AFib	Fibrinogen α-chain
Acys	Cystatin C
ALys	Lysozyme
AApoAI Apolipoprotein AI	AApoAI Apolipoprotein AI
AApoAII Apolipoprotein AII	AApoAII Apolipoprotein AII
ATTR Transthyretin	ATTR Transthyretin
AGel Gelsolin	AGel Gelsolin

Table 1. Amyloid proteins and their precursors

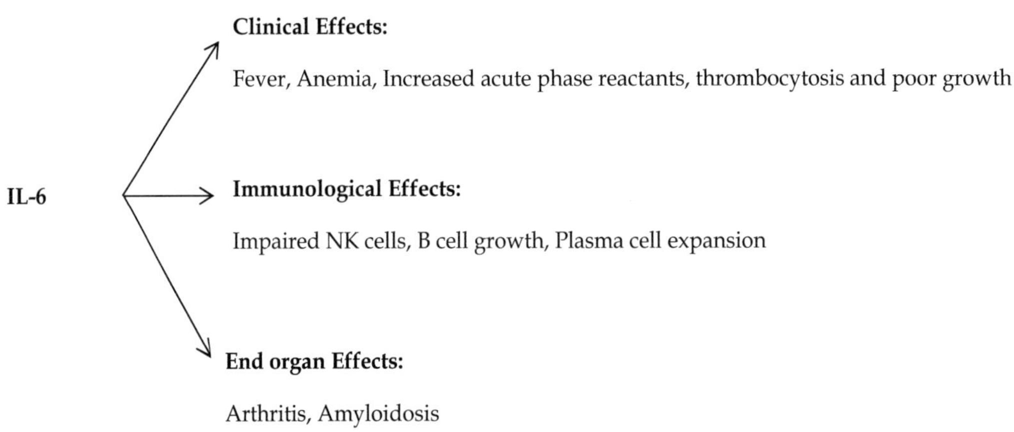

Fig. 1. IL-6 is an important mediator in systemic JIA and causes many different manifestation

AL amyloidosis is generally seen in the elderly. β2-microglobulin amyloidosis (Aβ2M amyloidosis) is seen in patients with renal failure. AFib and ACys amyloidoses are hereditary, autosomal dominant, and late-onset diseases having rarely been reported in children (6,7). Apart from the AL and AA amyloidosis, the kidney is also rarely affected by hereditary type amyloidoses, such as amyloid of fibrinogen (AFib), Apolipoprotein AI (AApoAI), and lysozymederived (ALys) amyloidosis (17).

This review discusses the pathogenesis, common causes clinical manifestations, diagnosis, and treatment of amyloidosis in children.

2. Pathogenesis

Amyloidosis is a general denominator for a group of diseases that are characterized by extracellular deposition of fibrils of aggregated proteins (18). These fibrils consist of polymers in a β sheet configuration of a precursor protein. SAA is a precursor protein in reactive amyloidosis and an acute phase protein that is mainly produced in the liver upon stimulation with various pro-inflammatory cytokines, interleukin (IL)-1β, tumor necrosis factor (TNF)-α, and IL-6. It is found in plasma as an apolipoprotein of HDL cholesterol. During active inflammation serum concentrations beyond 1000 mg/l can be reached, which is 1000-fold higher than the constitutional concentration (19-21). Although the size of the SAA protein produced by the liver is 104 amino acids, amyloid fibrils found in patients with AA amyloidosis mainly consist of an accumulation of the 76 N-terminal amino acids of this protein, although proteins of different length have been reported (22,23). Polymerization of SAA into amyloid fibrils requires removal of the C-terminal of the AA protein (24). The C-terminal portion of SAA is cleaved off by macrophages. The persistent augmentation of an inflammatory pathway through the innate immune system might be crucial in the deposition of the amyloid protein leading to the clinical picture of renal amyloidosis (25).

3. Clinical manifestations

Amyloidosis is a multisystemic disease. Therefore, clinical manifestations vary widely, nonspecific and depending on the involved organ(s) and the amount of amyloid fibrils deposited. Several organs can be affected by AA amyloidosis, but the kidneys are most frequently involved.

Reactive amyloidosis usually presents as proteinuria with or without renal impairment. Renal involvement is found in >90% of patients (26). In addition, other organs including heart, peripheral nerves, thyroid, gastrointestinal system, and bone marrow can be involved by the type of amyloid fibrils. Clinically, it is difficult to distinguish AA and AL amyloidosis from each other because of overlapping clinical presentations. Gastrointestinal involvement is seen in about 20% of patients with reactive amyloidosis, and may present as diarrea, malabsorption or gastrointestinal pseudo-obstruction (23,26).Amyloidotic goitre, hepatomegaly, splenomegaly and polyneuropathy are less frequently encountered features of reactive amyloidosis (27,28). Amyloidosis can cause bleeding diathesis due to factor X deficiency, liver disease, or infiltration of blood vessels (29). In contrast to other types of amyloidosis, cardiac involvement is rare in reactive amyloidosis (30). Involvement of heart and kidneys are the most important predictors affecting survival (25). Infiltration of amyloid fibrils may cause enlargement of muscles and arthropathy. The clinical manifestations of Aβ2M amyloidosis include carpal tunnel syndrome, bone cysts, spondyloarthropathy, pathologic fractures, and swollen painful joints (31).

In kidney involvement; asymptomatic proteinuria is the most common initial presentation, gradually progressing to nephrotic syndrome and/or renal dysfunction. In the series reported by the Turkish FMF study group, the presenting clinical features of the patients with amyloidosis secondary to FMF were as follows: 32% proteinuria, 40% nephrotic syndrome, and 28% chronic renal failure (24). The patients having glomerular amyloid deposition are more common and have a poorer prognosis than patients having vascular and tubular amyloid deposition in rheumatoid arthritis-related AA amyloidosis (32). Nishi et al. (33) showed that 10–30% of patients with renal amyloidosis might have only mild proteinuria and normal renal function.

4. Diagnosis

Suspicion is essential in subjects having an underlying disease with a potential to cause amyloidosis. Amyloidosis should be suspected typically in a patient who presents with proteinuria. In fact, in patients who are candidates for this complication, secondary amyloidosis should also be considered in the differential diagnosis of cardiomyopathy, peripheral neuropathy, hepatomegaly, or in the presence of symptoms related to the gastrointestinal tract. The diagnosis of amyloidosis is based on the demonstration of amyloid fibrils in the biopsy of the involved tissue. Renal, rectal or abdominal fat biopsies may also reveal amyloid deposition. The deposited amyloid fibrils are extracellular, eosinophilic, and metachromatic on light microscopy. Congo red staining is necessary for diagnosis. Amyloid fibrils appear faintly red on Congo red staining and show the characteristic apple-green birefringence under polarized light. Actually, infiltrative renal diseases including amyloidosis must be considered in the differential diagnosis of all patients having chronic kidney disease and normal or large sized kidneys. AA amyloidosis can also be diagnosed using serum amyloid P component scintigraphy (34).

5. Underlying causes of secondary amyloidosis

5.1 Familial mediterranean fever

FMF is characterized by recurrent periodic fever episodes and serositis along with an increased acute inflammatory response (35,36). FMF is the overall most common autoinflammatory disease and has prevalences as high as 1/ 1,000–1/250 among Jews, Turks, Armenians, and Arabs (37). The most seri o u s complication of the disease is the development of AA type amyloidosis, first diagnosed by Mamou and Cattan in 1952 (38). This is due to caused by accumulation of amyloid fibrils in the extracellular spaces of various organs and tissues, most notably the kidneys, liver and spleen, leading to organ failure (39). Several genetic and environmental factors modify the risk for reactive amyloidosis (23).

The typical manifestation of amyloidosis in a FMF patient is defined with nephrotic ranged proteinuria, and uremia, arising from deposition of amyloid fibrils in the kidneys. The phenotypic features of the disease and the frequency of amyloidosis differs among various ethnic groups and it was emphasized by several authors that Turks have more severe disease with a higher incidence of amyloidosis (40).

FMF is caused by a mutation in the *MEFV* (pyrin) gene. Although some mutations have been described, the four most prevalent ones (M694V, M680I, M694I and V726A) account for over 80% of cases (41-43).

Pyrin expressed primarly in the innate immune system (granulocyte, dendritic cell, etc.).

Both pyrin and a related gene, cryopyrin, contain an N- terminal domain that encodes a death domain –related structure, now known as the pyrin domain, or PyD. Both pyrin and cyropyrin interact through their PyDs with a common adaptor protein, apoptotic speck

protein (ASC). ASC itself participates in apoptosis, recruitment, and activation of pro-caspase-1 (also named as IL-1β converting enzyme) and nuclear factor -kB, a transcription factor involved in initiation and resolution of the inflammatory response (44).
Wild -type pyrin has been found either to inhibit or accentuate caspase-1 activity and it is key molecule in the inflammasome. The net effect of pyrin, and the molecular mechanisms of FMF-associated mutations, remains controversial. This results in clinical attacks of inflammation in the form of fever and serositis along with increased acute-phase reactants (APRs) (erythrocyte sedimentation rate (ESR), C-reactive protein (CRP), and SAA). The continuous elevation of these APRs during and even between attacks predisposes to the development of AA systemic amyloidosis. This inflammatory state is what probably results in the variety of problems related to clinical inflammation observed in patients with FMF (25). If the child has not been treated properly and if secondary amyloidosis develops, urinalysis will reveal proteinuria (45). If proteinuria is not diagnosed, it will progress to full-blown nephrotic syndrome.
Not all FMF patients having amyloidosis, suggests the presence of other contributing factors. The role of genetic background was established by comparing the incidence of amyloidosis in Jewish patients from different ethnic origins. Apart from ethnicity, several other genetic risk factors have been defined. The M694V mutation has been shown to be a strong risk factor of developing amyloidosis in different ethnic groups (46-49). We studied in 308 patients with FMF and detected amyloidosis 8 (2.6%) patients with amyloidosis homozygous for the M694V mutation had earlier onset and, a more severe course (50).
Another factor that modulates the risk of developing amyloidosis is the SAA1 gene haplotype. Single nucleotide polymorphisms in the gene coding for SAA define 3 haplotypes: 1.1, 1.3 and 1.5. Patients with a 1.1/1.1 genotype have an increased risk for amyloidosis of 3–7-fold, independent of MEFV genotype (40,51). In addition, there is 4.5-6-fold increased risk of developing amyloidosis in affected family members of FMF patients who have already developed amyloidosis (36,52).
Colchicine treatment has changed the course of FMF by both reducing attack frequency and severity and preventing amyloidosis. Goldinger first described its effectiveness in 1972 and since then colchicine became the drug of choice for FMF (53). Colchicine, an alkaloid, binds to β-tubulin hindering its polarization with consequent defective transfer and mitosis, inhibition of neutrophil chemotaxis, and reduced expression of adhesion molecules (24).
Before the advent of colchicine, amyloidosis was relatively frequent. It occurred in up to 60%–75% of patients over the age of 40, and the incidence varied among different ethnic groups (54). Akse Onal et al. (37) observed a dramatic decrease of secondary amyloidosis in Turkey. They think that the decrease of the rate of amyloidosis in childhood is due to better education of Turkish physicians on the subject and the improvement in the infectious milieu of young children.

5.2 TNF receptor-associated periodic syndrome

This dominantly inherited disorder was first described in a large family of Irish/Scottish ancestry and hence named familial Hibernian fever (55). It is the second most common periodic fever disorder. Dominantly inherited heterozygous mutations in TNFRSF1A, encoding the TNF receptor 1 cause TRAPS (56). Because all known mutations are in the extracellular domain of the receptor, it has been hypothesized that TRAPS mutations interfere with the shedding of the TNF receptor (57). Impaired receptor shedding might then lead to repeated signaling and prolongation of the immune response. TNFRSF1A mutations cause to reduced cell surface expression of mutant receptors. This would lead to deficiency of anti inflammatory soluble TNF receptors. Patients experience recurrent, often prolonged fevers that can be accompanied by severe abdominal pain, pleurisy, arthritis a migratory skin rash with underling fasciitis and/or periorbital edema (58,59). The age of onset varies widely, but most patients become symptomatic within the first decade of life. Attacks persist for a minimum of 3 days, but usually last longer, up to several weeks (60,61). Some TRAPS patients eventually develop systemic AA amyloidosis. An estimated 14%–25% of TRAPS patients develop reactive amyloidosis (57,62). The risk of amyloidosis appears to be greater among patients with cysteine mutations (63). Affected family members of TRAPS patients with amyloidosis are at increased risk and it is advisable to screen urine samples at regular intervals for proteinuria. Treatment depends on the severity of the disease. For patients with infrequent attacks and normal SAA, prednisone during attacks may be effective (61). For patients with more severe disease, etanercept or adalimumab as anti-TNF agents were found to be effective. IL-1 receptor antagonist has also shown to be effective in non-responsive patients (64).

5.3 Cryopyrin-associated periodic syndrome

Cryopyrin-associated periodic syndromes (CAPS) are a group of rare autoinflammatory diseases including familial cold urticaria (FCAS), Muckle-Wells syndrome (MWS), and chronic infantile neurologic cutaneous articular syndrome (CINCA), also known as neonatal onset multisystem inflammatory disease (NOMID). CAPS are all caused by mutations in CIAS1 encoding cryopyrin, which is a component of the IL-1β inflammasome (56). These are all transmitted in an autosomal-dominant fashion. FCAS is characterized by recurrent, short attacks of fever, urticarial skin rash, arthralgia and conjunctivitis after exposure to cold. The peak of the attack occurs at 6–8 h and lasts up to 24 h. Amyloidosis is a rare complication of FCAS (2–4%) (65). In MWS, the typical attack includes fever, rash, arthralgia, arthritis, myalgia, headaches, conjunctivitis, episcleritis, and uveitis lasting up to 3 days. Progressive sensorineural hearing loss develops in the second and fourth decades. Amyloidosis develops in 25% of the cases (66). The onset of CINCA-NOMID is at or within several weeks of birth. It is characterized by urticaria-like rash, fever, chronic aseptic meningitis, eye findings including conjunctivitis, uveitis, and papillitis of the optic nerve. Half of patients develop a severe arthropathy.Patients have typical morphological changes of short stature, frontal bossing, macrocephaly, saddle nose, short, thick extremities with clubbing of fingers, and wrinkled skin. If untreated, 20% die by age 20 years, and others develop amyloidosis (67). [In CINCA and MWS, corticosteroid therapy can be useful in selected patients. Anti-IL-1 agents are very effective in all CAPS patients.

5.4 Hyper IgD syndrome

HIDS was identified as a separate disease entity in 1984 (68). It is inherited as an autosomal recessive trait. HIDS is caused by mutations in the MVK gene, on chromosome 12, which encodes mevalonate kinase. Mutations associated with HIDS lead to markedly reduced mevalonate kinase enzymatic activity. Excessive production of pro inflammatory cytokines by HIDS mononuclear cells may result from excessive accumulation of mevalonic acid substrate, recent data support an alternative hypothesis related to deficiencies in nonsterol isoprenoids synthesized through the mevalonate pathway. This is characterized by fever, arthralgia, abdominal pain, diarrhea, maculopapular rash, and lymphadenopathy lasting 3-7 days. An attack can be provoked by minor trauma, vaccination or stress. The attacks usually recur every 4-6 weeks, but there is considerable inter- and intraindividual variation. Secondary amyloidosis has been reported in 3% of the patients, which is rarer than that reported for the other monogenic autoinflammatory syndromes (69). Corticosteroids are ineffective in preventing or treating attacks. A number of treatments have been tried including biologics. Simvastatin used because of its inhibition of HMG-CoA reductase, the enzyme proximal to mevalonate kinase in the isoprenoid pathway (70).

5.5 Deficiency of the Interleukin-1 receptor antagonist

DIRA is a rare autosomal recessive autoinflammatory disease caused by mutations affecting the gene *IL1RN* encoding the endogenous IL-1 receptor antagonist (9, 10). Children with DIRA present with strikingly similar clinical features including systemic inflammation in the perinatal period, bone pain, characteristic radiographical findings of multifocal sterile osteolytic bone lesions, widening of multiple anterior ribs, periostitis, and pustular skin lesions. Amyloidosis associated with this syndrome have been reported yet.

5.6 Juvenile idiopathic arthritis

Juvenile idiopathic arthritis is the most common rheumatic disease of childhood. The diagnostic criteria requires a child younger than 16 years of age with arthritis for at least 6 weeks' duration with exclusion of other identifiable causes of arthritis. Juvenile idiopathic arthritis has been classified into seven subtypes. Secondary amyloidosis used to be one of the most serious and fatal complications of JIA. The form of JIA is important; amyloidosis has been observed mainly in systemic and polyarticular forms. Amyloidosis is typically accompanied by elevated levels of SAA and CRP. The prevalence of secondary amyloidosis (SA) in juvenile idiopathic arthritis (JIA) varies between 1% and 10% (9-11) Secondary amyloidosis due to JIA has been decreasing dramatically in recent years, which is due to earlier recognition and better management of the disease and the introduction of new biologic agents. In this decade, amyloidosis is a rare entity in JIA.

5.7 Other diseases

Crohn's and Behçet's disease are known to be associated with secondary amyloidosis in severe cases. The mechanism may be speculated to be due to uncontrolled inflammation similar to that in monogenic autoinflammatory diseases. Also, sickle cell anemia, chronic granulomatous disease associated aspergillosis, and Hodgkin's disease are other diseases that have been very rarely associated with AA type of amyloidosis in children in the medical literature (71).

6. Treatment

The diagnosis of amyloidosis and typing are crucial for the patient. In practice, specific treatment of the underlying disorder, aiming to suppress the inflammatory activity is the major strategy.

Treatment options of amyloidosis will be discussed in three main headings:

1. *Reducing the production of amyloidogenic precursor protein (AA and AL amyloidosis) and enhancing the clearance of amyloidogenic precursor protein (Aβ2M amyloidosis) and trying to break down the amyloid deposits*:
   Colchicine is the prototype drug that decreases production of amyloidogenic precursor protein. Biologic treatment, such as anti-TNF, anti-IL-1 therapy, may have a beneficial effect on the suppression of inflammation on amyloidosis. There are reports suggesting the effectiveness of anti-TNF and anti IL-1 antagonists on regression of secondary amyloidosis in FMF (72).
2. *Specific treatment strategies for secondary amyloidosis*:
   New treatment options directed to affect the amyloid structure (e.g., diflunisal for hereditary amyloidosis) or to prevent fibrillogenesis (e.g., eprodisate for AA amyloidosis) or to weaken their structural stability (e.g., iododoxorubicin) are being investigated (73). Eprodisate inhibits polymerization of amyloid fibrils and deposition of the fibrils in tissues by interfere with interactions between amyloidogenic proteins and glycosaminoglycans. Eprodisate therapy slowed the progression of renal disease compared to placebo. However, the drug had no significant effect on progression to end-stage renal disease or risk of death (73).
3. *Renal replacement therapy.*

7. Conclusions

The chronic inflammatuar and autoinflammatory diseases occur with persistant inflammation therefore they are the most common cause of reactive amyloidosis in children. Understanding the pathophysiology of this group of diseases will improve our data on the mechanisms of amyloid formation and therapy options.

8. References

[1] Bugov B, Lubomirova M, Kiperova B (2008). Biopsy of subcutaneous fatty tissue for diagnosis of systmemic amyloidosis. Hippokratia 12,4: 236-239.

[2] Strege RJ, Saeger W, Linke RP (1998). Diagnosis and immunohistochemical classification of systemic amyloidoses. Report of 43 cases in an unselected autopsy series. Virchows Arch. Jul;433(1):19-27.

[3] Merlini G, Bellotti V (2003). Molecular mechanisms of amyloidosis. N Engl J Med. 349:583–596.

[4] Glenner GG (1980). Amyloid deposits and amyloidosis. The b- fibrilloses. Engl J Med 302: 1283–1292; 1333–1343.

[5] Kazatchkine M, Husby G, Araki S (1993). Terminology. Nomenclature of amyloid and amyloidosis. WHO-IUIS nomenclature sub-committe. Bull WHO 71: 105–108.

[6] Perfetto F, Moggi-Pignone A, Livi R, Tempestini A, Bergesio F, Matucci-Cerinic M (2010). Systemic amyloidosis: a challenge for the rheumatologist. Nat Rev Rheumatol 6:417–429.

[7] Picken MM (2007). New insights into systemic amyloidosis: the importance of diagnosis of specific type. Curr Opin Nephrol Hypertens 16:196–203.

[8] Andersson Gare B (1999). Juvenile arthritis: who gets it, where and when? A review of current data on incidence and prevalence. Clin Exp Rheumatol;17:367–74.

[9] David J, Vouyiouka O, Ansell BM, Hall A, Woo P (1993). Amyloidosis in chronic juvenile arthritis: a morbidity and mortality study. Clin Exp Rheum 11:85-90.
[10] Filipowicz-Sosnowska AM, Rozropwicz-Denisiewicz K, Rosenthal CJ, Baum J. (1978). The amyloidosis of juvenile rheumatoid arthritis: comparative studies in Polish and American children. Arthitis Rheum 37:699-703.
[11] Ozdogan H, Kasapcopur O, Dede H, Arisoy N, Beceren T, Yurdakul S Yazici H (1991). Juvenile chronic arthritis in a Turkish population. Clin Exp Rheumatol 9:431-5.
[12] Savolainen HA, Isomaki HA (1993). Decrease in the number of deaths from secondary amyloidosis in patients with juvenile rheumatoid arthritis. J Rheumatol 20:1201-3.
[13] Immonen K, Savolainen HA, Hakala M (2007). Why can we no longer find juvenile idiopathic arthritis-associated amyloidosis in childhood or in adolescence in Finland? Scand J Rheumatol 36:402-403.
[14] Cantarini L, Lucherini OM, Simonini G, Galeazzi M, Baldari CT, Cimaz R (2010). Systemic-onset juvenile idiopathic arthritis complicated by early onset amyloidosis in a patient carrying a mutation in the MEFV gene. Rheumatol Int. 2010 Jan 1.
[15] Woo P (1992). Amyloidosis in pediatric rheumatic diseases. J Rheumatol Suppl 35:10−16.
[16] Grateau G (2003). Musculoskeletal disorders in secondary amyloidosis and hereditary fevers. Best Pract Res Clin Rheumatol 17:929−944.
[17] Rysavá R (2007). AL amyloidosis with renal involvement. Kidney Blood Press Res 30:359-36.
[18] Merlini G, Bellotti V (2003). Molecular mechanisms of amyloidosis. N Engl J Med 349:583-596.
[19] Hoffman JS, Benditt EP (1982). Changes in high density lipoprotein content following endotoxin administration in the mouse. Formation of serum amyloid protein-rich subfractions. J Biol Chem 257:10510-10517.
[20] Marhaug G (1983). Three assays for the characterization and quantitation of human serum amyloid A. Scand J Immunol 18:329-338.
[21] Benson MD, Scheinberg MA, Shirahama T, Cathcart ES, Skinner M (1977). Kinetics of serum amyloid protein A in casein-induced murine amyloidosis. J Clin Invest 59:412-417.
[22] Husebekk A, Skogen B, Husby G, Marhaug G (1985). Transformation of amyloid precursor SAA to protein AA and incorporation in amyloid fibrils in vivo. Scand J Immunol 21:283-287.
[23] van der Hilst JC, Simon A, Drenth JP (2005). Hereditary periodic fever and reactive amyloidosis. Clin Exp Med. 2005 Oct;5(3):87-98.
[24] Ben Chetritt R (2003). FMF and renal amyloidosis. Phenotypegenotype correlation, treatment and prognosis. J Nephrol 16:431-434.
[25] Ozen S (2004). Renal amyloidosis in familial Mediterranean fever. Kidney Int 65:1118-1127.
[26] Gertz MA, Kyle RA (1991). Secondary systemic amyloidosis: response and survival in 64 patients. Medicine (Baltimore)70:246-256.
[27] Mainenti PP, Cantalupo T, Nicotra S, Camera L, Imbriaco M, Di Vizio D et al (2004). Systemic amyloidosis: the CT sign of splenic hypoperfusion. Amyloid 11:281-282.

[28] Tuglular S, Yalcinkaya F, Paydas S, Oner A, Utas C, Bozfakioglu S et al (2002). A retrospective analysis for aetiology and clinical findings of 287 secondary amyloidosis cases in Turkey. Nephrol Dial Transplant 17:2003–2005.
[29] Sucker C, Hetzel GR, Grabensee B, Stockschlaeder M, Scharf RE (2006). Amyloidosis and bleeding: pathophysiology, diagnosis, and therapy. Am J Kidney Dis 47:947–955.
[30] Dubrey SW, Cha K, Simms RW, Skinner M, Falk RH (1996). Electrocardiography and Doppler echocardiography in secondary (AA) amyloidosis. Am J Cardiol 77:313–315.
[31] Drüeke TB, Massy ZA (2009). Beta2-microglobulin. Semin Dial 22:378–380.
[32] Uda H, Yokota A, Kobayashi K, Miyake T, Fushimi H, Maeda A, Saiki O (2006). Two distinct clinical courses of renal involvement in rheumatoid patients with AA amyloidosis. J Rheumatol 33:1482–1487.
[33] Nishi S, Alchi B, Imai N, Gejyo F (2008). New advances in renal amyloidosis. Clin Exp Nephrol 12:93–101.
[34] Hawkins PN (2002). Serum amyloid P component scintigraphy for diagnosing and monitoring amyloidosis. Curr Opin Nephrol Hypertens 11:649–655.
[35] Ozen S, Berdeli A, Türel B et al (2006). Arg753Gln TLR-2 polymorphism in familial Mediterranean fever: linking the environment to the phenotype in a monogenic inflammatory disease. J Rheumatol 33:2498–2500.
[36] Saatci U, Bakkaloglu A, Ozen S et al (1993). Familial Mediterranean fever and amyloidosis in children. Acta Paediatr 82 (8):705–706.
[37] Akse-Onal V, Sağ E, Ozen S, Bakkaloglu A, Cakar N, Besbas N, Gucer S. (2010). Decrease in the rate of secondary amyloidosis in Turkish children with FMF: are we doing better? Eur J Pediatr. 169(8):971-4. .
[38] Mamou H, Cattan R. (1952). La maladie periodique sur 14 cas personnels dont 8 compliqués de nephropathies. *Semaine hop. Paris*; 28: 1062.
[39] Falk RH, Comenzo RL, Skinner M (1997). The systemic amyloidoses. N Engl J Med 337:898–909.
[40] Yalçinkaya F, Cakar N, Misirlioğlu M, Tümer N, Akar N, Tekin M, Taştan H, Koçak H, Ozkaya N, Elhan AH (2000). Genotype-phenotype correlation in a large group of Turkish patients with familial mediterranean fever: evidence for mutation-independent amyloidosis. Rheumatology (Oxford). Jan;39(1):67-72.
[41] The French FMF Consortium (1997). A candidate gene for familial Mediterranean fever. Nat Genet 17:25–31.
[42] The International FMF Consortium (1997). Ancient missense mutations in a new member of the RoRet gene family are likely to cause familial Mediterranean fever. Cell 90:797–807.
[43] Touitou I, Lesage S, McDermott M, Cuisset L, Hoffman H, Dode C (2004). Infevers: an evolving mutation database for auto-inflammatory syndromes. Hum Mutat 24:194–1.
[44] Padeh S, Berkun Y. Auto-inflammatory fever syndromes (2007). Rheum Dis Clin North Am. 33(3):585-623.
[45] Lidar M, Livneh A (2007). Familial Mediterranean fever: clinical, molecular and management advances. Neth J Med 65:318–324.

[46] Mimouni A, Magal N, Stoffman N, Shohat T, Minasian A, Krasnov M et al (2000). Familial Mediterranean fever: effects of genotype and ethnicity on inflammatory attacks and amyloidosis. Pediatrics 105:E70.
[47] Mansour I, Delague V, Cazeneuve C, Dode C, Chouery E, Pecheux C et al (2001). Familial Mediterranean fever in Lebanon: mutation spectrum, evidence for cases in Maronites, Greek orthodoxes, Greek catholics, Syriacs and Chiites and for an association between amyloidosis and M694V and M694I mutations. Eur J Hum Genet 9:51-55.
[48] Brik R, Shinawi M, Kepten I, Berant M, Gershoni-Baruch R (1999). Familial Mediterranean fever: clinical and genetic characterization in a mixed pediatric population of Jewish and Arab patients. Pediatrics 103:e70.
[49] Cazeneuve C, Sarkisian T, Pecheux C, Dervichian M, Nedelec B, Reinert P et al (1999). MEFV-gene analysis in Armenian patients with Familial Mediterranean fever: diagnostic value and unfavorable renal prognosis of the M694V homozygous genotype - genetic and therapeutic implications. Am J Hum Genet 65:88-97.
[50] Ozalkaya E, Mir S, Sozeri B, Berdeli A, Mutlubas F, Cura A (2010). Familial Mediterranean fever gene mutation frequencies and genotype-phenotype correlations in the Aegean region of Turkey.Rheumatol Int. Mar 9.
[51] Gershoni-Baruch R, Brik R, Zacks N, Shinawi M, Lidar M, Livneh A (2003). The contribution of genotypes at the MEFV and SAA1 loci to amyloidosis and disease severity in patients with familial Mediterranean fever. Arthritis Rheum 48:1149-1155.
[52] Tunca M, Akar S, Onen F, Ozdogan H, Kasapcopur O, Yalcinkaya F et al (2005). Familial Mediterranean fever (FMF) in Turkey: results of a nationwide multicenter study. Medicine (Baltimore) 84:1-11.
[53] Goldinger SE (1972). Colchicine for familial Mediterranean fever. N Engl J Med 287:1302.
[54] Gafni J, Ravid M, Sohar E (1968). The role of amyloidosis in familial Mediterranean fever. A population study. Isr J Med Sci 4:995-999.
[55] Williamson LM, Hull D, Mehta R, Reeves WG, Robinson BH, Toghill PJ (1982). Familial Hibernian fever. Q J Med 51:469-480.
[56] Masters SL, Simon A, Aksentijevich I, Kastner DL. (2009). Horror autoinflammaticus: the molecular pathophysiology of autoinflammatory disease (*).Annu Rev Immunol. 27:621-68.
[57] McDermott MF, Aksentijevich I, Galon J, McDermott EM, Ogunkolade BW, Centola M et al (1999). Germline mutations in the extracellular domains of the 55 kDa TNF receptor, TNFR1, define a family of dominantly inherited autoinflammatory syndromes. Cell 97:133-144.
[58] Hull KM, Drewe E, Aksentijevich I, Singh HK, Wong K et al., (2002). The TNF receptor-associated periodic syndrome (TRAPS): emerging concepts of an autoinflammatory disorder. Medicine 81:349-68.
[59] Hull KM, Wong K, Wood GM, Chu WS, Kastner DL (2002). Monocytic fasciitis: a newly recognized clinical feature of tumor necrosis factor receptor dysfunction. Arthritis Rheum 46:2189-94.
[60] McDermott EM, Smillie DM, Powell RJ (1997). Clinical spectrum of familial Hibernian fever: a 14-year follow-up study of the index case and extended family. Mayo Clin Proc 72:806-817.

[61] Hull KM, Drewe E, Aksentijevich I, Singh HK, Wong K, McDermott EM et al (2002). The TNF receptor-associate periodic syndrome (TRAPS) - emerging concepts of an autoinflammatory disorder. Medicine 81:349–368.
[62] Galon J, Aksentijevich I, McDermott MF, O'Shea JJ, Kastner DL (2000). TNF receptor-associated periodic syndromes (TRAPS): mutations in TNFR1 and early experience with Etanercept therapy. FASEB J 14:A1150.
[63] Aksentijevich I, Galon J, Soares M, Mansfield E, Hull K, Oh HH, Goldbach-Mansky R, Dean J, Athreya B, Regianato AJ, Henrickson M, Pons-Estel B, O'Shea JJ, Kastner DL (2001). The tumor necrosis factor receptor associated periodic syndrome: new mutations in TNFRSF1A, ancestral origins, genotypephenotype studies, and evidence for further heterogeneity of periodic fevers. Am J Hum Genet 69:301–314.
[64] Gottorno M, Pelagatti MA, Meini A, Obici L, Barcellona R, Federici S, Buoncompagni A, Plebani A, Merlini G, Martini A (2008). Persistent efficacy of anakinra in patients with tumor necrosis factor receptor associated periodic syndrome. Arthritis Rheum 58:1516–1520.
[65] Hoffman HM, Wanderer AA, Broide DH (2001). Familial cold autoinflammatory syndrome: phenotype and genotype of an autosomal dominant periodic fever. J Allergy Clin Immunol 108:615–620.
[66] Hawkins PN, Lachmann HJ, Aganna E, McDermott MF (2004). Spectrum of clinical features in Muckle-Wells syndrome and response to anakinra. Arthritis Rheum 50:607–612.
[67] Feldmann J, Prieur AM, Quartier P, Berquin P, Certain S, Cortis E, Teilac-Hamel D, Fischer A, de Saint BG (2002). Chronic infantile neurological cutaneous and articular syndrome is caused by mutations in CIAS1, a gene highly expressed in polymorphonuclear cells and chondrocytes. Am J Hum Genet 71:198– 203.
[68] van der Meer JWM, Vossen JM, Radl J, van Nieuwkoop JA, Meyer CJ, Lobatto S et al (1984). Hyperimmunoglobulinaemia D and periodic fever: a new syndrome. Lancet 1:1087–1090.
[69] Samuels J, Ozen S (2006). Familial Mediterranean fever and the other auto inflammatory syndromes: evaluation of the patient with recurrent fever. Curr Opin Rheumatol 18:108–117.
[70] Simon A, Bijzet J, Voorbij HA, Mantovani A, van der Meer JW, Drenth JP (2004). Effect of inflammatory attacks in the classical type hyper-IgD syndrome on immunoglobulin D, cholesterol and parameters of the acute phase response. J Intern Med 256:247–253.
[71] Bilginer Y, Akpolat T, Ozen S(2011).Renal amyloidosis in children.Pediatr Nephrol. Mar 1.
[72] Gottenberg JE, Merle-Vincent F, Bentaberry F, Allanore Y, Berenbaum F, Fautrel B, Combe B, Durbach A, Sibilia J, Dougados M, Mariette X (2003). Anti-tumor necrosis factor alpha therapy in fifteen patients with AA amyloidoses secondary to inflammatory arthritis. Arthritis Rheum 48:2019–20.
[73] Dember LM, Hawkins PN, Hazenberg BP, Gorevic PD, Merlini G, Butrimiene I, Livneh A, Lesnyak O, Puéchal X, Lachmann HJ, Obici L, Balshaw R, Garceau D, Hauck W, Skinner M (2007). Eprodisate for AA Amyloidosis Trial Group. Eprodisate for the treatment of renal disease in AA amyloidosis. N Engl J Med 356:2349–2360.

3

Intracardiac Thrombosis, Embolism and Anticoagulation Therapy in Patients with Cardiac Amyloidosis – Inspiration from a Case Observation

Dali Feng[1], Kyle Klarich[2] and Jae K. Oh[2]
[1]*The Metropolitan Heart and Vascular Institute, Minneapolis, Minnesota*
[2]*The Cardiovascular Division, Mayo Clinic, Rochester, Minnesota*
USA

1. Introduction

Amyloidosis is uncommon. Data from Olmsted County, Minnesota, report age-adjusted incidences between 6.1 and 10.5 per million person-years.[1] It is estimated that there are 1275 to 3200 new cases annually in the United States.[1, 2] Amyloidosis is classified by the precursor plasma proteins that form the extracellular fibril deposits. The primary systemic type, AL, is due to monoclonal immunoglobulin free light chains, the hereditary ("familial") type is due to mutant transthyretin deposition, the wild type transthyretin type (wild type TTR, or "senile" type) is due to normal wild-type transthyretin deposition, and the secondary type (AA type) is related to amyloid A protein.[2, 3] Amyloidosis, especially the AL type, frequently involves the heart and can cause arrhythmias, heart failure with left ventricular diastolic dysfunction, and sudden cardiac death.[4, 5] In part because of cardiac involvement, AL amyloidosis has the worst prognosis, with a median survival of 6 months when heart failure is present.[2, 5-7] Many patients with cardiac amyloidosis die suddenly, presumably related to either arrhythmia or electromechanical dissociation.[8] However, systematic studies evaluating the causes of death are lacking until recently.

2. Case reports of intracardiac thrombosis in cardiac amyloidosis

We initially saw a 58-year-old woman with primary amyloidosis who presented with biatrial thrombosis while in sinus rhythm. The patient presented with orthopnea, postural hypotension, epigastric pain, anorexia, nausea, vomiting, and lower extremity edema that had progressed for 5 months. Esophageal gastric endoscopy showed negative findings, but a gastric mucosa biopsy specimen was positive for amyloid deposition. Examinations from other institution included a transthoracic echocardiogram and a coronary angiogram 1 month earlier were unremarkable. She was referred to Mayo Clinic for further evaluation. Physical examination findings included a pulse rate of 106 beats per minute, blood pressure of 114/80 mm Hg, and an elevated jugular venous pressure. Her lungs were clear to auscultation. Her heart rate and rhythm were regular and had no appreciable murmur, rub, or gallop. She had mild hepatomegaly and moderate bilateral pitting edema in both lower extremities.

Immunoglobulin G gama monoclonal protein was detected in her serum and urine. The electrocardiogram showed sinus tachycardia and a heart rate of 104 beats per minute, low QRS voltage, and a Q wave in V_1 through V_4. A transthoracic echocardiogram showed a large mobile mass (32×17 mm) protruding from the left atrial appendage (Fig. 1) that was consistent with a thrombus. Concentric left ventricular wall thickening, right ventricular free wall thickening, and the granular "sparkling" appearance of the myocardium was noted. The generalized hypokinetic left ventricle had a mildly reduced ejection fraction of 45 %. Other characteristic findings of cardiac amyloidosis that also were present included thickened cardiac valves and atrial septum, moderately dilated atria, inferior vena cava and hepatic vein dilatation with systolic flow reversal, and small circumferential pericardial effusion. A restrictive left ventricle filling pattern was apparent and suggested considerably elevated left ventricular filling pressure (figure 2). There was minimal atrial reversal in the pulmonary vein. Tissue Doppler echocardiography showed only small mitral A waves but no A' waves in the mitral annulus (figure 3). These observations suggested atrial electromechanical dissociation, also termed atrial standstill.

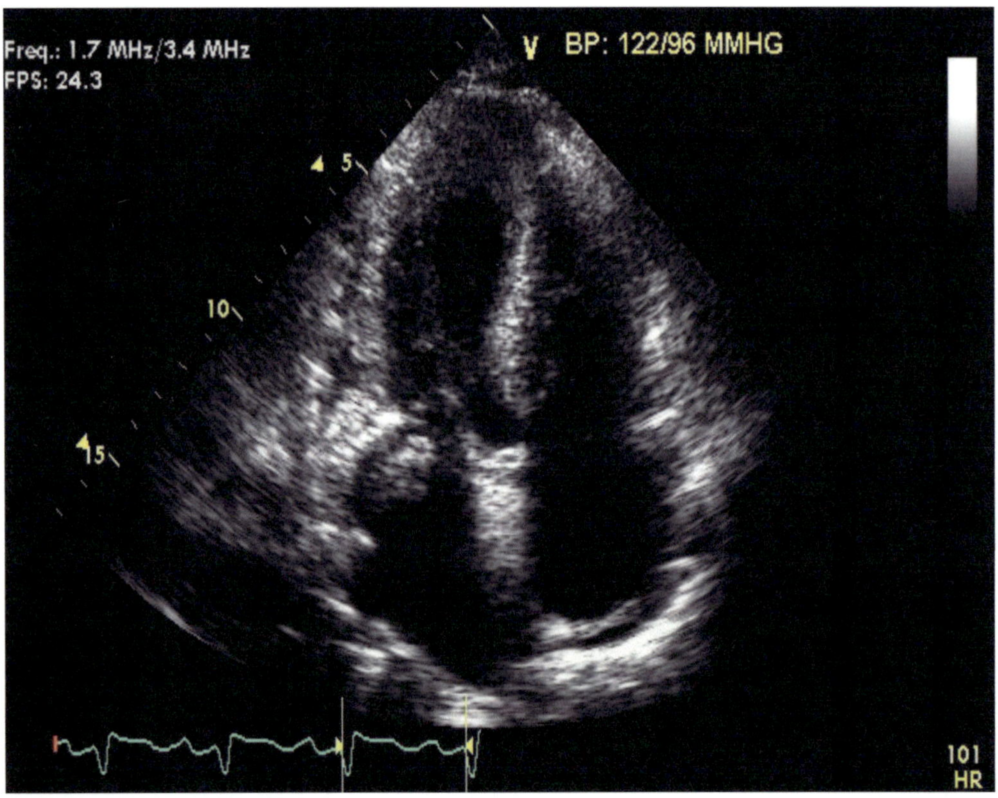

Fig. 1. A transthoracic echocardiogram of 4 chambers view showed a large mobile mass (32×17 mm) protruding from the left atrial appendage that was consistent with a thrombus. Concentric left ventricular wall thickening, right ventricular free wall thickening, and the granular "sparkling" appearance of the myocardium was noted

The patient was immediately hospitalized and received anticoagulation therapy with intravenous heparin. She quickly became confused and hypotensive, had decompensated

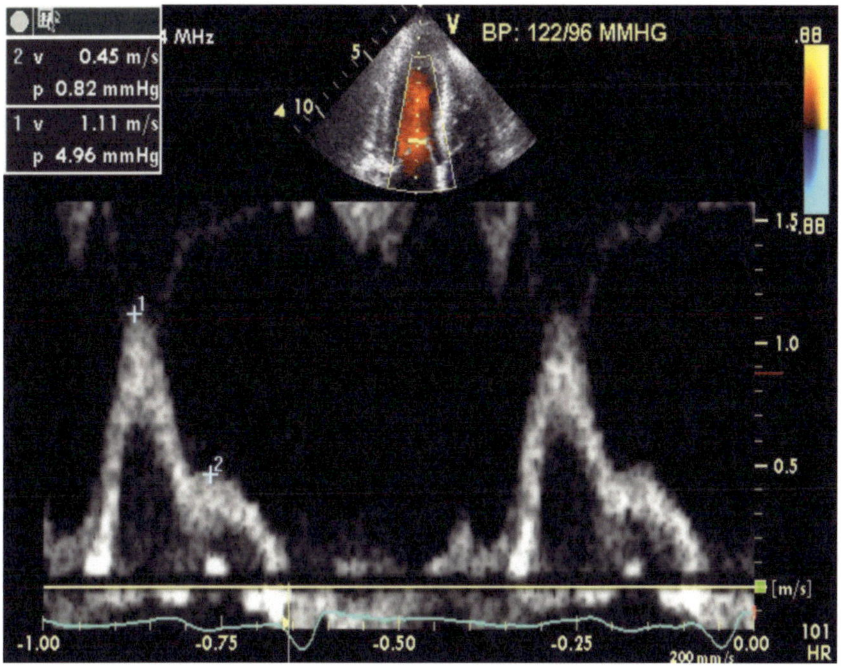

Fig. 2. A restrictive left ventricle filling pattern was apparent and suggested considerably elevated left ventricular filling pressure

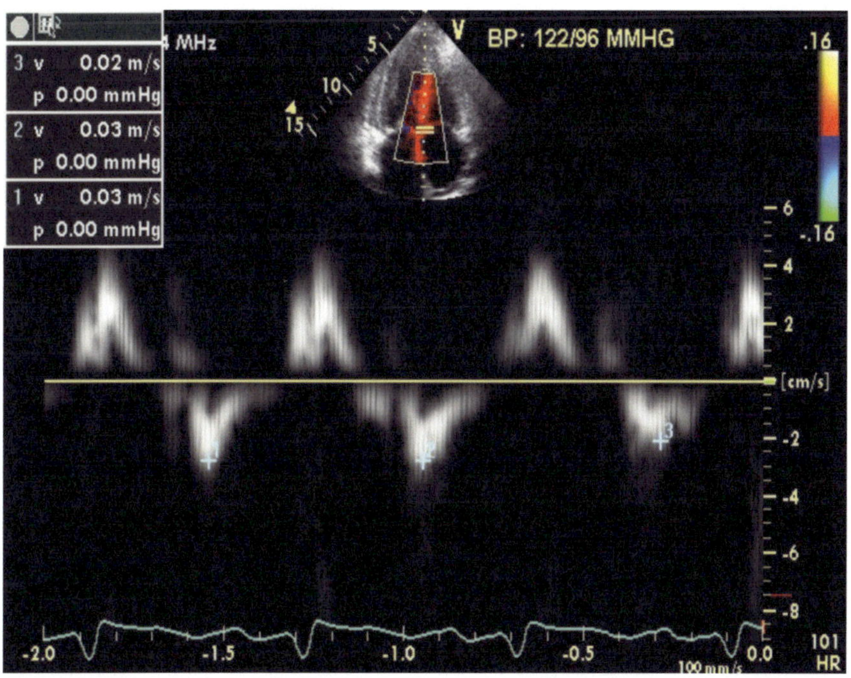

Fig. 3. Tissue Doppler echocardiography showed only small mitral A waves but no A′ waves in the mitral annulus

heart failure and then cardiogenic shock, and required inotropic support. On her third hospitalization day, she had a cardiac arrest and could not be resuscitated.

An autopsy confirmed thrombi in the left atrial appendage (Fig. 4) and right atrial appendage, and multiple infarctions were identified in the distal small bowel, ascending colon, bilateral kidneys, and spleen. Histologic studies showed extensive amyloid deposition in the heart, kidney, spleen, gastrointestinal tract, and pancreas (figure 5 a and b). Interestingly, the patient had not reported abdominal pain or other gastrointestinal symptoms, which could suggest that a mesenteric embolism occurred before death.

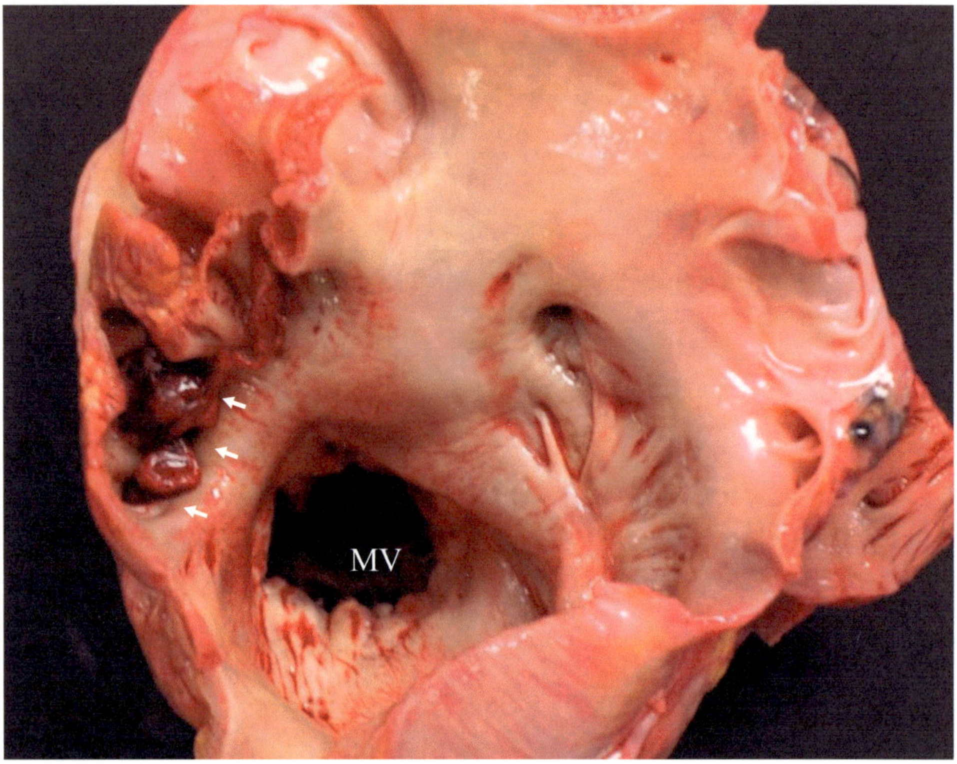

Fig. 4. An intracardiac thrombus in the left atrial appendage (LAA); MV: mitral valve

The mechanism underlying intracardiac thrombosis in sinus rhythm for a patient with cardiac amyloidosis was not clear. We postulated that severely reduced atrial contractility attributable to amyloid infiltrate, increased left atrial afterload, and left atrial enlargement with depressed left ventricle systolic and diastolic function may partially explain why the patient developed left atrial thrombosis in sinus rhythm.

There have been only a few similar case reports in the literature.[9-12] These cases shared some common salient clinical features. First, all the patients were in normal sinus rhythm, which is very rare for intracardiac thrombosis while in sinus rhythm. Second, their LVEF were normal or only mild depressed. Third, intracardiac thrombosis was often undiagnosed until the index catastrophic pulmonary or systemic embolism. Forth, very poor outcome with most patients died with in a few days and few months after the diagnosis. The characteristics of these subjects were summarized in the Table 1.

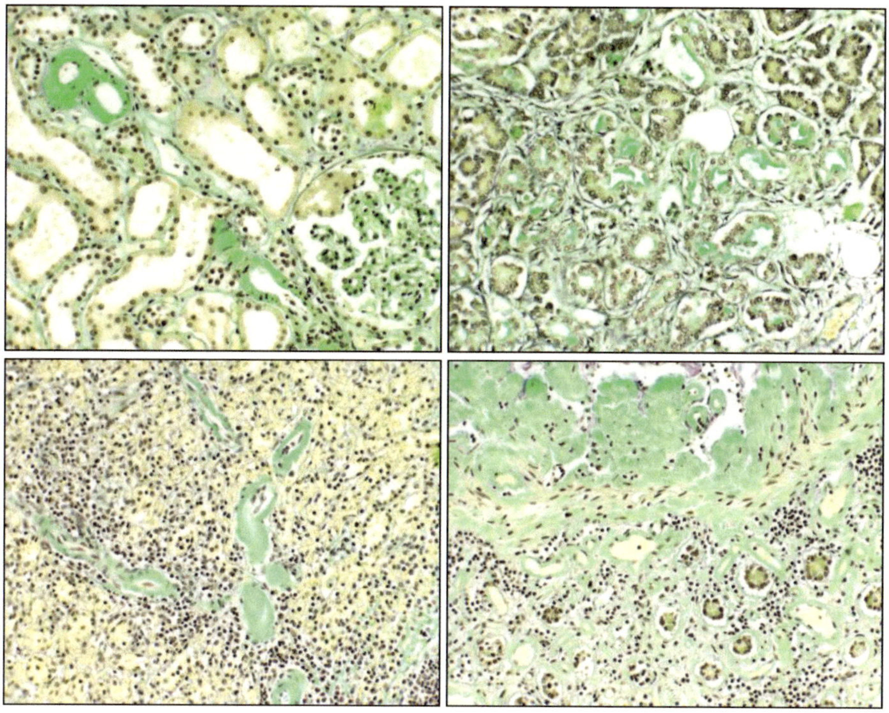

(a)

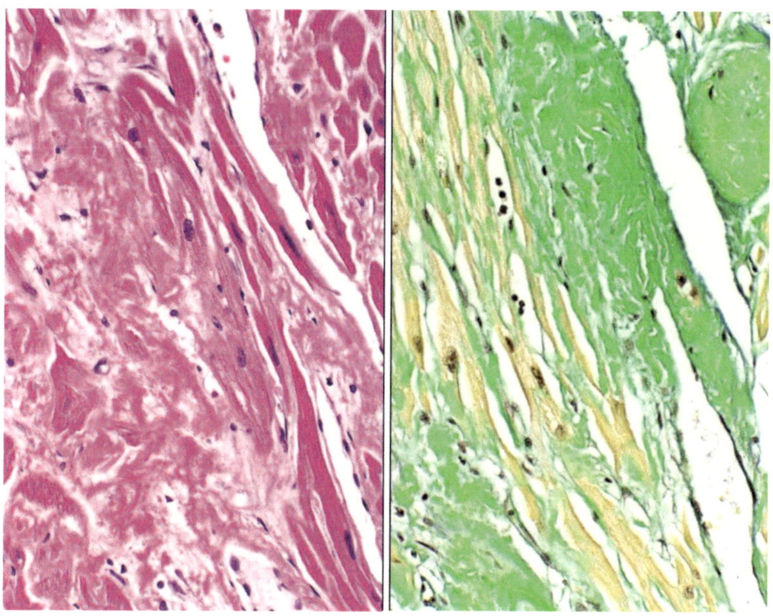

(b)

Fig. 5. Extensive interstitial amyloid deposition in the heart (figure a), kidney, spleen, gastrointestinal tract, and pancreas (figure b). The amyloid was stained as light pink on the Congo red stain and as green on sulfated Alcian blue stain

Authors	No	Presentation	Location	Rhythm	Method	Out come
Botker[9]	1	46 W, AL, recurrent stroke,	LA	SR	Autopsy	Died 1 m later of cardiac/renal failure
Plehn[24]	1	58 W; AL, CHF, LVEF 50%.	LAA	SR	TTE	Stroke/Heart Tx 4mons/died 14 mons
Browne[10]	2	66 M, MM, CHF, LVEF 46%, RLE embolism	Atria/LV	SR/PVC	Autopsy	Deceased in 3 days due to CHf/shock SCD 6
		54 M, AL, nephrotic syndrome, CHF, LVEF 57%, RLE embolism.	Unclear	SR/PAC	Autopsy	mons later
Willens[15]	1	74 W, CHF, LLE embolism. Mild LV systolic dysfunction.	L/RAA	SR	TEE	Deceased "several mons" later
Dubrey[17]	3	44/W; AL, CHF, EF 30%	L/RAA	SR	Autopsy	Died of CHF 4 m later
		52 W; AL, CHF,	LAA	SR	TTE	Died of CHF 1 m later
		58 W; AL, CHF, LVEF 50%	LAA	SR	TTE	Stroke/Heart Tx 4 m later /Died 14 m later
Cools[12]	1	64 M, MM, sever edema, and CHF no nephrotic syndrome ?LVEF	IVC	SR	CT/US	Deceased 4 mons later intestine infarction
Santarone[11, 16]	3	60 W, AL, CHF, nl LVEF	Atria	SR	TTE/TEE	SCD/PE 15 d later
		62 W, AL, CHF, nl LVEF	LAA	SR	TEE	Died of CHF 9 m later
		65 M, AL, SOB, nl LVEF	LAA	SR/PVC	TTE	SCD 4 m later

Table 1. Summary of the case report on intracardaic thrombosis and their clinical features in cardiac amyloidosis

3. Intracardiac thrombosis and embolism from autopsy data at the Mayo Clinic

The frequency of intracardiac thrombosis and its relationship to thromboembolic complications and mortality had been not well established. To clarify this issue, we reviewed autopsy and explanted hearts with various types of amyloidosis to determine how frequently intracardiac thrombi are present and how frequently they cause embolic events or death. We then elucidated the clinical and echocardiographic characteristics that predict intracardiac thrombosis and embolism. We searched the Mayo Clinic Tissue Registry database for cases of cardiac amyloidosis from1996 to 2005.[13] Of 142 cases, 26 were excluded because of inadequate tissue or incomplete clinical information. The remaining 116 cases included 112 autopsy cases and 4 surgically explanted hearts. A control group included 46 non-amyloid fatal trauma cases.

3.1 Transthoracic echocardiogram

Transthoracic echocardiograms (TTE) were obtained in 82/116 patients. The TTE was reviewed independently without knowledge of the clinical and pathological data. TTE parameters extracted included left ventricular (LV) ejection fraction (LVEF), LV end diastolic diameter (LVEDD), LV end systolic diameter (LVESD), stroke volume, ventricular septum thickness, LV posterior wall thickness, right ventricular (RV) free wall thickness, RV systolic pressure, left atrium (LA) volume index, right atrium (RA) enlargement (0=normal, 1=mild, 2=moderate, 3=severe), LV diastolic function grade,[14] mitral inflow E and A velocity, deceleration time, mitral septal annulus tissue Doppler velocity (early peak diastolic velocity: e′, late peak diastolic velocity: a′) and pulmonary venous flow profile [peak systolic velocity (S), peak diastolic velocity (D), D/S, and atrial contractile velocity], E/A, and E/e'.[14] HR and BP at the time of TTE were documented.

3.2 Pathology data

All cardiac chambers were examined for thrombi. Thrombi were characterized as to their exact anatomic location and size. The presence of cardiac amyloid was confirmed with Congo red or sulfated Alcian blue stain. Amyloid subtype was determined immunohistochemically with antibodies against serum amyloid P component, lambda and kappa free immunoglobulin light chains, transthyretin, amyloid A component, and beta-2 microglobulin.

3.3 Cause of death

The autopsy reports were evaluated by a pathologist and a cardiologist without knowledge of the patient's clinical diagnosis (i.e., trauma, amyloidosis, amyloidosis type, or cardiac rhythm). Death was due to a thromboembolic cause if: major acute pulmonary emboli were present, irrespective of pulmonary infarction; mesenteric artery embolism with bowel infarction was present; major embolic stroke with associated intracranial hemorrhage was present or if emboli were the cause of complications such as aspiration pneumonia and death; renal infarcts were present with renal failure; or death occurred during or shortly after surgical intervention for emboli.

3.4 Results

Age ranged from 31-101 years (mean of 72±16). Sixty-one percent were men. In the control group, mean age was 55±27 years; 69% were men. The demographic data for the amyloid patients are shown in Table 2. There were 55 AL cases, 55 wild type TTR cases, 4 AA types, and 2 familial types. Because AA and familial types are rare (n = 6), they were combined into one group with the TTR cases (called other, n=61). Results were similar with and without these. Compared with the other amyloid group, the AL was younger; had less AF; a shorter survival time from the onset of symptoms and less commonly had CAD (Table 2). They had thicker ventricular architecture. There were no significant difference in CHF history in two groups but the AL type had greater value for NYHA class. There were no differences in gender, ethnicity, creatine, and LVEF.

3.4.1 Intracardiac thrombus

Intracardiac thrombi were identified in 38/116 (33%) hearts. Twenty-three had 1 thrombus while 15 had 2-5 thrombi for a total of 63. Thirty-six were in the RA, 19 in the LA (Figure 1), 4 on the coronary sinus valve, 3 in the RV, and 1 in the LV. No intracardiac thrombus was identified in the 46 fatal trauma subjects. There were significant differences in the frequency of intracardiac thrombosis between the cardiac amyloid group and the control group (33% versus 0%, $p<0.0001$). The AL group had more intracardiac thrombi than the other amyloid group (51% versus 16%, $p<0.0001$). Of the 4 AA cases, 2 had intracardiac thrombus. There were none in the familial cases.

3.4.2 Embolic events and cause of death

There were 23 embolic events in patients with amyloid. There were 19 fatal and 4 non-fatal emboli. AL patients had more fatal thromboembolism (14/53; 26%) than the other amyloid patients (5/59; 8 %) and than the control group (1/46; 2%; p<0.001). Embolic fatalities for the AL group included 7 pulmonary emboli (PE), 1 mesentery artery embolus with bowel infarction, 1 iliac artery embolus and the patient died during attempted embolectomy, and 5 cases with multiple emboli. In addition, there were 4 non-fatal embolic events in the AL group including 3 found at autopsy and 1 with PE and brachial artery embolism who survived after cardiac transplant. Among the other amyloid group, there were 5 embolic fatalities, including 3 PEs, 1 mesenteric artery embolus with bowel infarction, and 1 case with multiple systemic emboli.

	AL (n=55)	Other Amyloid (n=61)	P value
Age, years	60 ± 11	83 ± 11	<0.0001
Gender, % male	61	62	=0.80
Ethnic, % Caucasian	100	100	=0.53
Atrial fibrillation, %	22	45	=0.008
Anticoagulation , %	26	37	=0.21
Survival time (months)	23 ± 25	63 ± 12	=0.01
CAD by autopsy, % *	10	90	<0.0001
CAD severity score (0 to 4) *	1.5 (1.2-1.5)	3.3 (2.9-3.5)	<0.0001
Cardiac mass, g	532±150	474±132	=0.017
LV septal thickness, mm	16.5±4.2	16.0±4.2	=0.26
LV posterior wall, mm	16.0±3.5	14.7±3.8	=0.029
RV free wall, mm	6.0±2.4	4.9±1.7	=0.006
CHF (%)	77	63	=0.10
NYHA class (1-4)	2.8±1.2	2.1±1.2	=0.01
LVEF (%)	50 ± 18	52 ± 16	=0.66
Creatine mg/dL	2.3 ± 1.5	1.8 ± 1.1	=0.07

CAD = coronary artery disease; CAD severity score at autopsy: 0 = none, 1 = minimal, 2 = mild, 3 = moderate, 4 = severe.

Table 2. Patient characteristics in AL and the other amyloid groups

3.4.3 Clinical characteristics, TTE and thromboembolism

Forty-five subjects (40%) had intracardiac thrombosis, embolism or both. Compared to the group without thromboembolism, they were younger, less often hypertensive, had more AL type, and lower systolic BP (Table 3). The thromboembolic group had less CAD and when present, less extensive involvement. Other demographic and clinical variables were similar. TTE features are in Table 3. Times from TTE to death were similar. The thromboembolic group had a higher HR at TTE, a smaller LVEDD, thicker LV posterior and RV walls, a smaller SV, a lower RV systolic pressure, a lower LVEF, worse LV diastolic function, a shorter deceleration time, poorer LA mechanical activity (a lower A and a′ velocity), and a higher E/A and E/e′ than the non thromboembolic group. Furthermore, PV peak systolic velocity and A velocity were significantly lower and D/S was higher. LA volume index and RA size were not different (Table 4). RV wall was thicker in subjects who had RA thrombosis compared with those who did not have RA thrombosis (7.9±2.7 mm vs. 6.6±3.1 mm, p=0.02).

3.4.4 Multivariate analysis and ROC

By multivariate analysis, AL type [OR=15.6 (2.8-117.6), p=0.001] and AF [OR=6.0 (1.7-26.7), p=0.004] were independently associated with thromboembolism in a model with clinical variables (Table 5) with high odds ratios for both [OR=55.0 (8.1-1131.5), p<0.0001]. For TTE

variables, RV wall thickness [OR=1.3 (1.0-1.7), p=0.03] with 1 mm increase in the wall, LV diastolic function [OR 8.8 (1.6-64.1), p=0.01] with restrictive pattern (grade 3 or 4) compared with grade 2 or less, and HR at echo [OR=1.7 (1.1-2.9), p=0.02] with 10 beats/minute of increase were independently associated with thromboembolism. There were no differences in thromboembolic risk between LV diastolic function grade 2 versus grade 1 or normal diastolic function. When both clinical and TTE variables were included in the analyses, AL type [OR 8.4 (1.8-51.2), p=0.006], LV diastolic function [OR=12.2 (2.7-72.7), p=0.0008] and a higher HR [OR=1.1 (1.0-1.2), p=0.048] were independently associated with thromboembolism (Table 5). Other variables were not associated with thromboembolism including atrial sizes.
The receiver operating characteristic curve (ROC) for using LV diastolic function grade to predict thromboembolism is shown in Figure 2. Grade 3 LV diastolic dysfunction had a sensitivity of 78% and a specificity of 79%. The area under curve was 0.81. Using amyloid type, LV diastolic function, and HR, the area under the curve was 0.87. Presence of both LV diastolic grade 3 or 4 and AL type increased specificity to 94 % but decreased sensitivity to 56 % as one would expect.

	With (n=45)	Without (n=71)	P value
Age, years	65 ± 2.2	77 ± 1.8	<0.0001
Gender, % male	58	62	0.67
Body mass index, kg/m2	26.0±0.9	26.7±0.8	0.54
Hypertension, %	17	41	0.008
Diabetes, %	7	19	0.08
CHF, %	65	71	0.55
NYHA class (1-4)	2.4±1.3	2.3±1.2	0.65
Atrial fibrillation, %	37	33	0.64
Anticoagulation , %	36	28	0.42
Cancer, %	15	22	0.41
Syncope, %	34	17	0.08
AL amyloidosis, %	73	31	<0.0001
Stem cell transplant, %	23	10	0.09
Recent operation, %	10	17	0.31
History of thrombosis, %	27	24	0.76
Systolic BP, mm Hg	111±18	128±24	0.0005
Diastolic BP, mm Hg	67±12	69±15	0.54
Creatinine, mg/dL	2.2±1.7	1.9±1.1	0.17
CAD by autopsy, %	29.3	55.4	0.008
CAD severity score (0 to 4) *	2.0±1.2	2.7±1.3	0.02

* CAD severity score: 0 = no, 1 = minimal, 2 = mild, 3 = moderate and 4 = severe.

Table 3. Characteristics in patients with and without Thromboembolism

3.5 Discussion

The Mayo autopsy study of patients with cardiac amyloidosis identifies a high frequency of intracardiac thrombosis, especially in AL patients, despite normal sinus rhythm and relatively preserved LVEF. Most thrombi arose in the atria. Thrombosis and embolism caused significant fatality. AL type, AF, poor LV diastolic function, RV wall thickness by TTE, and higher HR were independent predictors for thromboembolism. Many risk factors

	With (n=35)	Without (n=47)	P Value
Time (from TTE to death), day	15 (1-55)	43 (2-209)	0.12
HR at echo, beats/min	86±17	79±14	0.02
LV end diastolic diameter, mm	44.3±7.8	48.1±8.1	0.04
LV end systolic diameter, mm	32.4±9.3	33.1±9.8	0.76
LV septal thickness, mm	14.2±3.9	12.9±3.3	0.12
LV posterior wall thickness, mm	13.8±3.6	12.2±3.1	0.03
RV free wall thickness, mm	8.3±3.6	5.9±2.1	0.0007
LA volume index (cc/m^2)	40.1±14.9	48.2±35.2	0.21
RA enlargement (0-3)	1.8±1.2	1.4±1.1	0.08
Stroke volume, mL	51.1±20.9	67.6±23.4	0.002
RV systolic pressure, mm Hg	44.3±9.4	51.1±15.9	0.045
LVEF (%)	46±19	54±15	0.03
LV diastolic function grade (0-4)	3.1±1.1	1.9±0.8	0.0001
Mitral deceleration time (ms)	160±37	193±60	0.006
Mitral E velocity (m/s)	0.87±0.21	0.90±0.26	0.65
Mitral A velocity (m/s)	0.27±0.29	0.52±0.33	0.0008
E/A	3.4±2.6	2.0±1.9	0.03
Mitral annulus e' velocity (cm/s)	4.4±2.3	5.9±2.7	0.06
Mitral annulus a' velocity (cm/s)	2.3±3.3	6.6±4.7	0.003
E/e'	23±12	16±8	0.02
PV systolic velocity, m/s	0.32±0.18	0.48±0.20	0.002
PV diastolic velocity, m/s	0.65±0.20	0.60±0.18	0.37
PV A velocity, m/s	0.14±0.13	0.24±0.13	0.008
PV diastolic/systolic ratio	3.0±2.3	1.5±0.8	0.001

Table 4. TTE characteristics in subjects with and without Thromboembolism

Dependent Variate	Models *	Predictors	OR	95 % CI	P value
Thromboembolism	Model 1	AL type	15.6	2.8-117.6	0.001
		AF	6.0	1.7-26.7	0.004
		AL and AF	55.0	8.1-1131.5	0.0001
Thromboembolism	Model 2	RV free wall	1.3	1.0-1.7	0.03
		LV diastolic function	8.8	1.6-64.1	0.01
		Heart rate	1.7	1.1-2.9	0.02
Thromboembolism	Model 3	AL type	8.4	1.8-51.2	0.006
		LV diastolic function	12.2	2.7-72.7	0.0008
		Heart rate	1.1	1.0-1.2	0.048

CI = confidence interval.

* Model 1: Clinical variates included are age, amyloid type, AF, hypertension, and CAD.

Model 2: Echo variates included are RV wall thickness, LV diastolic function, LVEF, SV, mitral A velocity, and HR at TTE.

Model 3: Combined model with variates included amyloid type, AF, RV free wall, LV diastolic function, SV, and HR.

Table 5. Predictors for thromboembolism by multivariate analyses

in patients without amyloidosis such as age, CHF, hypertension and diabetes were not significantly associated with thromboembolism from the Mayo Autopsy study. Surprisingly, atrial size was not associated with thromboembolism despite the fact that most thrombi were found in the atria. Measures of atrial mechanical activity such as A velocity and a' velocity were different only in univariate analyses but not multivariate analyses.

3.5.1 Intracardiac thrombosis in cardiac amyloidosis

The high incidence of intracardiac thrombosis from Mayo autopsy study confirms the observations of Roberts.[4] AL type was associated with a 51% incidence compared to only 16% in the other amyloid groups despite the fact that these groups were older and more frequently had AF. Other than case reports and a small autopsy study,[10,12,15-17] the Mayo's investigation was the only systemic study to report the high frequency of intracardiac thrombosis and clinical thromboembolic complications resulting in mortality. Roberts et al retrospectively studied 49 AL and 5 familial type hearts and identified intracardiac thrombi in 26%. The clinical implications of these thrombi are unknown. Halligan et al. found 2% of biopsy-proven AL patients had clinically documented thromboembolism[18] and thrombosis was associated increased mortality. Common features of previous reports include middle-age years of patients, relatively preserved LVEF despite clinical CHF and multiple thrombi. A majority of the patients had a poor prognosis. Most patients were in sinus rhythm.

3.5.2 Intracardiac thrombosis and embolism

Twenty-six percent of our patients died from embolic complications in the AL group. Not all patients with documented embolism had intracardiac thrombosis at autopsy (30%) perhaps because some thrombi had been dislodged prior to death. Alternatively, some patients could have had other sources for thrombi.

3.5.3 Clinical variables and thromboembolism

Several studies show that advanced age, AF, CHF, diabetes, and hypertension are risk factors for thromboembolism in non amyloid patients.[19,20] In the Mayo autopsy investigation, the mean age was younger in patients with thromboembolism. This is because primary amyloid patients were much younger than the non primary patients and they were 8.4 times more likely to develop thromboembolism. Thromboembolic patients also had a fewer comorbidities because of their younger age. By multivariate analyses, only two clinical variables, AF and AL cardiac amyloidosis, were independently associated with thromboembolism. After TTE variables and clinical variables were introduced into the analysis, AF was no longer an independent risk factor. This is likely because AF was associated with poor atrial mechanical activity and LV diastolic dysfunction. Nonetheless, we suggest that when present, AF should be considered a marker of possible intracardiac thrombosis, especially in AL patients. On the other hand, higher heart rate at TTE is independently associated with increased risk for thromboembolism. Increased heart rate reflects the underline severity of disease and therefore indicates decompensation.

Of interest, the presence of CAD and the severity of CAD at autopsy were negatively associated with intracardiac thrombosis and embolic events. This is likely because CAD is associated with older age and the mean age in our study was significantly older in the other amyloid groups. After adjusting for age, amyloid type, and other variables, CAD was not associated with intracardiac thrombosis or embolism.

Clinical CHF and NYHA class were not significantly different in patients with or without thromboembolism. Multivariate analyses only confirmed an association between poor LV diastolic function, i.e., restrictive diastology (class 3 or 4) by TTE and intracardiac thrombosis and embolism. Because many patients were elderly with multiple comorbidities, the clinical diagnosis of CHF or NYHA class is subjective indicator of over all well being and may not be always accurate. TTE with structure and function evaluation (including diastolic measures) provides more comprehensive information and is more helpful for risk stratification.

3.5.4 TTE characters and thromboembolism

Multivariate analyses showed only LV diastolic function and higher HR at TTE, and to a lesser extent, RV wall thickness were significantly associated with thromboembolism. Poor atrial mechanical activity (mitral A and a′ velocity) was significant only in univariate analyses. The observation was not surprising because LV diastolic function was graded based on several echo features including mitral inflow profile and mitral tissue Doppler.

RV wall thickness is associated with abnormal RV diastolic function.[21] Advanced RV infiltrate by amyloid (≥7mm) was associated with a restrictive tricuspid inflow filling pattern; lesser thickness was associated with abnormal RV relaxation.[21] In the current study, the mean RV wall thickness was 8.3 mm in the thromboembolic group. A thickened RV wall therefore reflected more advanced amyloid deposition with a poor RV diastolic function and with consequent stasis and thrombosis.

The LA volume index and RA size were not significantly different in the patients with and without thromboembolism although the indexes were large in both (>40cc/m^2). One would speculate that atrial size should be bigger in the thromboembolic group because of poor LV diastolic function, higher LV/LA filling pressure as estimated by E/e′ and a thicker RV wall. In the study, 73% of thromboembolic patients had AL amyloid and thus a worse prognosis. It may be that patients with AL amyloidosis do not have time to develop atrial enlargement because of short survival times. In addition advanced age and comorbidities contribute to increased LA size[22] and thromboembolic patients were younger and had a fewer comorbidities. Finally, it is possible that amyloid infiltrate in the atria prevented them from being distended as suggested by Modesto et al with strain imaging.[23]

3.5.5 Mechanism for thromboembolism

Our TTE data support the concept stasis could lead to intracardiac thrombosis. Even though the mean LVEF was relatively-preserved, those with intracardiac thrombosis had lower LVEF. Furthermore, the LV diastolic function and atrial mechanical activity were more impaired. Reduced atrial contractility secondary to amyloid infiltration has been reported[17,24] and LV diastolic function is typically impaired before systolic function.[25] The combination of systolic and diastolic ventricular dysfunction, chronic amyloid infiltrate in the atria, and direct toxic effect on myocardium[26] could lead to atrial mechanical dysfunction, atrial enlargement, and blood stasis.[23,27] Such atrial electrical-mechanical dissociation may partially explain why many cardiac amyloidosis patients developed atrial thrombosis while in sinus rhythm.[17,24,28] It is possible that endomyocardial damage and endothelial dysfunction from amyloid depositions may be responsible.[29,30] Hypercoagulability may also contribute.[7,31]

3.5.6 Summary of the Mayo autopsy study

There was a high frequency of intracardiac thrombosis in patients with cardiac amyloidosis, especially the AL type, despite sinus rhythm and preserved LVEF. Intracardiac thrombosis leads to embolic events and mortality. The presence of AL type, AF, poor LV diastolic function, greater RV wall thickness, and higher heart rare were associated with thromboembolism. Poor LV diastolic function and atrial mechanical activity are likely contributory to the complication. Transesophageal echocardiography (TEE) may be indicated for earlier detection[11] in the high risk patients since TTE is well known for its insensitivity in detecting intracardiac thrombosis especially in the atria. If intracardiac thrombosis is detected, anticoagulation therapy may be indicated. However, anticoagulation may exacerbate the hemorrhagic tendency well known in amyloidosis because of fragile blood vessel walls secondary to amyloid deposition and the coexisting coagulopathy.[2,31] Three AL amyloid patients in this study died from massive gastrointestinal bleeding.

4. TEE, intracardiac thrombosis, embolism and anticoagulation therapy in patients with cardiac amyloidosis

The autopsy study have identified a high prevalence of intracardiac thrombosis in these patients at autopsy, especially in AL cardiac amyloidosis.[4,13] Furthermore, in our autopsy series, systemic embolism was a significant cause of mortality.[13] However, it is possible that autopsy series may over emphasize the frequency of intracardiac thrombosis and there only have been a few anecdotal reports in the literature on intracardiac thrombosis detected by TEE or TTE in live patients.[9-12,15-17] The prevalence of intracardiac thrombus and the effects of anticoagulation in living cardiac amyloid patients has not been reported. Accordingly, we evaluated both TTE and TEE studies from patients with various types of cardiac amyloidosis to determine how frequently detectable intracardiac thrombi are present; the clinical and echocardiographic characteristics associated with their presence; and the effects of therapeutic anticoagulation.

4.1 Study groups

We searched the Mayo Clinic Hematology Data base for all cases of amyloidosis from 1999 to 2007. There were 156 patients had cardiac amyloid who also had TEE. The detail of exclusion and inclusion criteria was reported elsewhere.[32]

Clinical information, including demographic data, comorbidities, presence of heart failure (HF), New York Heart Association (NYHA) functional class, the use of anticoagulants prior and at the time of TEE, ECG, TTE, TEE, MRI and other laboratory data were abstracted from clinical records. Cardiac rhythm was determined from the patient's ECG, Holter monitoring data, and medical records. INR and APTT around the time of TEE were charted. Therapeutic anticoagulation was defined as INR ≥ 2 at the time of TEE or documented two or more consecutive therapeutic INR 2-3 prior to TEE for those with long term anticoagulation, or at least 48 hours of intravenous heparin therapy or 48 hours of subcutaneous low molecular weight heparin therapy prior to TEE. Other abstracted information included results of tissue biopsies, urine and serum protein electrophoresis, immunofixation, serum free light chain assay, genetic testing, and family history.[13]

4.2 Echocardiograms

TTE and TEE studies were reviewed independently without knowledge of the clinical and pathological data and was reported previously[13] The TEE studies were reviewed for presence or absence of intracardiac thrombus and their location and size.[14] Left atrial appendage (LAA) and LA spontaneous contrast and their severity were semi-quantified as none, mild, moderate or severe (0, 1, 2, or 3 respectively).[33] Left atrial appendage emptying velocity was measured by pulse Doppler echocardiography as previously reported.[33] The degree of atherosclerosis in aorta was semi-quantified as none, mild, moderate or severe.[34 35] HR and BP at the time of TEE were documented.

4.3 Demographic data and amyloid subtypes

Amyloidosis was AL type in 80, 56 wild TTR type, 17 mutant TTR type, and 3 AA type (Table 6). Because AA are rare, they were combined into one group with the wild and mutant TTR cases (called other amyloidosis, n=76). Compared with other amyloid group, the AL group was younger; had fewer males, less AF, was less often receiving anticoagulation therapy and less often had a history of hypertension, and were more likely to be treated with stem cell transplantation, all $p \leq 0.05$ (Table 6). There was no significant difference in a history of HF, NYHA class or other variables between the two groups listed in Table 1 (all p>0.05).

	All Patients (n=156)	AL (n=80)	Other Amyloid (n=76)	P value
Age, years	67 ± 11	61 ± 10	74 ± 9	<0.0001
Gender, % male	77	65	89	0.0003
Body mass index, kg/m^2	26.1 ± 4.4	26.4±4.2	25.6±4.7	0.35
Heart Rate, bpm	81 ± 18	81 ± 19	80 ± 16	0.51
Systolic BP, mm Hg	118 ± 22	117±21	120±22	0.29
Diastolic BP, mm Hg	70 ± 14	71±13	69±14	0.34
Atrial fibrillation, %	64	56	72	0.03
Anticoagulation, %	43	33	54	0.007
Hypertension, %	39	30	49	0.02
Diabetes, %	5	4	7	0.43
NYHA class 1, %	21	20	22	0.95
NYHA class 2, %	35	34	36	
NYHA class 3, %	37	39	34	
NYHA class 4, %	8	9	8	
Median NYHA class	2 (1-3)	2 (1-3)	2 (1-3)	0.64
Syncope, %	24	21	26	0.46
Stem cell transplant, %	11	21	0	<0.0001
History of thromboembolism,%	22	24	21	0.69

Table 6. Patient characteristics in AL and the other amyloid groups in TEE study

4.4 Indications for TEE

TEE was performed in 57 patients (37%) for AF and/or prior to direct current cardioversion, in 33 patients (21%) searching for source for embolism, in 14 patients (9%) for evaluation of valvular heart disease, in 12 patients (8%) for rule out endocarditis, and in 6 patients (4%) for other reasons. TEE was performed prospectively in 34 cardiac amyloid patients (22%)

after our initial autopsy observations at the discretion of referral hematologists or cardiologists. All TEE studies were performed without major complications or mortality. All patients with TEE also had TTE studies with exception in one.

4.5 Intracardiac thrombus

There were 58 intracardiac thrombi identified in 42 (27%) of 156 patients by TEE. Most patients with thrombi (30 patients, 71%) had 1 thrombus while 8 patients (19%) had 2 thrombi, and 4 patients (10%) had 3. Most clots occurred in the left atrium/appendage (n=32) or in the right atrium/appendage (n=19). Of all of these thrombi detected by TEE, only 3 were detected by TTE. There was a significant difference in the frequency of intracardiac thrombosis between patients with AL amyloidosis and the other types (35% vs. 18%, p=0.02). The frequencies for intracardiac thrombosis were 18% for wild TTR type, 17% for mutant TTR type, and 33% for AA type.

The frequency of intracardiac thrombi in those receiving therapeutic anticoagulants was only 13%, much lower than in those not on therapeutic anticoagulant therapy at the time of TEE studies (37%, p=0.001). We further analyzed these patients on chronic anticoagulation with therapeutic INR at the time of TEE with stratifying findings according to persistent or permanent AF versus non AF. Chronic anticoagulation was associated with a significantly lower risk for intracardiac thrombosis [prevalence 18 % (6/33) versus 50 % (13/26) in those who were not on anticoagulation, p=0.01]. Similar trend was observed for patients who had no AF with respective intracardiac thrombosis prevalence 0 % (0/12) in chronic anticoagulation group versus 20 % (8/40) in the no anticoagulation group, p=0.09.

4.6 Clinical characteristics and thrombosis

Compared to the group without thrombosis, the intracardiac thrombosis group was younger, had more AF but was less apt to be receiving therapeutic anticoagulation (table 7). They were also more likely to have AL amyloidosis, had a lower systolic BP and faster heart rate, all $p \leq 0.05$. Similar results were obtained after the exclusion of patients who had AF. The prevalences of intracardiac thrombosis were 0% (0/21) in other types of cardiac amyloid patients who had no AF; 23% (8/35) in those with AL amyloidosis who had no AF, 25% (14/55) in other types with AF; and 44% (20/45) in AL patients with AF, p=0.0002. Other demographic and clinical variables were similar. Interestingly, the group with thrombosis did not have more frequent documented history of embolism. Furthermore, there was no significant difference in prevalence of intracardiac thrombosis between those patients studied retrospectively and those studied prospectively (31% vs. 25%, p=0.25).

4.7 TTE and thrombosis (table 8)

The group with thrombi had a smaller LV end diastolic dimension, a thicker LV posterior wall, a larger RA size, a smaller SV and CI, a lower LVEF, worse LV diastolic function, a shorter deceleration time, poorer LA mechanical activity (a lower A and a' velocity), and a higher E/A and E/e' than the non thrombotic group. Furthermore, PV peak systolic velocity and A velocity were significantly lower and D/S was higher (all $p \leq 0.05$). LA volume index was not statistically different. After exclusion of AF patients, the differences of several TTE parameters between the thrombosis group and the non thrombosis group were no longer statistically different although the trends were similar (table 8).

	All Patients				Patients without AF		
Thrombus status	All (n=156)	With (n=42)	Without (n=114)	P value	With (n=8)	Without (n=48)	P value
Age, years	67 ± 11	64 ± 12	69 ± 11	0.02	56 ± 9	65±12	0.04
Gender, % male	77	64	82	0.06	50	63	0.23
Body mass index, kg/m^2	26.1 ± 4.4	25.2±4.7	26.4±4.3	0.18	24.5±2.9	25.6±3.9	0.55
Hypertension, %	39	26	43	0.06	13	41	0.12
Diabetes, %	5	2	6	0.35	0	7	0.53
CHF, %	79	88	75	0.36	88	62	0.46
NYHA class 1, %	21	12	25	0.36	12	38	0.46
NYHA class 2, %	35	36	34		25	27	
NYHA class 3, %	37	43	34		50	29	
NYHA class 4, %	8	9	7		13	6	
Median NYHA class	2 (1-3)	3 (1-4)	2 (1-3)	0.10	3 (1-4)	2 (1-3)	0.11
Atrial fibrillation, %	64	81	58	0.008	0	0	--
Anticoagulation, %	43	21	51	0.001	0	29	0.05
Syncope, %	24	29	22	0.39	27	14	0.18
AL amyloidosis, %	51	67	46	0.02	100	56	0.01
Stem cell transplant, %	11	12	11	0.93	14	20	0.62
History of thromboembolism, %	22	24	22	0.92	32	30	1.00
Nephrotic Syndrome, %	17	24	15	0.23	25	27	0.90
Systolic BP, mm Hg	118 ± 22	110 ± 20	122 ± 22	0.002	91 ± 7	122 ± 21	0.0001
Diastolic BP, mm Hg	70 ± 14	68±13	71±14	0.18	57±10	71±15	0.02
Heart Rate, bpm	81 ± 18	86 ± 16	79 ± 18	0.01	87±14	78±14	0.13

Table 7. Characteristics in patients with and without Intracardiac Thrombosis in TEE study

4.8 TEE and thrombosis (table 9)

Those with intracardiac thrombi more frequently had spontaneous echo contrast in the LA, and also more severe spontaneous echo contrast in both the LA and LAA and, lower LAA emptying velocity compared to the non thrombotic group. There is no difference in the degree of atherosclerosis in aorta. Similar results were obtained after the exclusion of patients who had AF.

4.9 Multivariate analysis and ROC (table 10)

By multivariate analysis, AF, therapeutic anticoagulation, and lower systolic BP were independently associated with intracardiac thrombosis while there was a borderline trend for AL type in the model when only clinical variables were used. For TTE variables, LV diastolic function was the only variable independently associated with intracardiac thrombosis. Comparing restrictive filling with non restrictive filling LV diastolic function, the OR is 10.6 with 95% CI 1.5-220.3, p=0.04. For TEE variables, the only independent variable associated with intracardiac thrombosis was LAA emptying velocity. When clinical, TTE and TEE variables which were statistically significant by the above 3 models were included in the final model, AF, anticoagulation therapy, LV diastolic function, and LAA emptying velocity were independently associated with intracardiac thrombosis.

The receiver operating characteristic analysis for LAA emptying velocity to predict intracardiac thrombosis is performed. Using 15 cm/s as the cut off, LAA emptying velocity had a sensitivity of 70% and a specificity of 73%. By using 23 cm/s as the cut off, which is

		All Patients			Patients without AF		
Thrombus Status		With (n=42)	Without (n=114)	P value	With (n=8)	Without (n=48)	P value
LV end diastolic diameter, mm	45±8	43±8	46±7	0.02	44±9	45±8	0.77
LV end systolic diameter, mm	32±8	33±10	32±8	0.55	37±10	30±9	0.09
LV septal thickness, mm	15.7±3.9	16.3±3.6	15.3±3.9	0.20	15±3.7	14.9±3.6	0.95
LV posterior wall thickness, mm	14.8±3.3	15.8±3.2	14.4±3.2	0.02	14.4±3.1	13.9±3.1	0.67
RV free wall thickness, mm	8.8±2.5	9.5±2.9	8.5±2.3	0.08	9.8±2.3	8.6±2.5	0.33
LA volume index, ml/m^2)	48±22	51±17	47±23	0.38	43±7	41±29	0.90
RA enlargement (0-3)	2 (0-3)	3 (1-3)	2 (0-3)	0.008	2 (1-3)	1 (0-3)	0.10
Normal RA, %	15	5	19	0.04	0	40	0.20
Mild RAE, %	14	7	16		29	18	
Moderate RAE, %	26	29	25		29	12	
Severe RAE, %	45	59	40		42	30	
Stroke volume, mL	65±23	51±18	71±23	0.0009	40±11	73±26	0.001
CI, L/m^2/min	2.6±0.8	2.3±0.6	2.8±0.9	0.0002	1.9±0.5	2.9±1.0	0.008
LVEF, %	50.9±14.9	43.2±13.7	53.8±14.4	0.0001	37.8±15	56±15	0.002
Median LV diastolic function	3 (1-4)	3 (3-4)	2 (1-3)	0.0001	4 (3-4)	2(1-3)	0.0002
Normal LV diastolic function, %	1	0	1	0.0001	0	2	0.0001
LV diastolic function 1, %	14	0	18		0	35	
LV diastolic function 2, %	31	8	39		0	35	
LV diastolic function 3, %	43	59	38		43	26	
LV diastolic function 4, %	11	33	4		57	2	
Mitral deceleration time, ms	181±54	159±39	188±56	0.004	144±24	195±65	0.09
Mitral E velocity, m/s	0.94±0.29	0.93±0.26	0.94±0.31	0.85	0.90±0.24	0.96±0.33	0.70
Mitral A velocity, m/s	0.44±0.33	0.21±0.18	0.52±0.33	0.0001	0.28±0.10	0.64±0.35	0.0003
E/A	2.7±1.9	3.9±2.2	2.3±1.6	0.001	5.0±3.0	2.1±1.9	0.004
Mitral annulus s′ velocity, cm/s	4.6±1.8	3.7±1.8	4.9±1.7	0.008	3.0±1.0	5.3±1.6	0.01
Mitral annulus e′ velocity, cm/s	4.5±1.8	3.6±1.4	4.8±1.9	0.002	3.5±1.0	5.0±2.0	0.09
Mitral annulus a′ velocity, cm/s	3.0±2.6	1.8±2.1	3.6±2.9	0.01	2.0±1.0	4.6±3.1	0.11
E/e′	23±12	29±15	21±10	0.002	27±13	21±11	0.21
PV systolic velocity, m/s	0.35±0.18	0.28±0.18	0.38±0.18	0.009	0.22±0.11	0.46±0.18	0.007
PV diastolic velocity, m/s	0.62±0.20	0.64±0.18	0.61±0.20	0.45	0.67±0.23	0.55±0.22	0.23
PV A velocity, m/s	0.21±0.14	0.13±0.11	0.23±0.14	0.004	0.10±0.12	0.27±0.16	0.03
PV diastolic/systolic ratio	2.4±1.8	3.0±1.7	2.2±1.8	0.05	3.1±0.7	1.5±1.2	0.008
RV systolic pressure, mm Hg	42.7±12.3	44.4±11.6	42.1±12.6	0.33	40±9	41±14	0.89

Table 8. TTE characteristics in patients with and without intracardiac thrombosis

comparable as reported previously,[33] the sensitivity increased to 100% but specificity decreased to 53%. The area under curve was 0.81. Using grade 3 as a cut off value for LV diastolic function, it had a sensitivity of 92% and a specificity of 59%. The area under curve was 0.82.

No significant differences existed in intracardiac thrombosis between LV diastolic function grade 2 and grade 1 [0% (0/21) vs. 7% (3/46), p=0.49]. The prevalence of intracardiac thrombosis was 44% for grade 3 or 4. Comparing restrictive filling pattern (grade 3 or 4 diastolic function) with non restrictive filling pattern (grade 1 or 2), the OR for intracardiac thrombosis is 17.1 with 95% CI 5.9-73.8, p<0.0001, by univariate analysis.

	All Patients				Patients without AF		
Thrombus Status	All (n=156)	With (n=42)	Without (n=114)	P value	With (n=8)	Without (n=48)	P value
LAA emptying velocity, cm/s	23 ± 14	13 ± 5	27 ± 15	0.0001	11±2	35±17	0.03
LAA spontaneous contrast (%)	61	92	50	0.0001	100	30	0.004
No LAA spontaneous contrast (%)	39	8	50	0.0001	0	71	0.0001
LAA spontaneous contrast 1 (%)	8	0	11		0	11	
LAA spontaneous contrast 2 (%)	17	14	18		0	9	
LAA spontaneous contrast 3 (%)	36	78	22		100	9	
Medium LAA spontaneous contrast	2 (0-3)	3 (1-3)	1 (0-3)	0.0001	3 (3-3)	0 (0-2)	0.0001
No LA spontaneous contrast (%)	39	8	50	0.0001	0	73	0.001
LA spontaneous contrast 1 (%)	9	0	13		0	9	
LA spontaneous contrast 2 (%)	29	46	23		40	11	
LA spontaneous contrast 3 (%)	23	46	14		60	7	
Medium LA spontaneous contrast	2 (0-3)	2 (2-3)	0 (0-2)	0.0001	2 (2-3)	0 (0-2)	0.0001
Atherosclerosis (0-3)	1 (0-3)	1 (0-3)	1 (0-3)	0.63	1 (0-1)	1 (0-2)	0.96

Table 9. TEE characteristics in subjects with and without intracardiac thrombosis

Dependent Variate	Models *	Predictors	OR	95 % CI	P value
Thrombosis	Model 1	AL type	2.3	0.96-5.6	0.06
		AF	6.8	2.5-20.7	0.0001
		Anticoagulation	0.2	0.07-0.47	0.0003
		SBP	0.7	0.55-0.87	0.0008
	Model 2	LV diastolic function[@]	10.6	1.5-220.3	0.04
	Model 3	LAA emptying velocity[$]	0.2	0.05-0.57	0.002
	Model 4	AF	11.8	1.0-395.2	0.05
		Anticoagulation	0.09	0.01-0.51	0.006
		LV diastolic function[@]	15.2	7.5->999.9	0.008
		LAA emptying velocity[$]	0.1	0.01-0.32	0.0001

* Model 1: Clinical variates included are amyloid type, AF, anticoagulation, HR and SBP (with 10 mmHg increase).

Model 2: TTE variables included are LV diastolic function (@: grade 3 or 4 versus grade 2 or less), LVEF, SV, and mitral A velocity.

Model 3: TEE variables included are LAA emptying velocity ($: increase in 10cm/s in velocity), spontaneous echo contrast in LA and LAA (semi-quantification as 0-3).

Model 4: Combined model included amyloid type, AF, anticoagulation, SBP, LV diastolic function, and LAA emptying velocity.

Table 10. Predictors for thromboembolism by multivariate analyses

Multivariate analysis with AF, LAA emptying velocity, and LV diastolic function as dependent variables increased area under curve to 0.85. When further stratifying thrombosis risk based on LAA emptying velocity and LV diastolic function, we found 0% intracardiac thrombosis in patients with LAA emptying velocity > 15 cm/s and LV diastolic function grade ≤ 2, 26 % in patients with either LAA emptying velocity ≤ 15 cm/s or LV diastolic grade 3 or 4, and 67% in patients who had both ($p<0.0001$). Similar results were obtained after further stratification by AF. The respective prevalence of intracardiac thrombosis was 0%, 15%, and 50% for non AF patients ($p=0.02$), and 0%, 32%, and 72% for AF patients ($p=0.002$).

4.10 Clinical implications of TEE study

Our data from a large TEE study of patients with different types of cardiac amyloidosis confirms our previous autopsy study describing a high frequency of intracardiac thrombosis. We were able to identify that AF, poor LV diastolic function, and LA mechanical dysfunction as indicated by a low LAA emptying velocity were independent predictors of intracardiac thrombosis. Furthermore, it appears from our data that therapeutic anticoagulation therapy protects against intracardiac thrombosis. Low systolic blood pressure also was independently associated with increased risk for intracardiac thrombosis while AL type cardiac amyloidosis had a borderline trend when only clinical variables were considered for multivariates analyses.

4.11 Intracardiac thrombosis in cardiac amyloidosis

Our TEE study confirms the observations of Roberts and our prior autopsy study which showed a high prevalence of intracardiac thrombosis in cardiac amyloidosis.[4] AL type was associated with a 35% prevalence of intracardiac thrombosis compared to 18% in the other amyloid groups despite the fact that the other amyloid groups were older and more frequently had AF. The prevalence of intracardiac thrombosis in TTR related amyloid (either wild or mutant TTR) is comparable to that reported in the AF population without anticoagulation.[36-38] In comparison, AL patients have a higher prevalence of intracardiac thrombosis than that reported in the general non amyloid AF population.[36-38] In fact, the prevalence of intracardiac thrombosis is comparable to that reported in patients with severe mitral valve stenosis with AF, which had the highest prevalence of intracardiac thrombosis (33%).[39]

4.12 Clinical variables and intracardiac thrombosis

In our current study, AF and low systolic BP were independently associated with thrombosis. A low SBP may reflect a low cardiac out put status and severe amyloid heart disease with cardiac decompensation. Most importantly, we identified that therapeutic anticoagulation was significantly associated with a decreased risk for intracardiac thrombosis by both univariate and multivariate analyses.

Clinical HF and NYHA class were not significantly different in patients with or without thrombosis as observed in the Mayo autopsy study.[13] Because many patients were elderly with multiple comorbidities, the clinical diagnosis of HF or NYHA class is a subjective indicator of over all well being and may not be always accurate for grading the severity of heart failure. Moreover, other traditional risk factors for thromboembolism such as age, diabetes and hypertension were not significantly associated with intracardiac thrombosis.

We speculated that risk factors with only modest effect could not be detected in this special study population, in which overwhelming effects from AL type, AF, and anticoagulation therapy are likely to have masked their modest effects.

4.13 TTE, TEE characters and intracardiac thrombosis

Univariate analysis showed that the group with thrombi had evidence of more advanced cardiac amyloid deposition as indicated by a smaller LV end diastolic dimension, a thicker LV wall, and also poorer LV systolic and diastolic function, a higher LV filling pressure estimated by E/e′ as well as less LA mechanical activity than the group without thrombi. Furthermore, LA and LAA spontaneous contrast were more often present and more pronounced in those with intracardiac thrombi. Similar TTE and TEE results were obtained after exclusion of AF patients. Therefore, AF only plays a partial role for intracardiac thrombosis. Multivariate analyses showed that the only two echo variable: i.e. LV diastolic dysfunction and low LAA emptying velocity, in addition to AF, were independently associated with intracardiac thrombosis. The Mayo autopsy and TEE studies and prior study support the hypothesis that the combination of systolic and diastolic ventricular dysfunction and chronic amyloid infiltrate in the atria lead to atrial mechanical dysfunction,[17,24] atrial enlargement, and blood stasis.[23,27] Such atrial electrical-mechanical dissociation at least partially explains why some cardiac amyloid patients developed atrial thrombosis while in sinus rhythm.[17, 24, 28]

4.14 Anticoagulation and intracardiac thrombosis

We identified that therapeutic anticoagulation therapy at the time of TEE was associated with a significant lower risk for intracardiac thrombosis. Thus, effective anticoagulation might reduce thromboembolism, which is a significant contributor for mortality in cardiac amyloid patients.[13] However, anticoagulation may exacerbate the hemorrhagic tendency, which is a well known complication of amyloidosis because of fragile blood vessel walls secondary to amyloid deposition and the coexisting coagulopathy in such patients.[2,31] In our prior autopsy series, three cardiac amyloid patients died from massive gastrointestinal bleeding.[13] Therefore, the potential benefits of anticoagulation must be carefully weighed against possible hemorrhagic complications before anticoagulation is initiated.

5. Further directions

A recent study suggests that chemotherapy in AL patients with cardiac involvement results in a clinical improvement despite an unchanged TTE appearance.[40] Improvement may be due to the abolition of the production of new light chains, which are toxic to myocardium by increasing oxidant stress and causing diastolic dysfunction.[26,41] Furthermore, there has been report of echocardiographic improvement and decreased amyloid accumulation by 99m Tc-PYP scintigram after chemotherapy and stem cell transplant.[42] Therefore, it is possible that early detection of amyloidosis, vigilant screening for intracardiac thrombosis with early anticoagulation, and more aggressive treatment of the underlying plasma dyscrasia might improve the prognosis. [3,23,43,44] Because of retrospective study design and limited number of patients on anticoagulation, we could not evaluate whether anticoagulation will prevent thromboembolism. Further prospective study is needed to specifically answer this question.

6. Summary

We demonstrated a high frequency of intracardiac thrombosis in patients with cardiac amyloidosis from both autopsy study and from TEE study. The risk for intracardiac thrombosis and thromboembolism is especially high in patients who had the AL type, presented with AF, had poor LV diastolic function, and poor atrial mechanical function were independently associated with increased risk. Importantly, therapeutic anticoagulation therapy appeared protective against intracardiac thrombosis. Early screening for intracardiac thrombosis by TEE, especially in the high risk patient as identified in our studies, may be indicated. If intracardiac thrombosis or severe LAA mechanical dysfunction (especially with coexisting restrictive LV filling) is detected, anticoagulation should be carefully considered.

7. References

[1] Kyle RA, Linos A, Beard CM, Linke RP, Gertz MA, O'Fallon WM, Kurland LT. Incidence and natural history of primary systemic amyloidosis in Olmsted County, Minnesota, 1950 through 1989.[see comment]. Blood. 1992;79(7):1817-1822.

[2] Falk RH, Comenzo RL, Skinner M. The systemic amyloidoses [see comment]. New England Journal of Medicine. 1997;337(13):898-909.

[3] Falk RH. Diagnosis and management of the cardiac amyloidoses. Circulation. 2005; 112(13):2047-2060.

[4] Roberts WC, Waller BF. Cardiac amyloidosis causing cardiac dysfunction: analysis of 54 necropsy patients. American Journal of Cardiology. 1983;52(1):137-146.

[5] Skinner M, Anderson J, Simms R, Falk R, Wang M, Libbey C, Jones LA, Cohen AS. Treatment of 100 patients with primary amyloidosis: a randomized trial of melphalan, prednisone, and colchicine versus colchicine only. American Journal of Medicine. 1996;100(3):290-298.

[6] Kyle RA, Greipp PR. Amyloidosis (AL). Clinical and laboratory features in 229 cases. Mayo Clinic Proceedings. 1983;58(10):665-683.

[7] Park MA, Mueller PS, Kyle RA, Larson DR, Plevak MF, Gertz MA. Primary (AL) hepatic amyloidosis: clinical features and natural history in 98 patients. Medicine. 2003; 82(5):291-298.

[8] Chamarthi B, Dubrey SW, Cha K, Skinner M, Falk RH. Features and prognosis of exertional syncope in light-chain associated AL cardiac amyloidosis. American Journal of Cardiology. 1997;80(9):1242-1245.

[9] Botker HE, Rasmussen OB. Recurrent cerebral embolism in cardiac amyloidosis. International Journal of Cardiology. 1986;13(1):81-83.

[10] Browne RS, Schneiderman H, Kayani N, Radford MJ, Hager WD. Amyloid heart disease manifested by systemic arterial thromboemboli. Chest. 1992;102(1):304-307.

[11] Santarone M, Corrado G, Tagliagambe LM, Manzillo GF, Tadeo G, Spata M, Longhi M. Atrial thrombosis in cardiac amyloidosis: diagnostic contribution of transesophageal echocardiography. Journal of the American Society of Echocardiography. 1999; 12(6):533-536.

[12] Cools FJ, Kockx MM, Boeckxstaens GE, Heuvel PV, Cuykens JJ. Primary systemic amyloidosis complicated by massive thrombosis. Chest. 1996;110(1):282-284.

[13] Feng D, Edwards WD, Oh JK, Chandrasekaran K, Grogan M, Martinez MW, Syed, II, Hughes DA, Lust JA, Jaffe AS, Gertz MA, Klarich KW. Intracardiac thrombosis and embolism in patients with cardiac amyloidosis. Circulation. 2007; 116(21):2420-2426.
[14] Oh JK. The Echo Manual. Philadelphia: Lippincott Wlliams & Wilkins; 1999.
[15] Willens HJ, Levy R, Kessler KM. Thromboembolic complications in cardiac amyloidosis detected by transesophageal echocardiography. American Heart Journal. 1995; 129(2):405-406.
[16] Santarone M, Corrado G, Tagliagambe LM. Images in cardiology: Biatrial thrombosis in cardiac amyloidosis. Heart. 1999;81(3):302.
[17] Dubrey S, Pollak A, Skinner M, Falk RH. Atrial thrombi occurring during sinus rhythm in cardiac amyloidosis: evidence for atrial electromechanical dissociation.[see comment]. British Heart Journal. 1995;74(5):541-544.
[18] Halligan CS, Lacy MQ, Vincent Rajkumar S, Dispenzieri A, Witzig TE, Lust JA, Fonseca R, Gertz MA, Kyle RA, Pruthi RK. Natural history of thromboembolism in AL amyloidosis. Amyloid. 2006;13(1):31-36.
[19] Risk factors for stroke and efficacy of antithrombotic therapy in atrial fibrillation. Analysis of pooled data from five randomized controlled trials. Arch Intern Med. 1994;154(13):1449-1457.
[20] Predictors of thromboembolism in atrial fibrillation: I. Clinical features of patients at risk. The Stroke Prevention in Atrial Fibrillation Investigators. Ann Intern Med. 1992;116(1):1-5.
[21] Klein AL, Hatle LK, Burstow DJ, Taliercio CP, Seward JB, Kyle RA, Bailey KR, Gertz MA, Tajik AJ. Comprehensive Doppler assessment of right ventricular diastolic function in cardiac amyloidosis. J Am Coll Cardiol. 1990;15(1):99-108.
[22] Vaziri SM, Larson MG, Lauer MS, Benjamin EJ, Levy D. Influence of blood pressure on left atrial size. The Framingham Heart Study. Hypertension. 1995;25(6):1155-1160.
[23] Modesto KM, Dispenzieri A, Cauduro SA, Lacy M, Khandheria BK, Pellikka PA, Belohlavek M, Seward JB, Kyle R, Tajik AJ, Gertz M, Abraham TP. Left atrial myopathy in cardiac amyloidosis: implications of novel echocardiographic techniques. Eur Heart J. 2005;26(2):173-179.
[24] Plehn JF, Southworth J, Cornwell GG, 3rd. Brief report: atrial systolic failure in primary amyloidosis.[see comment]. New England Journal of Medicine. 1992;327(22):1570-1573.
[25] Klein AL, Hatle LK, Burstow DJ, Seward JB, Kyle RA, Bailey KR, Luscher TF, Gertz MA, Tajik AJ. Doppler characterization of left ventricular diastolic function in cardiac amyloidosis. Journal of the American College of Cardiology. 1989; 13(5):1017-1026.
[26] Liao R, Jain M, Teller P, Connors LH, Ngoy S, Skinner M, Falk RH, Apstein CS. Infusion of light chains from patients with cardiac amyloidosis causes diastolic dysfunction in isolated mouse hearts. Circulation. 2001;104(14):1594-1597.
[27] Murphy L, Falk RH. Left atrial kinetic energy in AL amyloidosis: can it detect early dysfunction? American Journal of Cardiology. 2000;86(2):244-246.
[28] Stables RH, Ormerod OJ. Atrial thrombi occurring during sinus rhythm in cardiac amyloidosis: evidence for atrial electromechanical dissociation.[comment]. Heart. 1996;75(4):426.

[29] Berghoff M, Kathpal M, Khan F, Skinner M, Falk R, Freeman R. Endothelial dysfunction precedes C-fiber abnormalities in primary (AL) amyloidosis. Annals of Neurology. 2003;53(6):725-730.
[30] Inoue H, Saito I, Nakazawa R, Mukaida N, Matsushima K, Azuma N, Suzuki M, Miyasaka N. Expression of inflammatory cytokines and adhesion molecules in haemodialysis-associated amyloidosis. Nephrology Dialysis Transplantation. 1995; 10(11):2077-2082.
[31] Yood RA, Skinner M, Rubinow A, Talarico L, Cohen AS. Bleeding manifestations in 100 patients with amyloidosis. JAMA. 1983;249(10):1322-1324.
[32] Feng D, Syed IS, Martinez M, Oh JK, Jaffe AS, Grogan M, Edwards WD, Gertz MA, Klarich KW. Intracardiac thrombosis and anticoagulation therapy in cardiac amyloidosis. Circulation. 2009;119(18):2490-2497.
[33] Mugge A, Kuhn H, Nikutta P, Grote J, Lopez JA, Daniel WG. Assessment of left atrial appendage function by biplane transesophageal echocardiography in patients with nonrheumatic atrial fibrillation: identification of a subgroup of patients at increased embolic risk. J Am Coll Cardiol. 1994;23(3):599-607.
[34] Atherosclerotic disease of the aortic arch as a risk factor for recurrent ischemic stroke. The French Study of Aortic Plaques in Stroke Group. N Engl J Med. 1996; 334(19):1216-1221.
[35] Amarenco P, Duyckaerts C, Tzourio C, Henin D, Bousser MG, Hauw JJ. The prevalence of ulcerated plaques in the aortic arch in patients with stroke. N Engl J Med. 1992;326(4):221-225.
[36] Manning WJ, Silverman DI, Keighley CS, Oettgen P, Douglas PS. Transesophageal echocardiographically facilitated early cardioversion from atrial fibrillation using short-term anticoagulation: final results of a prospective 4.5-year study. J Am Coll Cardiol. 1995;25(6):1354-1361.
[37] Weigner MJ, Thomas LR, Patel U, Schwartz JG, Burger AJ, Douglas PS, Silverman DI, Manning WJ. Early cardioversion of atrial fibrillation facilitated by transesophageal echocardiography: short-term safety and impact on maintenance of sinus rhythm at 1 year. Am J Med. 2001;110(9):694-702.
[38] Klein AL, Grimm RA, Murray RD, Apperson-Hansen C, Asinger RW, Black IW, Davidoff R, Erbel R, Halperin JL, Orsinelli DA, Porter TR, Stoddard MF. Use of transesophageal echocardiography to guide cardioversion in patients with atrial fibrillation. N Engl J Med. 2001;344(19):1411-1420.
[39] Srimannarayana J, Varma RS, Satheesh S, Anilkumar R, Balachander J. Prevalence of left atrial thrombus in rheumatic mitral stenosis with atrial fibrillation and its response to anticoagulation: a transesophageal echocardiographic study. Indian Heart J. 2003;55(4):358-361.
[40] Dubrey S, Mendes L, Skinner M, Falk RH. Resolution of heart failure in patients with AL amyloidosis. Annals of Internal Medicine. 1996;125(6):481-484.
[41] Brenner DA, Jain M, Pimentel DR, Wang B, Connors LH, Skinner M, Apstein CS, Liao R. Human amyloidogenic light chains directly impair cardiomyocyte function through an increase in cellular oxidant stress. Circulation Research. 2004;94(8):1008-1010.
[42] Yagi S, Akaike M, Ozaki S, Moriya C, Takeuchi K, Hara T, Fujimura M, Sumitomo Y, Iwase T, Ikeda Y, Aihara K, Kimura T, Nishiuchi T, Abe M, Matsumoto T.

Improvement of cardiac diastolic function and prognosis after autologous peripheral blood stem cell transplantation in AL cardiac amyloidosis. Intern Med. 2007;46(20):1705-1710.
[43] Dubrey SW, Burke MM, Hawkins PN, Banner NR. Cardiac transplantation for amyloid heart disease: the United Kingdom experience. Journal of Heart & Lung Transplantation. 2004;23(10):1142-1153.
[44] Merlini G, Bellotti V. Molecular mechanisms of amyloidosis. New England Journal of Medicine. 2003;349(6):583-596.

4

Cardiovascular Complications in Patients with AL Amyloidosis

Maurizio Zangari[1], Tamara Berno[2], Fenghuang Zhan[1], Guido Tricot[1] and Louis Fink[3]
[1]*University of Utah, Division of Hematology, Myeloma Program, Salt Lake City, Utah;*
[2]*University of Padua;*
[3]*Laboratory Medicine, Nevada Cancer Institute, Las Vegas, Nevada;*
[2]*Italy*
[1,3]*USA*

1. Introduction

Amyloidosis is a disease characterized by aberrant precursor molecules whose misfolded intermediate forms aggregate and are deposited as interstitial fibrils. The most common type of systemic amyloidosis is immunoglobulin light-chain amyloidosis (AL). Less common types of systemic amyloidosis are the transthyretin (ATTR) types caused by either mutant (hereditary) variants or wild-type ("senile systemic") transthyretin. Although rare in developed countries secondary amyloidosis is associated with autoimmune or inflammatory diseases, chronic infections and malignancies. Different precursor proteins can coexist in the same patient as in the African-American population, which has a 4% incidence of an hereditary ATTR variant (Val122Ile) and a significant incidence of monoclonal gammopathy (1, 2).
The amyloids are highly ordered cross-β sheet protein with extra cellular deposition in single or multiple organs. Cardiac deposition, leading to an infiltrative/restrictive cardiomyopathy, is a common feature and may be present at the diagnosis or discovered while investigating a patient presenting with non-cardiac amyloidosis.
AL amyloidosis, is associated with clinical cardiac involvement in about half of all cases, although subclincal involvement may be detected in almost every case at autopsy on endomyocardial biopsy. Laser micro dissection with mass spectrometry assessing the constituents of the Congophilic deposits is now the gold standard for amyloid typing, obtaining protein type identification in over 98% of cases (3).
Evaluation for cardiac involvement is a critical step of the initial staging of amyloidosis. Criteria for the assessment of organ involvement at baseline and after treatment have been standardized (4). In systemic AL amyloidosis the extent of cardiac involvement has prognostic indications, with a median survival of 6 months for untreated or non-responding patients (5, 6).

2. Clotting alterations

The cardiovascular complications observed in patients with amyloidosis range from myocardial involvement to haemostatic dysfunctions leading to thrombotic or hemorrhagic complications. At presentation, 15-40% of patients with AL amyloidosis experience hemorrhagic manifestations (7, 8). Petecchiae, purpura in periorbital and facial areas ecchymosis and bleeding tendencies are common clinical features and severe hemorrhages may contribute to worsening the clinical course and lead to death. Increased fragility of blood vessels and impaired vasoconstriction, caused by deposition of insoluble fiber, are frequent causes of bleeding (9, 10). Acquired coagulation factor deficiency, most commonly factor X, is a unique feature of AL amyloidosis. In a reported large series of patients with primary amyloidosis, 8.9% showed factor X deficiency (defined as factor X activity < 50%); about half of them experienced bleeding episodes and the severity and frequency of these episodes was most pronounced with the lowest factor X levels(11). Absorption of the coagulation factor by AL fibrils, primarily in the liver and spleen is the proposed pathogenetic mechanism. Deficiency of factor X in patients with splenic amyloid in some cases has been corrected by splenectomy wich can produce resolution of the bleeding diathesis (12). Normalization of factor X levels has been reported after oral melphalan chemotherapy. Resolution of the bleeding episode was also described in five of 10 patients treated with high dose melphalan followed by autologous stem cell transplantation although bleeding complications in the peritransplant period were fatal in two patients (13). Perivascular amyloid deposition, inhibition of fibrinogen conversion to fibrin, and specific deficiencies of factor X, IX, and V along with circulating heparin-like anticoagulants play important roles in determing the haemostatic abnormalities.

Prolongation of pro-thrombin time (PT), thrombin time (TT), reptilase time (RT) and Russell's viper venom time (RVVT) are the most common coagulation abnormalities. Abnormal fibrinogen and/or elevated fibrinogen/fibrin degradation products (FDP) are considered to be the main factors that affect both TT and RT. It has been postulated that inhibitors must be present in plasma of patients with AL amyloidosis and the inhibitory activity persists in the supernatant even after fibrinogen precipitation (14). Several pathologic conditions other than the presence of a plasma thrombin inhibitor could explain the prolongation of aPTT and PT in AL patients e.g. malabsorption associated with amyloid deposits in the gastrointestinal tract, reduced food intake due to macroglossia or vomiting, liver failure and plasma deficiencies of some clotting factors due to their affinity for amyloid deposits.

Although TT and RT prolongations are peculiar features of AL Amyloidosis, they do not predict bleeding manifestations. Other coagulation abnormalities such as factor X deficiency, enhanced fibrinolysis, and amyloid angiopathy seem to correlate better with clinical symptoms (15).

Deficiencies in specific coagulation factors in have long been recognized and along with factor X, acquired deficiencies in factor IX, factor II and factor VII have also been described (16). Hypofibrinogenemia has also been observed in systemic AL amyloidosis in association with disseminated intravascular coagulation and increased fibrinolysis (17).

Hyperfibrinolysis related to a reduced level of α2-antiplasmin or to a complex formed with plasmin can be associated with either bleeding manifestations or abnormal coagulation tests in patients with amyloidosis. Bleeding diathesis associated with a shortened clot lysis time and elevated FDP is pathognomonic. The pathogenesis appears to be related to a reduced level of α2-antiplasmin, often secondary to complex formation with plasmin (18, 19).

Increased urokinase plasminogen activator activity also has been observed a patient with primary amyloidosis. Immunoprecipitation studies showed that single-chain urokinase plasminogen activator was the main fibrinolytic agonist in the patient's plasma. Treatment with ε-amino-caproic acid was effective in controlling bleeding symptoms in some patients, even when accelerated fibrinolysis is not demonstrable (20). Standard chemotherapy and new novel agents can also induce bleeding complications by multiple mechanisms. Drugs with anti-angiogenic activity may be associated with vascular complications in amyloidosis patients and their use should be closely monitored as these patients could have pre-existing haemostatic abnormalities associated with their paraproteins.

3. Cardiac amyloidosis

Definition of cardiac involvement (cardiomegaly, pleural effusions, and Kerley B lines on the chest radiograph) (21) over the past three decades has been supplanted by echocardiography. A granular sparkling appearance with wall thickening, diastolic relaxation abnormalities, right ventricular dysfunction and abnormal echocardiography strain have all been shown to be associated with prognosis (22). Serum cardiac biomarkers have been recently introduced and serum troponin T and N-terminal pro-brain natriuretic peptide (NT-proBNP) are now widely available. Using a cutoff value of 0.035 mcg/L Troponin T and 332 pg/mL NT-proBNP, patients can be classified into three stages: Stage I both biomarkers low (33% incidence); Stage II, only 1 marker high (37%); Stage III both values high (30% incidence) . The reported median survivals are 26.4, 10 and 3.5 months, respectively for Stages I, II, III (23).
The cardiac biomarkers values have been validated in different cohorts of patients treated with either conventional chemotherapy or stem cell transplantation (SCT) (24). Stage III patients are at high mortality risk in SCT studies and also are poor candidates for clinical trials of standard agents (25).
Echocardiography is one of the earliest tests employed in the investigation of suspected heart disease. The specificity of the echocardiographyc findings increases in the presence of the clinical manifestations suggestive of myocardial amyloidosis. The earliest finding in cardiac amyloidosis is suggested by reduced diastolic mitral inflow velocities upon Doppler imaging (26, 27).
A granular sparkling texture of the myocardium with increased thickness is strongly suggestive of cardiac amyloid infiltration with a specificity approaching 81%. The addition of the finding of increased septal diameter remarkably increases the specificity of ventricular wall thickness parameter; an interventricular septum thickness of more than 15 mm is also considered a poor prognostic sign (28).The thickness of the left ventricular walls correlates with reduced survival. Low voltage/mass ratio strongly favors the diagnosis of amyloid myocardial infiltration (29). Typical clinical presentation of cardiac amyloidosis with specific echocardiographyc findings such as dilated atria, interatrial septal hypertrophy > 7 mm, thickened valves and right ventricular free wall has been proposed as diagnostic of cardiac amyloidosis even without an endomyocardial biopsy (30).
The diagnosis can be confirmed by endomyocardial biopsy and the extent of involvement appears as the most important determinant of clinical outcome as cardiac troponin and NT-proBNP have been shown to be potent prognostic indicators, the suppression of amyloidogenic serum light chains by treatment and reductions in NT-proBNP have been associated with improved outcome.
Circulating amyloidogenic light chains interact with cardiac cell membrane constituents and other local matrix components. Extracellular space amyloid deposition causes myocardial damage by direct cell toxicity mediated by the formation of light chain oligomers (31). The

pathologic features are thickening of all four chambers, biatrial dilatation, a normal or mildly dilated right ventricle and a left ventricular cavity that is normal or small. Myocardial cells are separated and distorted by amyloid deposition. Intramyocardial vessels are frequently infiltrated by amyloid, resulting in impaired vasodilatation, which may result in myocardial ischemia. Rarely amyloid deposits have been found in epicardial vessels resulting in obstructive coronary artery disease indistinguishable on coronary angiography from cholesterol-laden plaques. The predominant manifestation of amyloid heart disease is congestive failure (32).

Accumulation of amyloid in the myocardial interstitium results in late gadolinium enhancement, often with a predominant diffuse, global and subendocardial distribution that matches the distribution of amyloid on histology although other more focal patterns have also been reported. This is associated with substantial alteration in gadolinium kinetics, with faster washout of gadolinium from blood and myocardium than normal (33). Some studies have suggested that gadolinium kinetics may be even more predictive than echocardiography or serum markers. The value of the Cardiovascular Magnetic Resonance (CMR) measurements may in part be due to the fact that cardiac amyloid burden cannot be measured satisfactorily by other techniques, and therefore CMR may offer a fundamental new window into the cardiac pathology in this disease (34). Recognition that T1 mapping in cardiac amyloidosis may be significantly more predictive of poor prognosis than the other currently used measures ,its use may be justified when early and more intensive chemotherapy is planned .

A number of the gadolinium kinetics parameters have been significantly associated with mortality, but the one with greatest discriminatory value was the intra-myocardial T1 gradient after gadolinium injection, with 95% accuracy at a threshold value of 23 ms (Kaplan Meier analysis $P = 0.002$). Although further experience and reproduction of these results by other centers is necessary, the technique is in principle straightforward and could be implemented on most 1.5T scanners (35).

4. Gene expression and cytogenetic abnormalities

Gene expression profiling studies have revealed subsets of genes associated with the development of amyloidosis. A unique molecular profile for AL amyloidosis may be relevant to the development of disease.

The comparison of gene expression profiles between AL, normal BM and myeloma plasma cells has revealed that AL plasma cells had an intermediate transcription profile. A few genes may be of particular relevance in understanding the differences in the pathobiology of these two disease entities. One of these, TNFRSF7, a member of the tumor necrosis factor (TNR) receptor superfamily which codes for CD27, a marker expressed on memory B cells and is important in controlling maturation and apoptosis of plasma cells, has a higher average expression in AL plasma cells. CD27 has been postulated to be important in the oncogenesis of myeloma, since MM plasma cells (PC) do not express this marker, whereas normal PCs do, and the expression of CD27 declines with the more advanced stages of MM. CD27 interacts with its ligand CD70, and this interaction is thought to be important in the differentiation of plasma cells. Interestingly, the tail of CD27 binds a proapoptotic protein, Siva, and CD27-70 interaction may activate a death signal that determines the life span of PCs.

CD27 expression is progressively down regulated in the transition from normal plasma cells to MGUS to MM to myeloma cell lines suggesting that molecular mechanism in AL disease is an early event. Another gene that was significantly different between AL and MM was the chemokine SDF-1, which is comparatively more highly expressed in AL PCs. However, SDF-1 levels in normal PCs are higher than those expressed in AL (36, 37). Whereas over expression of SDF-1 has been implicated in preventing apoptosis, promoting proliferation and metastatic spread in a number of neoplastic diseases through interactions with CXCR4, it is apparent that the relatively high levels of SDF-1 in normal and AL PCs have a paradoxical effect. This paradox can be explained by the binding of SDF-1 to CXCR4 which results in activation of the suppressors of cytokine signaling (SOCS) proteins, in particular, SOCS-3, which can negatively regulate CXCR4 function without interfering with surface receptor expression.

Clonal AL plasma cells express recurring cytogenetic abnormalities, including t(11,14), gain 11q, del 13q, and gain 1q.Interestingly, t(11;14) was associated with worse overall survival in a recent study of AL patients (38). Over expression of cyclin D1 (CCND1 located on chromosome 11q13) in purified AL plasma cells occurs in one-half of AL patients and is associated with unique pathobiologic characteristics at diagnosis: including high frequencies of light-chain only M proteins and kappa light chains, increased cardiac biomarker levels, and poorer overall survival (39).

5. Therapy

The therapy aim for AL amyloidosis is to eliminate the clonal plasma cells producing the toxic precursor protein. Once a case of amyloidosis is recognized, it is vital to precisely determine the type of amyloid as the prognosis and treatment differ considerably among the various types. The management of heart failure in patients with amyloidosis remains challenging. Judicious diuretics use and salt restriction with avoidance of intravascular volume depletion remains the mainstay of the treatment. Angiotensin-converting enzyme inhibitors and Angiotensin-II receptor blockers are poorly tolerated in cardiac amyloidosis. The role of calcium channel blockers and digoxin is limited and probably detrimental. This is due to an exaggerated negative inotropic effect. A high incidence of sudden death in patients treated with digoxin has been reported (40).

Heart transplantation remains a controversial option because of the systemic involvement and the potential recurrence of graft Amyloidosis (41). In primary amyloidosis, heart transplantation is only a palliative procedure and consequent supportive chemotherapy should be considered. The long-term prognosis is poor (39% survival at 4 years in one study and 30% at 5 years in another, even with adjuvant chemotherapy. Sequential heart and autologous stem cell transplantation for primary amyloidosis has been reported (42).

Active agents in the treatment of the amyloid include corticosteroids (prednisone, dexamethasone), alkylating agents (melphalan, cyclophosphamide), immunomodulatory drugs (thalidomide, lenalidomide) and proteasome inhibitors (bortezomib).Conventional chemotherapy based on melphalan and prednisone was introduced in 1972 can achieve a median survival of 12 to 18 months and in patients with severe cardiac failure, continuous, oral, daily melphalan has been used as palliative method (43). Based on the observation that dexamethasone as single agent was able to produce hematological and organ responses, melphalan and dexamethasone have been later used in combination in this setting (44). Melphalan and dexamethasone is still now considered a front-line therapy, inducing a hematological response of 67% of the time with a 33% of CR and an organ response rate of 48% in a phase II study of 45 patients. A 5-year follow-up the study showed a median PFS of

3.8 years and OS of 5.1 years. Subsequent studies have later confirmed the efficacy of this combination (45).

Amyloid therapy remained unchanged until the introduction of stem cell transplantation (SCT) wich was designed to target rapidly the amyloidogenic light chain production by the clonal plasma cell populations. High rates of hematological and organ response have now been documented in multiple centers with long-term data reported and median survivals of over a decade for SCT patients achieving complete response. The high rate of treatment-related mortality (5 to 10% even at experienced centers) would explain the failure to show a survival advantage when compared to standard therapy in a large prospective randomized trial (46). Risk-adapted SCT, which tailors the melphalan dose according to age and risk status of the patient, may improve early survival (47). To compensate for the loss of efficacy due to attenuated conditioning, adjuvant therapy post SCT for patients not achieving a CR has been tested. Thalidomide and dexamethasone or bortezomib and dexamethasone has been used as adjuvant therapy post SCT with CR rates at 12 months post SCT of 39% and 65% of evaluated patients (48).

The propensity for sudden cardiac death, the frequency of multi-organ involvement and the problem of progressive organ disease and drug-related side effects has limited clinical research in amyloid. The first novel agent to be tested in relapsed AL was thalidomide. Initially it was poorly tolerated at high doses but showed efficacy at moderate doses in combination with dexamethasone and alkylating agents (melphalan or cyclophosphamide) resulting in hematological and organ responses. Current reccomendations suggest to start with thalidomide at a dose of 50 mg daily and it can be increased if tolerated (49).

Lenalidomide has been combined with dexamethasone in two studies with hematological response of 41% and 67% respectively. Several phase I/II combining Lenalidomide and dexamethasone with an alkylating agent (melphalan or cyclophosphamide) have been recently completed. In a phase 1/2 dose-escalation study of lenalidomide in combination with melphalan and dexamethasone. A complete hematological response was achieved in 42% at the dose of 15 mg of lenalidomide per day. After a median follow-up of 19 months, estimated 2-year overall survival (OS) and event-free survival (EFS) were 80.8% and 53.8% respectively (50).

In a preliminary report on a phase II study of the thalidomide derivative pomalidomide with weekly dexamethasone in AL amyloidosis patients previously treated with SCT and alkylating agents lenalinamide or thalidomide one-third achieved a hematological response by 6 months, highlighting the promising anti amyloid effect of this potent immunomodulatory drug (51).

Bortezomib is a selective inhibitor of the 26S proteasome, a protein complex involved in the regulation of degradation of aberrant proteins as well as for the regulation of other proteins involved in the regulation of apoptosis, and cell-cycle progression.

Single agent Bortezomib in a phase I dose escalation study achieved hematological responses in 50% of patients and CR in 20%. A multicenter study of 94 AL amyloid patients treated with bortezomib with or without dexamethasone has reported hematological responses in 71% and CR in 25% of patients; cardiac response was documented in 29% of subjects (52). Bortezomib is currently being evaluated in combination with melphalan and dexamethasone in 2 trials in Europe and USA.

The past decade has seen significant advances in the treatment of patients with AL, leading to improvement s in both quality of life and survival. The novel agents have significantly expanded the armamentarium against AL. The central challenges of this decade will be how to combine these agents and how to bring forth new ones for approval.

6. References

[1] Lachmann HJ, Booth DR, Booth SL, et al. Misdiagnosis of hereditary amyloidosis as AL (primary) amyloidosis. *N Engl J Med.* 2002;346:1786-1791.
[2] Comenzo RL, Zhou P, Fleisher M, Clark B, Teruya-Feldstein J. Seeking confidence in the diagnosis of systemic AL (Ig light-chain) amyloidosis: patients can have both monoclonal gammopathies and hereditary amyloid proteins. *Blood.* 2006;107:3489-3491.
[3] Vrana JA, Gamez JD, Madden BJ, Theis JD, Bergen HR 3d, Dogan A. Classification of amyloidosis by laser microdissection and mass spectrometry-based proteomic analysis in clinical biopsy specimens. *Blood.* 2009;114:4957-4959.
[4] Gertz MA, Comenzo R, Falk RH, et al. Definition of organ involvement and treatment response in immunoglobulin light chain amyloidosis (AL): a consensus opinion from the 10th International Symposium on Amyloid and Amyloidosis, Tours, France, 18-22 April 2004. *Am J Haematol.* 2005;79:319-328.
[5] Lebovic D, Hoffman J, Levine BM, et al. Predictors of survival in patients with systemic light-chain amyloidosis and cardiac involvement initially ineligible for stem cell transplantation and treated with oral melphalan and dexamethasone. *Br J Haematol.* 2008;143:369-373.
[6] Kyle RA, Gertz MA. Primary systemic amyloidosis: clinical and laboratory features in 474 cases. Seminar Hematol. 1995;32:45-49.
[7] Kyle RA, Gertz MA. Primary systemic amyloiodosis: clinical and laboratory features in 474 cases. Semin Hematol. 1995;32:45-59.
[8] Mumford A, O'Donnell J, Gillmore J, et al. Bleeding symptoms and coagulation abnormalities in 337 patients with AL-amyloidosis. *Br J Hematol.* 2000;110:454460.
[9] Sucker C, Hetzel GR, Grabensee B, et al. Amyloidosis and bleeding: pathophisiology, diagnosis and therapy. *Am J Kidney Dis.* 2006;47(6):947-55.
[10] Hoshino Y, Hatake K, Muroi K, et al. Bleeding tendency caused the deposit of amyloid substance in the perivascular region. *Intern Med.* 1993;32(11):879-881.
[11] Choufani E, Sanchowarala V, Ernst T, et al. Acquired factor X deficiency in patients with amyloid light-chain amyloidosis: incidence, bleeding manifestations, and response to high dose chemotherapy. *Blood.* 2001; 97:1885-1887.
[12] Greipp PR, Kyle RA, Bowie EJ. Factor X deficiency in primary amyloidosis:resolution after splenectomy. *N Engl J Med.* 1979;301(19):1050-1051.
[13] Rosenstein ED, Itzkowitz SH, Penziner AS, et al. resolution of factor X deficiency in primary amyloidosis following splenectomy. *Arch Intern Med.* 1983;143(3):597-599.
[14] Gamba G, Montani N, Anesi E, et al. Clotting alterations in primary systemic amyloidosis. *Haematologica.* 2000;85(3):289-92.
[15] Galbraith PA, Sharma N, Parker WL, et al. Acquired factor X deficiency. Altered plasma antithrombin activity and association with amyloidosis. *JAMA.* 1974;230(12):1658-1660.
[16] Korsan-Bengsten K, Hjort PF, Ygge J. Acquired factor X deficiency in a patient with amyloidosis. *Thromb Diath Haemorragh.* 1962;7:558-566.

[17] McPherson RA, Onstad JW, Ugoretz RG, Wolf PL. Coagulopathy in amyloidosis: combined deficiency of factors IX and X. *Am J Hematol.* 1977;3:225-35.
[18] Liebman H, Chinowsky M, Valdin J, et al. Increased fibrinolysis and amyloidosis. *Arch Intern Med.* 1983; 143(4):678-82.
[19] Takahashi H, Koike T, Yoshida N, et al. Excessive fibrinolysis in suspected amyloidosis: demonstration of plasmin-alpha 2-plasmin inhibitor complex and von Willebrand factor fragment in plasma. *AM J Hematol.* 1986;23(2):153-66.
[20] Liebman HA, Crfagno MK, Weitz IC, et al. Excessive fibrinolysis in amyloidosis associated with elevated plasma single-chain urokinase. *Am J Clin Pathol.* 1992; 98(5):534-541.
[21] Desai HV, Aronow WS, Peterson SJ, Frishman WH. Cardiac amyloidosis: Approaches to diagnosis and management. *Cardiol Rev.* 2010;18:1-11.
[22] Koyama J, Falk RH. Prognostic significance of strain Doppler imaging in light-chain amyloidosis. *JACC Cardiovasc Imaging.* 2010;3:333-342.
[23] Dispenzieri A, Gertz MA, Kyle RA, et al. Serum cardiac troponins and N-terminal pro-brain natriuretic peptide: A staging system for primary systemic amyloidosis. *J Clin Oncol.* 2004;22:3751-3757.
[24] Kumar S, Dispenzieri A, Gertz MA. High dose melphalan versus melphalan plus dexamethasone for AL amyloidosis. *N Engl J Med.* 2008;358:91.
[25] Dispenzieri A, Lacy MQ, Zeldenrust SR, et al. The activity of lenalidomide with or without dexamethasone in patients with prmary systemic amyloidosis. *Blood.* 2007; 109:465-470. Epub 2006 Sep 28.
[26] Cueto-Garcia L, Tajik AJ, Kyle RA, et al. Serial echocardiographic observations in patients with primary systemic amyloidosis: an introduction to the concept of early (asymptomatic) amyloid infiltration of the heart. *Mayo Clin Proc.* 1984;59:589-97.
[27] Koyama J, Ray-Sequin PA, Davidoff R, et al. Usefulness of pulsed tissue Doppler imaging for evaluating systolic and diastolic left ventricular function in patients with Al (primary) amyloidosis. *Am J Cardiol.* 2002;89:1067-71.
[28] Selvanaygam JB, Hawkins PN, Paul B, Myerson SG, Neubauer S. Evaluation and management of the cardiac amylodosis. *J Am Coll Cardiol.* 2007;50:2101-10 [PubMed]
[29] Kothari SS, Ramakrishnan S, Bahl VK. Cardiac Amyloidosis- An Update. *Indian Heart J.* 2004;56:197-203.
[30] Simons M. Amyloid cardiomyopathy in Updateonline 12.3
[31] Koyama J, Ray-Sequin PA, Falk RH. Longitudinal myocardial function assessed by tissue velocity, strain, and strain rate tissue Doppler Echocardiography in patients with AL (primary) Cardiac amyloidosis. *Circulation.* 2003;107:2446-2452.
[32] Maceira Am, Joshi J, Prasad SK, et al. Cardiovascular Magnetic resonance in cardiac amyloidosis. *Circulation.* 2005;111:186-193.
[33] Sueyoshi E, Sakamoto I, Okimoto T, Hayashi K, Tanaka K, Toda G. Cardiac amyloidosis: typical imaging findings and diffuse myocardial damage demonstrated by delayed contrast-enhanced MRI. *Cardiovasc Intervent Radiol.* 2006;29:710-2.
[34] Cheng AS, Banning AP, Mitchell AR, Neubauer S, Selvanayagam JB. Cardiac changes in systemic amyloidosis: visualisation by magnetic resonance imaging. *Int J Cardiol.* 2006;113:E21-3.

[35] Moon JC, McKenna WJ, McCrohon JA, Elliott PM, Smith GC, Pennell DJ. Toward clinical risk assessment in hyperthophic cardiomyopathy with gadolinium cardiovascular magnetic resonance. *J Am Coll Cardiol.* 2003;41:1561-7.

[36] Guikema JE, Hovenga S, Vellenga E, et al. CD27 is heterougeneously expressed in multiple myeloma: low CD27 expression in patients with high-risk disease. *Br J Haematol* 2003;121:3643

[37] Zhan F, Barlogie B, Arzoumanian V, Huang Y, Williams DR, Hollmig K, Pineda-Roman M, Tricot G, van Rhee F, Zangari M, Dhodapkar M, Shaughnessy JD Jr. Gene-expression signature of benign monoclonal gammopathy evident in multiple myeloma is linked to good prognosis. *Blood.* 2007 15;109(4):1692-700.

[38] Bochtler T, Hegenbart U, Cremer FW, et al. Evaluation of the cytogenetic aberration pattern in amyloid light-chain amyloidosis as compared with monoclonal gammopathy of undetermined significance reaveals common pathways of karyotypic instability. *Blood.* 2008;111:4700-4705

[39] Comenzo RL, Hofman JE, Hassoun H, Landau H, Iyer L, Zhou P. Pathobiologic associations of plasma cell (PC) overexpression of *Cyclin D1 (CCND1)* in systemic AL amyloidosis (AL) [abstract]. *Amyloid.* 2010;17(s1):61.

[40] Falk RH. Diagnosis and management of the cardiac amyloidoses. *Circulation.* 2005;112:2047-60. [PubMed]

[41] Shan KB, Inoue Y, Mehra MR. Amyloidosis and the heart. A comprehensive review. *Arch Intern Med.* 2006;166:180-1813. [PubMed]

[42] Kholovà I, Kautzner J. Current treatment in cardiac amyloidosis. *Curr Treat Options Cardiovasc Med.* 2006;8:468-473. [PubMed]

[43] Kyle RA, Bayrd ED. Amyloidosis: Review of 236 cases. *Medicine.* 1975;54:271-299.

[44] Palladini G, Perfetti V, Obici L, et al. Association of melphalan and high-dose dexamethasone is effective and well tolerated in patients with AL (primary) amyloidosis who are ineligible for stem cell transplantation. *Blood.* 2004;103:2936-2938. Epub 2003 Dec 18.

[45] Palladini G, Russo P, Nuvolone M., et al. Treatment with oral melphalan plus dexamethasone produces long-term remissions in AL amyloidosis. *Blood.* 2007; 110:787-788.

[46] Mhaskar R, Kumar A, Behera M, et al. Role of high-dose chemotherapy and autologous hematopoietic cell transplantation n primary systemic amyloidosis: A systematic review. *Biol Blood Marrow Transplant.* 2009;15:893-902. Epub 2009 Apr 2.

[47] Cohen AD, Zhou P, Chou J, et al. Risk-adapted autologous stem cell transplantation with adjuvant dexamethasone +/- thalidomide for systemic light chain amyloidosis: results of a phase II trial. *Br J Haematol.* 2007;139:224-233.

[48] Landau H, Hassoun H, Bello C, et al. Adjuvant bortezomib and dexamethasone following risk-adapted melphalan and stem cell transplant in systemic AL amyloidosis [abstract]. *Amyloid.* 2010;17(s1):80.

[49] Palladini G, Perfetti V, Perlini S, et al. The combination of thalidomide and intermediate-dose dexamethasone is an effective but toxic treatment for patients with primary amyloidosis (AL). *Blood.* 2005;105:2949-2951.

[50] Moreau P, Jaccard A, Benboubker L, et al. Lenalidomide in combination with melphalan and dexamethasone in patients with newly AL amyloidosis: a multicentre phase I/II dose escalation study [abstract]. *Blood.* 2010 Dec 2;116(63):4777-82. Epub 2010 Aug 19.

[51] Dispenzieri A, Gertz MA, Hayman SR, et al. A pilot study of pomalidomide and dexamethasone in previously treated light chain amyloidosis patients [abstract 3854]. *Blood.* 2009;114.

[52] Kastritis E, Wechalekar AD, Dimopoulos MA, et al. Bortezomib with or without dexamethasone in primary systemic (light-chain) amyloidosis. *J Clin Oncol* 2010; 28:1031-1037. Epub 2010 Jan 19.

[53] Wechalekar AD, Lachmann HJ, Offer M, et al. Efficacy of bortezomib in systemic AL amyloidosis with relapsed/refractory clonal disease. *Haematologica.* 2008;93:295-298.

5

Pulmonary Manifestations of Amyloidosis

Mark E. Lund[1,2], Priya Bakaya[2] and Jeffrey B. Hoag[1,2]
[1]*Cancer Treatment Centers of America, Eastern Regional Medical Center,*
[2]*Drexel University College of Medicine,*
Philadelphia, PA,
USA

1. Introduction

Amyloidosis is a disease characterized by the deposition of abnormal proteins in extracellular tissue. The deposits originate from serum derived or locally produced proteins. (Sipe et al., 2010) The term "amyloid" was first used by Rudolph Virchow in 1854. (Saleiro et al., 2008) According to the Nomenclature Committee of the International Society of Amyloidosis 2010 recommendations, an amyloid fibril protein must occur in tissue deposits and exhibit affinity for Congo red and green birefringence when viewed by polarization microscopy. Furthermore, the protein must have been unambiguously characterized by protein sequence analysis (DNA sequencing in the case of familial diseases). In this chapter, we will focus on the pulmonary manifestations of amyloid. We will discuss the classification, presentation, symptoms, diagnostic testing and therapeutic options with regards to amyloid in the respiratory tract.

Amyloidosis had been classified over the years based on the site of deposition and presence or absence of other diseases. (Thompson & Citron, 1983) The term "Generalized" or "Systemic" had been used to describe deposition in multiple anatomic sites and "localized" used to describe deposition in one anatomic site. The term "secondary" used to describe patients with coexistent disease like multiple myeloma and "primary" for patients with no such coexistent disease. (Utz et al., 1996)

2. Classification of pulmonary amyloidosis

Amyloid in the respiratory tract has been classified by authors at The Mayo Clinic as associated with systemic amyloidosis and localized pulmonary disease. (Utz et al., 1996) The most common cause of the respiratory amyloid disease is secondary to systemic AL Amyloidosis which accounts for up to 80% of pulmonary amyloid. (Pitz et al., 2006) Moreover, it has been reported that 88% of patients with systemic amyloid have pulmonary disease. (Smith et al., 1979)

Amyloidosis localized to the respiratory tract was first recognized by Lesser in 1877. (Lesser, 1877) Amyloidosis at present is best classified by the protein fibrils and then by the location of sites involved clinically. To date, there are 27 known extracellular fibril proteins identified in humans. Table 1 lists some of the common protein subunits. Clinically there are three broad classifications of pulmonary involvement. The amyloid deposition may predominantly involve the tracheobronchial tree with nodules or submucosal infiltration. There can also be predominant interstitial localization. A third presentation is with single or multiple pulmonary parenchymal nodular deposits. A combination of radiographic and bronchoscopic studies provides this classification of pulmonary amyloidosis. Interestingly, it is uncommon for interstitial and tracheobronchial involvement to develop in the same patient.

Classification	Amyloid Protein Fibril Type	Symptoms	Imaging	Treatment
Nodular	AL	Incidental Finding Cough Dyspnea	Round nodules with sharp margins, subpleural and peripheral, may be cavitary, can be PET avid	Observation Local treatment Bronchoscopic (if in larynx) Lobectomy (very rarely)
Tracheo-bronchial	AL, Rare AA	Cough Dyspnea Hemoptysis	Tracheal and bronchial wall thickening, post-obstructive pneumonia, atelectasis	Observation Local treatment with laser therapy External Beam Radiation Surgery (rarely)
Diffuse Alveolar-Septal	AL, AA, ATTR	Cough Dyspnea Lethargy	Interlobular septal thickening, traction bronchiectasis	Usually requires systemic treat-ment with chemotherapy and/or stem cell transplant
Adenopathy	AL	Incidental Finding Compression of the airway Wheezing Cough Dyspnea	Extrathoracic nodes more common, often calcify with an eggshell or popcorn pattern	Observation Bronchoscopic (Stenting) Surgical (rarely)
Pleural Effusion	AL	Dyspnea, cough, lethargy	Opacity on CXR Pleural studing on CT	Thoracentesis Chest tube PleurX catheter Chemical or Mechanical pleurodesis

Table 1. Classification of Pulmonary Amyloidosis with Commonly Encountered Symptoms, Radiographic Findings, and Treatment Modalities

2.1 Tracheobronchial amyloidosis

Pulmonary nodules of amyloid deposits can be found in the larynx, tracheobronchial tree and lung parenchyma. Discrete nodular deposits in the larynx were described in 1919 (New, 1919). Tracheobronchial amyloidosis is characterized by deposits in the trachea and large bronchi. This is the most common form of primary pulmonary amyloidosis. (Sugihara et al., 2006) Isolated tracheal disease is very rare with less than 20 cases reported in the literature as of 2006. (Sharma & Katlic, 2006) It typically presents in the fifth and sixth decade of life and is slightly more common in females than males. (Berk et al., 2002) As previously mentioned, tracheobronchial amyloid deposition can occur in two forms: nodular or unifocal disease and diffuse submucosal disease. Tracheobronchial amyloidosis has been associated with tracheobronchopathia osteochondroplastica (TBO) by some authors. (Jones & Chatterji, 1977) Tracheobronchopathia osteochondroplastica is a disorder characterized by the deposition of calcified or cartilaginous submucosal nodules in the airways. (Capizzi et al., 2000) The uncertainty is related to the fact that most patients with TBO do not show evidence of amyloid deposition. (Mimori et al., 1998)

In a retrospective review of a series at The Mayo Clinic of 17 patients with biopsy proven tracheobronchial amyloidosis concluded that this form of pulmonary amyloid appeared to be a type of localized amyloid, with protein fibril deposition only present in the tracheobronchial tree. (Utz et al., 1996) This form is quite rare with less than 150 cases published in the medical literature. Although tracheobronchial amyloidosis often follows a relatively stable course, it can present with significant morbidity in patients with extensive airway involvement. It may require repeated therapeutic bronchoscopies in an attempt to prevent progression of airway involvement. Three patterns of airway involvement have been described by Berk et al: (1) proximal, (2) mid or main bronchial, and (3) distal disease. (Berk et al., 2002) Although tracheobronchial amyloidosis is most commonly caused by the AL form of amyloid fibril deposition, AA amyloidosis has also been reported in a case of tracheobronchial amyloidosis complicating mediastinal fibrosis. (Hoag & Yung, 2008)

2.2 Diffuse interstitial amyloid

Diffuse amyloid deposition in the lung parenchyma is usually associated with systemic AL amyloidosis. It is characterized by widespread amyloid deposition involving small vessels and the interstitium. There is little association between the extent of amyloid deposition in the lung and level of functional compromise. A Mayo clinic series included 35 patients who had pulmonary involvement with primary systemic amyloidosis. Celli and coauthors reported case series of 12 patients with AL lung disease, of which only 1 patient his clinical outcome dictated by his pulmonary involvement. (Celli, 1978) Cordier and colleagues reported that only 10% of patient deaths were due to AL lung disease in their series. (Cordier, 1986) Pathologists at John Hopkins have examined the association between cardiac and pulmonary amyloid. (Smith et al., 1979) They found that all patients with pulmonary amyloid deposition had cardiac amyloid disease. They concluded that histologic and clinical pulmonary disease in AL patients was principally a marker of severe cardiac infiltration.

2.3 Nodular amyloidosis

Amyloid nodules in the lung parenchyma are usually incidental findings on chest radiographs and usually need to be differentiated from neoplastic lesions. These nodules are typically located peripherally or subpleurally, and they can also be bilateral in some cases. If these lesions are located more centrally, airflow limitation may occur leading to symptomatic presentations. Moreover, these amyloid lesions may cavitate. (Cordier et al., 1986) AL amyloidosis is a well recognized complication of Sjogren's syndrome and is most often associated with localized nodular pulmonary amyloidosis. An association with benign hypergammaglobulinemic purpura has been reported in one patient. (Bignold et al., 1980)

3. Other manifestations of thoracic amyloidosis

3.1 Adenopathy

Hilar and mediastinal adenopathy are commonly associated with the AL form of systemic amyloidosis, and rarely adenopathy is present in localized pulmonary disease. (Lachmann & Hawkins, 2006) The majority of patients with amyloid-associated lymphadenopathy have detectable circulating monoclonal immunoglobulin which are typically associated with very low grade lymphoplasmacytic lymphoma or Waldenstrom's macroglobulinemia. (Plockinger et al., 1993) Plockinger et al. reported a case of nodular amyloidosis of hilar lymph nodes with no evidence of a paraprotein immunoglobulins or light chains present on immunoelectrophoretic analyses of the plasma and urine. Amyloid infiltrated nodes frequently calcify in a "popcorn" pattern or an "eggshell" conformation. (Gross, 1981)

3.2 Pleural effusions

Pleural effusions have also been reported in patients with systemic amyloid disease. The incidence of pleural effusion in amyloidosis is not known. Effusions can be unilateral or bilateral, and they can present with either exudative or transudative chemistries. (Berk et al., 2003) One of the first reports of amyloid-associated pleural effusion included five patients by Kavuru and colleagues. (Kavuru et al., 1990) These authors found that pleural effusions in the majority of their patients (60%in their series) were believed related to either congestive heart disease or nephrotic syndrome, and only 40% of pleural effusions were "idiopathic". Despite this they found that even those patients with transudative effusions had pleural infiltration with amyloid on biopsy. The Amyloid Program at Boston University reported their 7 year experience with 636 patients. (Berk et al., 2003) Thirty five patients in this series (6%) had large recurrent pleural effusions along with another 10-15% with less significant effusions. They compared patients with primary systemic amyloidosis and coincident cardiomyopathy without pleural effusions and patients with recurrent large pleural effusions. They noted exudative chemistries in pleural fluid of 37% of their patients along with chylothorax in another two patients. In contrast to the conclusions drawn by Kavuru et al., their hypothesis was that direct amyloid infiltration of the parietal pleural was responsible for large recurrent pleural effusions. Their claim was supported by thoracoscopic descriptions of pleural studding and histologic evidence of amyloid infiltrating pleural surfaces on biopsy. (Kavuru et al., 1990) After extensive comparisons between the two groups using echocardiography, they concluded that cardiac dysfunction alone was not sufficient to produce the pleural effusions in their cohort. The paucity of chylous effusions in patients with AL amyloid despite the propensity of mediastinal lymphadenopathy points towards direct amyloid infiltration of lymph nodes by amyloid as the cause of chylothorax as opposed to a compression of lymph nodes. Although uncommon, pleural effusions in patients with primary pulmonary amyloidosis can be hemorrhagic. (BoydKing et al., 2009)

4. The clinical presentation of pulmonary amyloidosis

Pulmonary amyloid may present with symptoms or may be found as an incidental finding on thoracic imaging. Patients present to pulmonologists in a number of ways: patients with systemic amyloidosis may present with respiratory symptoms; localized forms of amyloid may be detected incidentally on imaging or biopsy; and patients may present with respiratory symptoms that warrant pulmonary workup leading to the diagnosis of amyloidosis. (Lachmann & Hawkins, 2006; Sipe et al., 2010; Thompson & Citron, 1983) Tracheobronchial amyloidosis usually presents in fifth decade of life with symptoms of cough, dyspnea, wheezing, and hemoptysis. (Berk et al., 2002) In addition, hoarseness is frequently reported.

The most common symptoms of amyloid involvement with the respiratory system are cough, wheezing, dyspnea on exertion, and hemoptysis; none of which are uniquely specific to the diagnosis of pulmonary amyloidosis. One elderly male presented with diffuse alveolar hemorrhage. (Shenin et al., 2010) Amyloid nodules in the lung parenchyma are most often asymptomatic and are usually incidental findings on imaging studies; however, they sometimes can produce space occupying effects, most often if they limit either air or blood flow in the lungs. These nodules tend to calcify, and sometimes they may cavitate. They can cause lumenal narrowing of the airways and thus may lead to post obstructive atelectasis and/or pneumonia. Diffuse alveolar-septal amyloidosis related to systemic AL disease may present with symptoms of dyspnea or even more frightening symptoms of hemoptysis due to dissection of pulmonary arteries infiltrated by amyloid protein deposits (Cools et al., 1996; Road et al., 1985) or massive pulmonary embolism related to thrombosis of inferior vena cava. Mediastinal or hilar adenopathy is less common than extrathoracic adenopathy in patients with systemic AL disease. However, these patients may sometimes present with cervical nodes that may enlarge, become tender or recede in periods mimicking sarcoidosis. Pleural effusions in patients with amyloidosis will cause dyspnea and may at times require repeated thoracenteses to relieve symptoms.

5. Diagnosis of pulmonary amyloid

5.1 General considerations for diagnosis

When systemic amyloid disease is present, consideration for pulmonary evaluation for amyloid involvement should be based upon symptoms and clinical suspicion. The delay from time of presentation to the diagnosis of pulmonary involvement has been up to 17 months in some series. (O'Regan et al., 2000) In a patient with systemic amyloidosis, exercise limitation or cough should prompt an evaluation for lung involvement. In the setting of isolated pulmonary disease, amyloid is often low on the differential diagnosis. Pulmonary amyloidosis can be evaluated with plain films, computed tomography, bronchoscopy and pulmonary function testing. Figure 1 depicts an algorithm of a diagnostic approach for patients with systemic amyloidosis.

5.2 Radiographic evaluation

As previously described, the nodular form amyloidosis is most often an incidental finding on thoracic imaging. The plain chest radiograph can be normal in as many as half of patients with pulmonary nodular amyloidosis. (O'Regan et al., 2000) Amyloid nodules are generally described as rounded with sharp, discreet margins, and they are occasionally cavitary

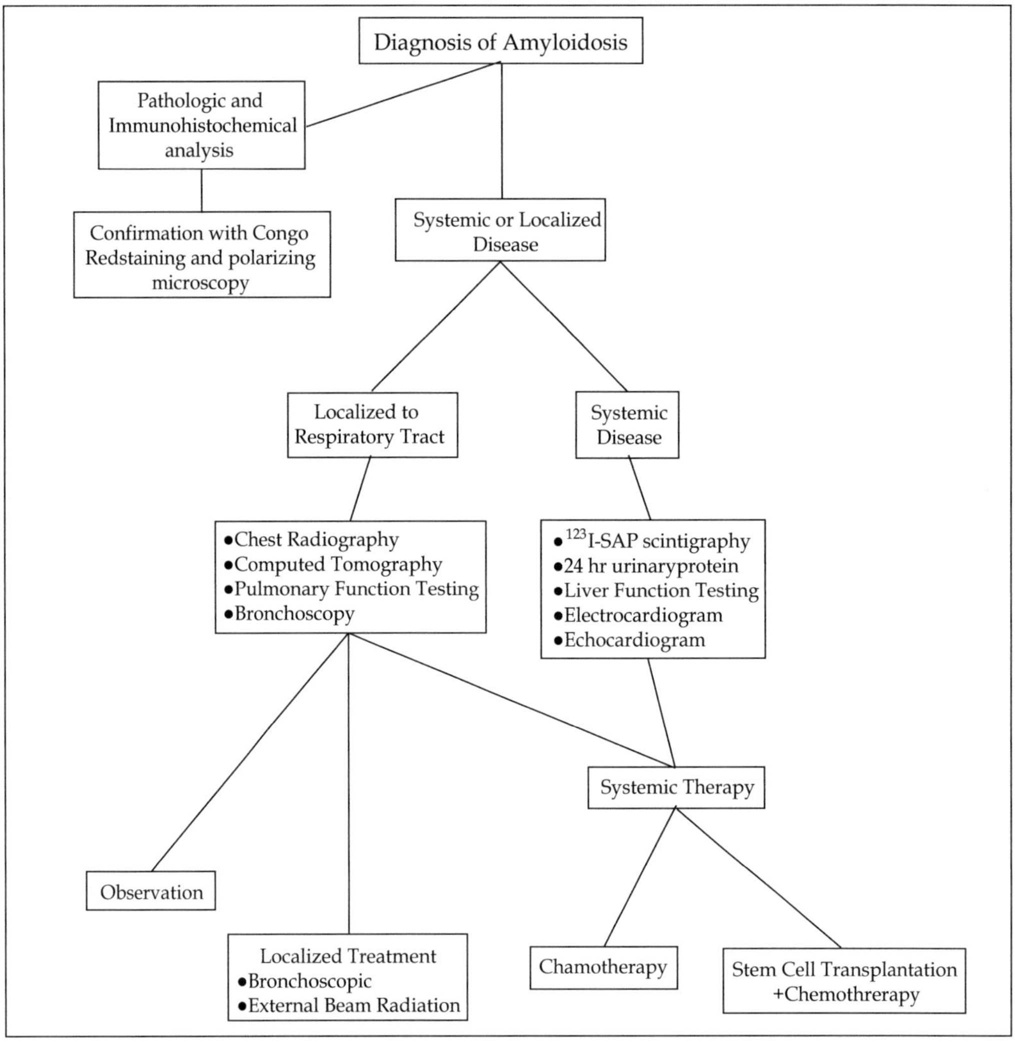

Fig. 1. Flow diagram of a decision pathway for the evaluation and treatment of respiratory amyloidosis

in appearance. One case report found that a lesion of amyloid measured 282 Hounsfield units, which is significantly less dense than blood. (M'Rad et al., 1988) Pulmonary nodular amyloidosis are predominantly subpleural and peripheral with a random distribution.

Imaging of patients with diffuse alveolar-septal disease may show infiltrative opacities on chest plain radiographs. In systemic amyloidosis, diffuse interstitial disease is most common. This may be reticular nodular on computed tomography imaging. Interlobular septal thickening and diffuse irregular lines with some honeycombing can be seen at the lung bases peripherally, and traction bronchiectasis can also be seen. Some report that diffuse cystic changes may predominate. (Wink, 2003)

Tracheal and bronchial wall thickening or discrete tumor masses may be a CT finding of tracheobronchial amyloid. The presence of multifocal masses with calcification should prompt a differential diagnosis of carcinoma, Wegener's Granulomatosis, relapsing

polychondritis, tracheobronchial tuberculosis, pulmonary hyalinizing granuloma, tracheobronchopathia osteochondroplastica along with tracheobronchial amyloidosis. (Bhadra et al., 2010; Carter & Patchefsky, 1998; Gibbaoui et al., 2004) Circumferential calcification involving the membranous airway should suggest amyloidosis as other forms of airway thickening do not involve this portion.
Positron emission tomography (PET) may demonstrate increased uptake of ^{18}F-flourodeoxyglucose (FDG) in patients with nodular amyloidosis. (Currie et al., 2005; Kung et al., 2003; Seo et al., 2010) From the studies of PET with pathology confirming amyloidosis, the standardized uptake value (SUV) ranged from 1.8 to 6.81, suggesting the need for biopsy to exclude malignancy. Coincident pulmonary nodular amyloid and adenocarcinoma has been reported in a patient with systemic AL amyloidosis. (Miyazaki et al., 2011) An uncharacteristic speculated appearance of the nodule in question in this case highlights the need for careful review of thoracic imaging in conjunction with a high index of suspicion. Coincident carcinoma and amyloid deposits have been described in thyroid medullary carcinoma. (Westermark et al., 2007)

5.3 Pulmonary function testing

Pulmonary function testing (PFT) in patients with pulmonary involvement of amyloidosis is similarly variable due to the variety of presentations. Overall, pulmonary functions can be normal or exhibit obstructive or restrictive disease. When tracheobronchial amyloidosis is present, the most common finding is airflow limitation as demonstrated by a reduced ratio of forced expiratory volume in the 1st second (FEV_1) to forced vital capacity (FVC) of less than 70%. The severity is dependent on the degree and location of amyloid deposition. In as series of patients with tracheobronchial amyloidosis from Boston, those with proximal disease tended to have more severe airflow limitation than those with more distal disease, although both groups had significant air trapping present with elevated residual volumes. (O'Regan et al., 2000) With the nodular form of pulmonary amyloidosis, direct compression of central airways may lead to obstructive patterns on PFTs. Evidence of a fixed upper airway obstruction not only suggests central airway disease but also portends a higher probability of progressive central obstructive disease. (Bhadra et al., 2010)
Restriction may be present as would be expected in patients with significant pleural effusion, or in very severe cases of diffuse alveolar-septal disease. Diffusing capacity for carbon monoxide is most often preserved.

5.4 Diagnostic bronchoscopic findings

The bronchoscopic findings of pulmonary amyloidosis vary with the classification of disease. In patients with interstitial or pulmonary nodular disease the endobronchial appearance on bronchoscopy may be entirely normal. In contradistinction to the interstitial variety, those with tracheobronchial amyloidosis commonly have significant visible pathology. The lesions of tracheobronchial amyloid can be nodular, sessile, or polyploidy. The sessile lesions have been described as hard yellow plaques that may be expansive or thinner longitudinal irregularities. Cobblestoning of the mucosa may be present. The sessile lesions may cause significant airway stenosis, and these regions of stenosis can be diffuse.
The nodules or polypoid lesions may suggest endolumenal carcinoma to both the experienced and inexperienced bronchoscopist. These nodules are usually firm, non mobile, and covered with hypervascular mucosa. Because of the hypervascularity in conjunction with the infiltrated submucosa, the endobronchial lesions in tracheobronchial amyloidosis

are quite friable, and bleed easily with minimal bronchoscopic contact. (Hoag & Yung, 2008) In contradistinction to tracheobronchopathia osteochondroplastica (TBO), the membranous trachea and mainstem airways are not spared. Tracheobronchial amyloidosis was associated with TBO in 22% in one series. (Piazza et al., 2003)

Ultimately, the diagnosis of pulmonary amyloidosis requires histologic confirmation. An excellent overview of the pathologic features of pulmonary amyloidosis has been published. (Katzenstein, 1997) Congo red staining that produces green birefringence under polarized light remains the gold standard for diagnosis. Classic teaching is that these lesions have a tendency to bleed. An increased risk of hemorrhage during biopsies of amyloidotic tissues may result from increased fragility of involved blood vessels, reduced elasticity of tissues and rarely to an acquired deficiency of clotting factors 9 or 10. So while endolumenal forceps biopsy is required, preparation for potential airway bleeding is advisable. Strange et al. reported on the fatal hemorrhage and air embolism complicating a routine transbronchial biopsy of a patient with pulmonary amyloidosis. (Strange et al., 1987) Treatment with low level Neodymium: Yttrium Aluminum Garnet (Nd:YAG) laser or argon plasma coagulation (APC) can be effective in controlling bleeding from the central airway amyloid lesion. Both approaches offer non contact therapy. Application of electrocautery can create rebleeding by disruption of the coagulum. The non-contact therapies (APC and Nd:YAG Laser) does not disrupt the bleeding site and remove the coagulum created by its application. Pretreatment with endobronchial epinephrine injections into the lesions may decrease the bleeding risk.

Effective biopsy may be obtained by the use of Wang needle or endobronchial forceps. Biopsy of the lesions may be difficult due to calcifications, and small biopsy specimens are open to sampling errors. False positive results also do occur in routine practice, usually as a result of poor Congo red staining. A confirmatory stain with Thioflavine T, which fluoresces yellow-green, may be helpful. (Saleiro et al., 2008) Any bronchoscopic finding suggesting tracheobronchopathia osteochondroplastica should be stained with Congo red due to the similarity of endobronchial appearance. (Bhadra et al., 2010) When the tissue is too calcified or when the operator feels uncomfortable with handling larger volume bleeding open surgical biopsy may be warranted.

Like any tumor mass, malignant or non-malignant, post obstructive pneumonia can develop in pulmonary amyloidosis. Protected brush samples or clean bronchoalveolar lavage for culture should be obtained when there is a high grade stenosis or evidence of mucopurulent drainage.

Once histologic evaluation with Congo red staining has been performed, immunochemistry to determine protein fibril type should be performed. Anatomical and functional evaluation of the various organs involved in systemic amyloidosis should also be performed. (Hawkins et al., 1990) Radiolabeled Serum Amyloid P (SAP) component localizes specifically to amyloid deposits *in vivo* in proportion to the amount of amyloid present and enables diagnosis, quantification and monitoring of amyloid to be performed scintigraphically. (Hazenberg et al., 2007)

6. Follow up of the patient with pulmonary amyloid

Several non-invasive methods of surveilling the progress of disease include computed tomography imaging and pulmonary function testing, especially serial spirometry. Proximal disease can present as pattern of fixed airway obstruction on flow volume loops, (Lachmann et al., 2006) or progression of disease may be apparent with progression flow limitation as demonstrated by decreasing FEV_1. Radiographic imaging may show areas of atelectasis or hyperinflation due to progression of obstructing endobronchial disease. Due to the relative rarity of this condition the most appropriate method of surveillance is not known.

7. Management of pulmonary amyloidosis

The outcome of patients with pulmonary amyloidosis reported in the literature is variable. From a series of 21 patients with primary pulmonary amyloidosis, the median survival was 16 months and no patients were alive at five years. (Utz et al., 1996) The survival of this cohort was much shorter than would be expected in comparison to patients with systemic amyloidosis without pulmonary involvement. As some have suggested that respiratory failure is rarely the direct cause of death in patients with amyloidosis, it seems that its presence is a marker of more severe disease. In contrast, in another series over 15 years with 10 patients reported survival averaged 8 years. (O'Regan et al., 2000) In this series death was predominantly caused by respiratory complications.

Due to the variability of amyloid involvement in the pulmonary system, the treatment for respiratory amyloidosis ranges from observation to bronchoscopic or surgical resection based on severity and symptomatology. Management decisions are mostly based on an individual basis. Systemic amyloidosis can be treated with chemotherapy while localized forms are typically treated with local interventions.

7.1 Chemotherapy

Infiltrative and systemic disease has been amenable to chemotherapy with oral melphalan and prednisone. (Kyle et al., 1997) A prospective study done at The Mayo Clinic in patients with systemic amyloidosis showed that combination therapy with melphalan, prednisone and colchicine or melphalan and prednisone resulted in prolonged survival compared to colchicine alone. The median duration of survival after randomization was 8.5 months in the colchicine group, 18 months in the group assigned to melphalan and prednisone, and 17 months in the group assigned to melphalan, prednisone, and colchicine ($p<0.001$). (Wechalekar et al., 2008) The National Amyloidosis Center in The United Kingdom has divided its treatment strategies for systemic AL disease into low dose, intermediate and high dose regimens. They recommend one of the intermediate dose regimens involving risk-adapted CTD (cyclophosphamide, thalidomide and dexamethasone) or oral mel-dex (melphalan, dexamethasone) as first line therapy, and autologous stem cell transplantation as an alternative treatment. (Cohen et al., 2007) Stem cell transplantation has been attempted with variable success in more severe disease. Recent phase 2 trials in systemic amyloidosis showed that risk-adapted Stem Cell Transplant with adjuvant thalidomide and dexamethasone is feasible and results in low treatment related mortality and high hematological and organ response rates in patients. (Cohen et al., 2007) There are several ongoing trials at amyloid centers in the United States and internationally, and physicians are encouraged to refer their patients to be enrolled in these studies in order to determine best practices.

7.2 Therapeutic bronchoscopy

In light of poor responses of tracheobronchial amyloid to systemic therapy, the majority of these patients will require endobronchial therapy. Bronchoscopic therapies remain the key to airway management in these patients.

Ablative therapy with Neodymium: Yttrium Aluminum Garnet (Nd:YAG) or Carbon Dioxide (CO_2) laser has been fairly successful. It appears that amyloid is very sensitive to photoablation. (Saleiro et al., 2008) Nd:YAG laser therapy is the most commonly utilized and is not only ablative but has significant hemostatic effects which is of particular benefit in these friable lesions. Laser ablation is the standard of care for endobronchial amyloidosis. In a retrospective series of 32 patients over 19 years, sixteen had persistent asymptomatic endolumenal disease. (Piazza et al., 2003) Two patients had endolumenal procedures with subsequent requirement of surgical resection. Each patient had no evidence of recurrent endolumenal amyloid after 5 to 8 years. Herman et al. reported on 13 cases of tracheobronchial amyloid successfully treated with Nd:YAG laser. (Herman et al., 1985) Follow up of another patient with CT imaging showed stabilization of the lesions after laser resection. (M'Rad et al., 1988) In a series by Diaz-Jimenez three of 11 laser ablations required termination because of significant hemorrhage. (Diaz-Jimenez et al., 1999)

In addition to photoablative strategies, cryotherapy has also been utilized to treat tracheobronchial amyloidosis. (Maiwand et al., 2001) Like other endolumenal therapies, multiple treatments (21 procedures over an 11 year follow up) over the patient's disease course are often required.

Rigid bronchoscopy has been utilized to mechanically debulk the amyloid lesions and for serial dilation of stenotic airways. In addition, the rigid bronchoscope has been used to help with potential bleeding when undergoing biopsy or laser photoablation. Placement of silicone stents has been utilized in conjunction with the ablative therapies to help prolong the airway stability. (Yang et al., 2003)

The use of airway stents after dilation may also be considered in select patients. Serial therapeutic bronchoscopies are not uncommon. (Gibbaoui et al., 2004) If large mediastinal amyloid masses or lymphadenopathy cause central airway obstruction airway stenting is an option. As in all benign airways disease it is always preferential to implant a silicone stent. If a self expanding metallic stent is the only option, the authors recommend a fully covered stent. Operator experience should not be the determinant of the type of stent placed. Because of the complex nature of these patients, the high risk of significant bleeding, and the potential for repeated procedural requirements, it is recommended that these patients be referred to a formally trained interventional pulmonologist or thoracic surgeon with significant experience in managing high grade central airway obstruction.

Localized tracheobronchial amyloidosis can cause post obstructive pneumonia. (Daniels et al., 2007) When evidence suggests a post obstructive state, appropriate empiric antibiotics should be started. Once bronchoscopic cultures are obtained, a strategy of proper de-escalation of therapy should be employed based upon the culture results.

7.3 Radiation therapy

External beam radiotherapy has been successfully utilized in tracheobronchial amyloidosis in a patient believed not to be a candidate for endolumenal therapy due to the diffuse nature of the airways disease. (Monroe et al., 2004) A total of 24 Gy was delivered in 12 fractions, and colchicine was given as an adjunctive therapy. Improvements were measured by sequential pulmonary function testing, radiographic imaging, bronchoscopic evaluation, and performance status.

Kurrus et al. published a case report demonstrating a benefit of external beam radiation (20 Gy in 10 fractions) in causing local response in a patient with localized tracheobronchial disease. (Kurrus et al., 1998) The authors noted decreased thickness of the airway wall and less friable and erythematous airway post radiation on a subsequent bronchoscopy. They treated the patient based on the hypothesis that plasma cells that secrete amyloidogenic protein are radiosensitive. Other hypotheses proffered include radiation injures cells other than plasma cells that may secrete amyloidogenic proteins, and free radicals generated by radiation may modify and enhance the degradation of amyloid protein deposits. Combined endobronchial and radiation therapy have demonstrated a similar beneficial effect. (Kalra et al., 2001). The authors know of no reports utilizing high dose rate brachytherapy for endobronchial disease. It stands to reason that this too would be a potentially viable option.

7.4 Pleural drainage

Large recurrent pleural effusions in patients with amyloidosis will often require repeated thoracenteses followed by pleurodesis. (Berk et al., 2003; Berk et al., 2005) In a case series reporting on 35 patients with recurrent amyloid pleural effusions at Boston University, chest tubes were placed in 18 patients after a failure of diuresis and intermittent thoracenteses. Seven patients had the chest tube removed without chemical pleurodesis because of unremitting large volume drainage. Eight patients underwent talc slurry pleurodesis via chest tube with symphysis achieved in those with output less than 100 ml/day while in those patients with more than 200 ml/day, the pleurodesis failed uniformly. Video-assisted thoracoscopic surgery with talc insufflation achieved success in 2 patients, and another 2 patients had PleurX™ catheters placed for continued intermittent drainage.

8. Conclusions

In conclusion, although amyloid in the respiratory tract is not a common occurrence, physicians should be aware of the various manifestations. Symptoms of pulmonary amyloidosis are very non specific and hence require a high degree of clinical suspicion. The workup should include a complete physical examination, pulmonary function testing, appropriate clinical imaging followed by biopsies and pathology confirmation of amyloid. The treatment strategy needs to be individualized to the particular patient's clinical status and symptomatology, and may range from close observation to locally directed and systemic therapeutic options. Airway interventions, including debulking of amyloidomas with rigid bronchoscopy, laser photoablation, or airway stents should be performed by an experienced interventional pulmonologist or thoracic surgeon. This will help reduce the risks of these therapies and allow the most expansive treatment options in a rare condition with un-defined best practices.

Future therapies will focus on strategies that involve preventing formation or propagation of insoluble beta-pleated sheets and/or enhance their degradation. Two ubiquitous molecules, serum amyloid P (SAP) and heparin sulfate proteoglycan (HSP), promote beta pleated sheet formation and inhibition of proteolytic degradation. (Gillmore et al., 2010) Drugs that target these molecules may be of interest in the future.

9. References

Berk JL, O'Regan A, Skinner M. (2002). Pulmonary and tracheobronchial amyloidosis. Semin Respir Crit Care Med. Vol 23, No. 2, (Apr 2002), pp. 155-65

Berk JL, Keane J, Seldin DC, Sanchorawala V, Koyama J, Dember LM, Falk RH. (2003). Persistent pleural effusions in primary systemic amyloidosis: etiology and prognosis. *Chest.* Vol. 124, No. 3, (Sep 2003), pp. 969-977

Berk JL. (2005). Pleural effusions in systemic amyloidosis. *Curr Opin Pulm Med.* Vol. 11, No. 4, (Jul 2005), pp. 324-8

Bhadra K, Butnor KJ, Davis GS. (2010). A Bronchoscopic Oddity Nodular Tracheobronchial Amyloid. *J Bronhcol Interven Pulmonol.* Vol. 17, No. 3, (Jul 2010), pp. 248-52

Bignold LP, Martyn M, Basten A. (1980). Nodular pulmonary amyloidosis associated with benign hypergammaglobulinemic purpura. *Chest.* Vol. 78, No. 2, (Aug 1980), pp. 334-6

BoydKing A, Sharma O, Stevenson K. (2009). Localized interstitial pulmonary amyloid: a case report and review of the literature. Curr Opin Pulmon Med. Vol. 15, No. 5, (Sep 2009), pp. 517-20

Capizzi SA, Betancourt E, Prakash UB. (2000). Tracheobronchial amyloidosis. *Mayo Clin Proc.* Vol. 75, No. 11, (Nov 2000), pp. 1148–52

Carter, D., Patchefsky,AS. (1998) Chapter 9 Spindle Cell Tumors of the Lung, In: Tumors and Tumor-like Lesions of the Lung, pp.(286-365) W.B. Saunders, 0-7216-3312-9, Philadelphia

Celli BR, Rubinow A, Cohen AS, Brody JS. (1978). Patterns of pulmonary involvement in systemic amyloidosis. *Chest.* Vol. 74, No. 5, (Nov 1978), pp. 543-547

Cohen AD, Zhou P, Chou J, Tenuya-Feldstein J, Reich L, Hassoun H, Levine B, Filippa DA, Riedel E, Kewalrammani T, Stubblefield MD, Fleisher M, Nimer S, Comenzo RL. (2007). Risk-adapted autologous stem cell transplantation with adjuvant dexamethasone + thalidomide for systemic light-chain amyloidosis: results of phase II trial. *Br J Haematol.* Vol. 139, No. 2, (Oct 2007), pp. 224-33

Cools FJ, Kockx MM, Borchxstaens GE, Heuvel PV, Cuykens JJ. (1996). Primary systemic amyloidosis complicated by massive thrombosis. *Chest.* Vol. 110, No. 1, (Jul 1996), pp. 282-4

Cordier JF, Loire R, Brune J. (1986). Amyloidosis of the lower respiratory tract. Clinical and pathologic features in a series of 21 patients. *Chest.* Vol. 90, No. 6, (Dec 1986), pp. 827-831

Currie GP, Rossiter C, Dempsey OJ, Legge JS. (2005). Pulmonary amyloid and PET scanning. *Respir Med.* Vol. 99, No. 11, (Nov 2005), pp. 1463-4

Daniels JT, Cury JD, Diaz J. (2007). An unusual cause of postobstructive Pneumonia. *Chest.* Vol. 131, No. 3, (Mar 2007), pp. 930-933

Diaz-Jimenez JP, Rodriguez A, Ballarin JIM, Castro MJ, Argemi TM, Manresa F. (1999). Diffuse tracheobronchial amyloidosis. *J Bronchol.* Vol. 6, No. 1, (Jan 1999), pp. 13-7

Gibbaoui H, Abouchacra S, Yaman M. (2004). A case of primary diffuse tracheobronchial amyloidosis. Ann Thorac Surg. Vol. 77, No. 5, (May 2004), pp. 1832-4

Gillmore JD, Tennent GA, Hutchinson WL, Gallimore JR, Lachmann HL, Goodman HJB, Offer M, Millar DJ, Petrie A, Hawkins PN, Pepys MB. (2010). Sustained pharmacological depletion of serum amyloid P component in patients with systemic amyloidosis. Br J Haematol. Vol. 148, No. 5, (Mar 2010), pp. 760-7

Gross BH. (1981). Radiographic manifestations of lymph node involvement in amyloidosis. *Radiology.* Vol. 138, No. 1, (Jan 1981), pp. 11-14

Hawkins PN, Lavender JP, Pepys MB. (1990). Evaluation of systemic amyloidosis by scintigraphy with ^{123}I -labelled serum amyloid P component. *N Engl J Med.* Vol. 323, No. 8, (Aug 23, 1990), pp. 508-513

Hazenberg BP, van Rijswijk MH, Lub-de Hooge MN, Vellenga E, Haagsma EB, Posthumus MD, Jager PL. (2007). Diagnostic performance and prognostic value of extravascular retention of ^{123}I-labeled serum amyloid P component in systemic amyloidosis. J Nucl Med. Vol. 48, No. 6, (Jun 2007), pp. 865-72

Herman DP, Colchen A, Milleron B, Bentata-Pessayre M, Personne C, Akoun G. (1985). The treatment of tracheobronchial amyloidosis using a bronchial laser. Apropos of a series of 13 cases. Rev Mal Respir. Vol. 2, No. 1, pp. 19-23

Hoag JB, Yung RC. (2008). An unexpected finding of endobronchial amyloidosis in a patient with mediastinal fibrosis. *J Bronchol.* Vol. 15, No. 1, pp. 61-3

Jones AW, Chatterji AN. (1977). Primary tracheobronchial Amyloidosis with tracheobronchopathia osteoplastica. Br J Dis Chest. Vol. 71, No. 4, (Oct 1977), pp. 268-72

Kalra S, Utz JP, Edell ES, Foote RL. (2001). External-beam radiation therapy in the treatment of diffuse tracheobronchial amyloidosis. *Mayo Clin Proc.* Vol. 76, No. 8, (Aug 2001), pp. 853-6

Katzenstein, A. (1997) Chapter 7 Systemic Diseases involving the Lung, In: Katzenstein and Askins Surgical Pathology of Non-neoplastic Lung Disease , pp.(168-192) W.B. Saunders, 0-7216-5575-9, Philadelphia

Kavuru MS, Adamo JP, Ahmad M, Mehta AC, Gephardt GN. (1990). Amyloidosis and Pleural Disease. *Chest.* Vol. 98, No. 1, (Jul 1990), pp. 20-3

Kung J, Zhuang H, Yu JQ, Duarte PS, Alavi A. (2003). Intense flourodeoxyglucose activity in pulmonary amyloid lesions on positron emission tomography. *Clin Nucl Med.* Vol. 28, No. 12, (Dec 2003), pp. 975-6

Kurrus JA, Hayes JK, Hoidal JR, Menendez MM, Elstad MR. (1998). Radiation therapy for tracheobronchial amyloidosis. *Chest.* Vol. 114, No. 5, (Nov 1998), pp. 1489-92

Kyle RA, Gertz MA, Greipp PR, Witzig TE, Lust JA, Lacy MQ, Therneau TM. (1997). A trial of three regimens for primary amyloidosis: colchicine alone, melphalan and prednisone, and melphalan, prednisone and colchicine. *N Engl J Med.* Vol. 336, No. 17, (Apr 24, 1997), pp. 1202-7

Lachmann HJ, Hawkins PN. (2006). Amyloidosis and lung. *Chron Respir Dis.* Vol. 3, No. 4, pp. 203-214Lesser A. (1877). Ein Fall von Enchondroma osteiodes mixtum der lunge mit partieller amyloid Entortung. *Virchows Arch (Path Anat)* Vol. 69, pp 404-408

M'Rad S, Le Thi Huong D, Wechsler B, Monsigny M, Buthiau D, Colchen A, Godeau P. (1988). Localized tracheobronchial amyloidosis. A new case studies with x-ray computed tomographic and nuclear magnetic resonance. Review of the literature. *Rev Pneumol Clin.* Vol. 44, No. 6, pp. 260-5

Maiwand MO, Nath AR, Kamath BSK. (2001). Cryosurgery in the treatment of tracheobronchial amyloidosis. *J Bronchol.* Vol. 8, No. 2, (Apr 2001), pp. 95-7

Mimori Y, Rikimaru T, Mitsui T, Shiraishi T, Kinoshita M, Oizumi K. (1998). Localized amyloidosis of the lower respiratory tract. *J Bronchol.* Vol 5, No. 4, (Oct 1998), pp. 316-8

Miyazaki D, Yazaki M, Ishii W, Matsuda M, Hoshii Y, Nara K, Nakayama J, Ikeda SI. (2011). A rare lung nodule consisting of adenocarcinoma and amyloid deposition in a patient with primary systemic AL amyloidosis. *Intern Med.* Vol. 50, No. 3, (Feb 2011), pp. 243-6

Monroe AT, Walia R, Zlotecki RA, Jantz MA. (2004). Tracheobronchial Amyloidosis: A case report of successful treatment with external bean radiation therapy. Chest. Vol. 125, No. 2, (Feb 2004), pp. 784-789

New GB. (1919). Amyloid Tumors of the upper air passages. *Laryngoscope.* Vol. 29, No. 6, pp. 327-41

O'Regan A, Fenlon HM, Beamis JF Jr., Steele MP, Skinner M, Berk JL. (2000). Tracheobronchial amyloidosis: The Boston University experience from 1984 to 1999. *Medicine.* Vol. 79, No. 2, (Mar 2000), pp 69-79

Piazza C, Cavaliere S, Foccoli P, Toninelli C, Bolzoni A, Peretti G. (2003). Endoscopic management of laryngo-tracheobronchial amyloidosis: as seroes of 32 patients. *Eur Arch Otorhinolaryngol.* Vol. 260, No. 7, (Aug 2003), pp. 349-54

Pitz MW, Gibson IW, Johnston JB. (2006). Isolated Pulmonary Amyloidosis: Case report ande review of the Literature. *Am J Hematol.* Vol. 81, No. 3, (Mar 2006), pp. 212-3

Plockinger B, Muller MR, Eskersberger F. (1993). Isolated amyloidosis of hilar lymph node. *Langenbecks Arch Chir.* Vol. 378, No. 3, pp. 167-70

Road JD, Jacques J, Sparling JR. (1985). Diffuse alveolar septal amyloidosis presenting with recuurent hemoptysis and medial dissection of pulmonary arteries. *Am Rev Respir Dis.* Vol. 132, No. 6, (Dec 1985), pp. 1368-70

Saleiro S, Hespanhol V, Magalhaes A. (2008). Endobronchial amyloidosis. J Bronchol. Vol. 15, No. 2, (Apr 2008), pp. 95-99

Seo JH, Lee SW, Ahn BC, Lee J. (2010). Pulmonary amyloidosis mimicking multiple metastatic lesions on F-18 FDG PET/CT. *Lung Cancer.* Vol. 67, No. 3, (Mar 2010), pp. 376-9

Sharma D, Katlic MR. (2006). Localized Tracheal Amyloidosis. *J Bronchol.* Vol. 13, No. 1, (Jan 2006), pp. 19-20

Shenin M, Xiong W, Naik M, Sandorfi N. (2010). Primary amyloidosis causing diffuse alveolar hemorrhage. *J Clin Rheumatol.* Vol. 16, No. 4, (Jun 2010), pp. 175-7

Sipe JD, Benson MD, Buxbaum JN, Ikeda S, Merlini G, Saraiva MJ, Westemark P. (2010). Amyloid fibril protein nomenclature: 2010 recommendations from the nomenclature committee of the International Society of Amyloidosis. *Amyloid.* Vol. 17, No. 3-4, (September–December 2010) pp. 101–104

Smith RR, Hutchins GM, Moore GW, Humphrey RL. (1979). Type and distribution of pulmonary parenchymal and vascular amyloid: Correlation with cardiac amyloid. *Am J Med.* Vol. 66, No. 1, (Jan 1979), pp. 96-104

Strange C, Heffner JE, Collins BS, Brown FM, Sahn SA. (1987). Pulmonary hemorrhage and air embolism complicating transbronchial biopsy in pulmonary amyloidosis. Chest. Vol. 92, No. 2, (Aug 1987), pp. 367-9

Sugihara E, Dambara T, Okamoto M, Sonobe S, Koga H, Inui A, Aiba M, Isonuma H, Hayashida Y. (2006). Clinical features of 10 patients with pulmonary amyloidosis. *J Bronchol.* Vol. 13, No. 4, (Oct 2006), pp. 191-3

Thompson PJ, Citron KM. (1983). Amyloid and the lower respiratory tract. *Thorax.* Vol. 38, No. 2, (Feb 1983), pp. 84-87

Utz JP, Swensen SJ, Gertz MA. (1996). Pulmonary Amyloidosis. The Mayo Clinic Experience from 1980 to 1993. *Annals of Internal Medicine.* Vol. 124, No. 4, (Feb 15, 1996), pp. 407-413

Wechalekar AD, Hawkins PN, Gillmore JD. (2008). Perspectives in treatment of AL amyloidosis. *Br J Haematol.* Vol. 140, No. 4, (Feb 2008), pp. 365-77

Westermark P, Benson MD, Buxbaum JN, (2007). A primer of amyloid nomenclature. *Amyloid.* Vol. 14, No. 3, (Sep 2007), pp. 179-83

Wink JS. (2003). An unusual presentation of an uncommon disease: A diffuse cystic radiologic pattern in a patient with localized pulmonary amyloidosis. Chest. Vol. 124, No. 4 suppl, (Oct 2003), pp. 280S

Yang S, Chia SY, Chuah KL, Eng P. (2003). Tracheobronchial amyloidosis treated with rigid bronchoscopy and stenting. Surg Endosc. Vol. 17, No. 4, (Apr 2003), pp. 658-9

6

Causal or Causal Relationship Between Oral Diseases and Systemic Amyloidosis – From Inflammation to Amyloidosis – A Trouble Connection

Murat İnanç Cengiz[1] and Kuddusi Cengiz[2]
[1]*Zonguldak Karaelmas University, Faculty of Dentistry, Department of Periodontology*
[2]*Ondokuz Mayıs University, Faculty of Medicine, Department of Nephrology*
Turkey

1. Introduction

Although recent decades have provided significant advances in our understanding of the pathology and pathogenesis of AA amyloidosis, the mechanism and etiopathological factors promoting amyloidosis are largely unknown (Elimowa et al., 2009). Its pathogenesis is multifactorial, involving many variables such as primary structure of the precursor protein, acute-phase response, the presence of non-fibril protein, receptors, lipid metabolism and proteases (Röcken and Shakespeare, 2002). This pathogenetic process centers on the conversion of normally soluble proteins into insoluble fibrillar aggregates that disrupt tissue structure and cause disease. The organ distribution pattern of amyloid deposits and the resulting disease outcome depend on the origin and type of fibrillar protein deposited (Glenner, 1980; Kisilevski, 1992). Hence, amyloidosis is classified on the basis of the origin and biochemical composition of the precursor proteins that form the fibrillar deposits. The two most common forms of systemic amyloidosis are light-chain (AL) amyloidosis and reactive (AA or secondary) amyloidosis due to chronic inflammatory diseases. Beta-2 microglobulin amyloidosis is a common complication associated with long term hemodialysis. Hereditary systemic amyloidoses are a group of autosomal dominant disorders caused by mutations in the genes of several plasma proteins. In this section, we focus on the more common of these conditions, which are systemic AA amyloidosis, oral focal infections especially chronic periodontitis, and familial amyloidosis especially auto-inflammatory diseases (Glenner, 1980; Kisilevski, 1992; Grateau et al., 2005).

Systemic AA amyloidosis, representing approximately 45 percent of generalized amyloidoses are inflammatory arthritis (Rheumatoid arthritis), chronic infections (Bronchiectasis, tuberculosis, chronic cutaneous infections, osteomyelitis), Immunodeficiency status, other conditions predisposing to chronic infections (Injected drug abuse, epidermolysis bullosa, paraplegia), Hereditary periodic fevers (Familial Mediterranean fever, Hyperimmunglobulin D syndrome, TNF receptor-associated periodic syndrome), Inflammatory bowel disease (Crohn's disease, ulcerative colitis), Neoplasia, Systemic vasculitis (Behçet's disease, systemic lupus erythematosis), others (Sarcoidosis). Reactive systemic AA amyloidosis is a potential complication of any disorder that gives rise to a sustained acute-phase response, and the list of chronic inflammatory, infective or neoplastic disorders that can underlie it is almost without limit (Lachmann and Hawkins, 2006).

Amyloid fibrils are derived from the cleavage fragments of the circulating acute-phase reactant (APR) serum amyloid A protein (SAA) (Pras et al., 1968). SAA is an apolipoprotein of high-density lipoprotein (HDL) which, like C-reactive protein (CRP), is synthesized by hepotocytes under the transcriptional regulation of cytokines including interleukin (IL)-1, IL–6, tumor necrosis factor (TNF)-alfa, beta and acute-phase reactants (APRs), either alone or combination, have been shown to affect SAA synthesis at the transcriptional level (Yamada, 1998). In the circulation, SAA levels may increase by 1000-fold in response to injury, infection, and inflammation, and thus SAA has properties resembling a classical positive APR. Because concentration of APRs may be correlated with the amount of damaged tissue, measurements of SAA are of value in the assessment of acivity and response to therapy during several inflammatory diseases (Malle and De Beer, 1996; Lachmann et al., 2005). Although AA amyloid can develop rapidly, the median latency between presentation with a chronic inflammatory disorder and clinically significant amyloidosis is almost two decades (Lachmann et al., 2005). The prognosis of AA amyloidosis depends on the degree of renal function and whether the underlying inflammatory disease can be suppressed. AA amyloidosis does not occur in the absence of an acute-phase response or without elevated SAA levels (Lachmann et al., 2007; Röcken and Shakespeare, 2002).

The theory of focal infection to explain various inflammatory disease was first suggested by Hippocrates and was widely propagated in the first three decades of the 20th Century. It was thought that foci of infection, which themselves might go unnoticed because of lack of symptoms, initiated the seeding of pathogenic microorganisms or their products to distant body sites.

Later, the concept of focal infection (i.e systemic effects from oral bacteria) is being changing and mostly relies on the correlation between chronic periodontitis and systemic diseases (Offenbacher, 1996; Scannapieco, 1998). At present it is generally agreed on that oral status is connected with systemic health, since poor oral health may occur concomitantly with more serious underlying diseases and/or it may predispose to other systemic diseases (Seymour et al, 2007). The pioneering approach of periodontal medicine has helped to renew attention on the theory of focal infection and the deepening of the relationship between chronic periodontitis and systemic health. Periodontal evaluations are normally not performed as part of medical assessment. Hence, periodontal diseases may be an overlooked source of inflammation in amyloid patients. However, the anagrommatic question of causal or causal association between infectious diseases and inflammatory changes is distant body sites was never satisfactorily addressed.

Various hypotheses, including common susceptibility, systemic inflammation, direct bacterial infection and cross-reactivity, or molecular mimicry, between bacterial antigens and self-antigens, have been postulated to explain these relationships. In this scenario, the association of periodontal disease with systemic diseases has set the stage for introducing the concept of periodontal medicine.

Obviously, cross-sectional clinical studies cannot determine whether periodontal disease is the cause of or is inconsequential to medical diseases, nor may longitudinal studies alone resolve the issue of causality. If periodontal disease and a given medical disease share etiological components, periodontal disease might appear earlier than the medical disease without having caused the disease, simply because periodontal disease develops faster than many medical diseases of complex multifactorial etiology. Although a number of studies have presented evidence of close relationships between periodontal and systemic diseases, the majority of findings are limited to epidemiological studies, while the etiological details remain unclear (Inaba and Amano,2010). Hence, periodontal diseases may be an overlooked source of inflammation in amyloid patients. Because of APRs that increase during the course of periodontal diseases is the cause of the etiopathogenesis of AA amyloidosis. Prior to, periodontal disease have not been investigated in the secondary amyloidosis with unknown etiology. Furthermore, in approximately 6 to 11.84% of causes of systemic AA amyloidosis no underlying disease can be found (Lachmann et al., 2007; Paydaş, 1999).

Clarification of the importance of oral focal infection requires controlled epidemiological studies and, probably, a better understanding of the etiology and the clinicopathological features of periodontal disease and medical diseases. Before adequate data are available, caution should be exercised in implicating periodontal disease or any other oral infection in the causation of major medical disorders like mortal systemic AA amyloidosis. Thus, the aim of this chapter is to emphasize that periodontal diseases may be considered as an etiological factor for amyloidosis. It is hereby suggested that periodontal evaluation should be performed as part of a routine medical assessment process. Preventing or treating periodontal disease might prevent or at least alleviate the progression of systemic AA amyloidosis. In terms of medical economics, understanding of the relationship between chronic periodontitis and systemic diseases has potential to change health policy, with ensuing economic benefits.

This chapter reviews the periodontal disease, auto-inflammatory syndromes relevant to oral health and suggested association of familial Mediterranean fever (FMF) and Behçet's disease

2. Periodontal infection and systemic health

Periodontal diseases are a group of bacterial inflammatory diseases of the supporting tissues of the teeth, in 1999, a classification of periodontal diseases has been proposed (Armitage, 1999). Periodontal diseases are common, initially bacteria-driven, chronic inflammatory condition leading to the formation of infected periodontal pockets, destruction of deep collagenous structures of the periodontium and alveolar bone, excessive mobility of the teeth and then their premature loss (Pihlstrom et al., 2005).

The cause of these common inflammatory conditions is the dental plaque. In 1 mm^3 of dental plaque weighing approximately 1mg. more than 10^8 bacteria are present and over 300 species have been isolated and characterized in these deposits. Normally, the oral microbial community and the host immune response are in equilibrium which allows for periodontal health to the maintained, but pathology can occur when the balance is compromised for several causes:

a. modification of the environmental conditions of the site, caused by either bacterial interactions or accumulation of dental plaque;
b. reduction in the proportion of benefical bacteria, such as those producing inhibitory substances, caused by bacterial interactions or the use of systemic antibiotics; and
c. deficit of the host immune system.

The progression from gingivitis to periodontitis is characterized by periodontal pocket development, which favours further plaque accumulation and a shift in its qualitative composition (Pizzo et al., 2010). In July 1998, the American Academy of periodontology launched an effort to educate the public about new discoveries: infections in the mouth may play an important role in disorders involving other parts of the body (Scannapieco, 1998). At present it is generally agreed on that oral status is connected with systemic health, since poor oral health may occur concomitantly with more serious underlying diseases and/or it may predispose to other systemic diseases (Seymour et al., 2007). The pioneering approach of periodontal medicine has helped to renew attention on the theory of focal infection and the deepening of the relationship between chronic periodontitis and systemic health (Pizzo et al., 2010). The oral cavity is an open system exposed to the environment. It has been estimated that, in an individual with moderate to severe periodontitis, the total surface area of the inflammed periodontal pockets can range from 8 to 20 cm^2 depending upon the number of teeth affected (Craig et al., 2007; Hujoel et al., 2001). Therefore, the large surface area of the aggregate periodontal lesion can potentially become a significant source of inflammation in individuals with moderate to severe periodontitis.

3. Periodontal disease and systemic amyloidosis

Periodontal pathogens, as well as their toxins, such as cytolitic enzymes and lypopolisaccharide (LPS) may have access to the blood stream through the compromised and/or ulcerated epithelium of the periodontal pocket. Moreover, within the inflammed gingival tissue a number of inflammatory mediators, such as tumor necrosis factor (TNF)-alpha, interleukin (IL)-1 beta, prostaglandin E_2 (PGE_2), and gammainterferon are produced; these can enter the blood stream and contribute to the global inflammatory burden. Thus, the systemic exposure to periodontal pathogens, their toxins, and periodontal derived/ elicited inflammatory mediators may determine pathologic consequences in different organ or system. Three mechanisms by which periodontal infection may influence systemic health have been described.

1. metastatic infection caused by translocation of Gram-negative bacteria from the periodontal pocket to the bloodstream;
2. metastatic injury, such as vascular lesions from the effects of circulating microbial toxins and pro-inflammatory mediators;
3. metastatic inflammation due to the immunological response to the periodontal pathogens and their toxins (Li et al., 2000).

A cross-sectional study has demostrated that plasma levels of inflammatory markers such as CRP, fibrinogen, interleukins and leucocyte counts increase in periodontitis patients when compared to periodontally healthy patients (Craig et al., 2003). Studies reported decrease in both IL-6 and CRP six months after initial periodontal therapy alone (D'Aiuto et al., 2004; 2005). Taken together, these studies suggest that not only can periodontitis elevate APRs and other systemic markers of inflammation but effective periodontal therapy may decrease acute-phase response values, as well.

Periodontal infections are polymicrobial and result from the accumulation of bacterial plaque and dental calculus at the gingival margin (Pihlstrom et al., 2005). These infections develop within several years and are often asymptomatic and painless, but may eventually lead to loss of teeth. It is widely regarded as one of the most common diseases worldwide, with a prevalence of 10%-15%. A recent health examination survey from Finland involving 6300 participants revealed that up to 64 % of the adult population had deepened gingival pockets associated with periodontitis, and nearly 20 % had a severe form of this disease with pocket deeper than 6 mm (Knuuttila, 2004). One cubic millimeter of dental plaque contains about 100 milion bacteria and may serve as a persistent reservoir for potential pathogenic bacteria (Thoden et al., 1984). Subgingivally located bacteria and bacterial components and products, especially endotoxins, may easily enter the blood circulatory system via the infected and injured epithelium of deepened gingival pockets as well as after daily oral hygiene routines. Even gentle mastication leads to increased release of bacterial endotoxins into the peripheral blood (Geerts et al., 2002). Such bacterial release as well as systemic inflammation induced by local inflammation mediators, very likely occurs in periodontitis patients, not just transiently but also long-term. Continuous exposure to several periodontal pathogens fits well with the theory of the role of infections in systemic AA amyloidosis. Total pathogen burden, the number of pathogens, and endotoxemia, the concentration and activity of endotoxins, to which an individual has been exposed, may contribute to amyloidosis. The systemic immune response, genetic factors, and environmental factors also affects the risk of developing periodontitis (Agrawal et al., 2006) and systemic AA amyloidosis (Elimova and Kisilevski, 2009; Röcken and Shakespeare, 2002).

4. Chronic periodontitis as a risk factor for systemic AA amyloidosis

Systemic AA amyloidosis does not occur in the absence of acute-phase response or without SAA levels. The serum concentration of SAA closely reflects the activity of chronic inflammatory diseases, and persistently high concentration is a prerequisite for the development of AA amyloidosis (Lachmann et al., 2007; Röcken and Shakespeare, 2002). The natural history of AA amyloidosis is typically progressive, leading to organ failure and death among patients whose underlying inflammatory disease remained active. By contrast, there was regression of amyloid deposits, stabilisation or recovery of amyloidotic organ function, and excellent long-term survival among patients in whom the SAA concentration fell within the normal limit as a result of anti-inflammatory therapy (Röcken and Shakespeare,2002; Lachmann et al., 2007). However, in approximately 6 to 11.84 % of causes of AA amyloidosis, no underlying disease could be found (Lachmann et al., 2007; Paydaş, 1997). The concept of focal infection (i.e systemic effects from oral bacteria) is being changing and mostly relies on the correlation between chronic periodontitis and systemic diseases (Offenbacher, 1996; Scannapieco, 1998; Seymour et al., 2007). Periodontal evaluations are normally not performed as part of a medical assessment. Hence, periodontal diseases may be an overlooked source of inflammation in amyloid patients. Prior to our study (Cengiz et al., 2010 a,b), periodontal diseases have not been investigated in the secondary amyloidosis with unknown etiology. Moderate to severe periodontitis is prevalent in the general population and may be more prevalent in the systemic AA amyloid population (Cengiz et al., 2010 b). Periodontitis has been associated with increased markers of systemic inflammation. Therefore, periodontitis and AA amyloid populations may be a covert source of systemic inflammation that can be managed through effective periodontal therapy. Patients with chronic periodontal diseases have higher levels of SAA-the precursor protein of amyloid fiber in AA amyloidosis-than do the patients without periodontal disease (Glurich et al., 2002). Also, it has been reported that SAA and other APR levels were elevated in response to intravenous challenge with live porphyromonas gingivalis (P. gingivalis), an important periodontal pathogen (Li et al., 2002).

In recent years, a study was published by Cengiz et al (2010b), analysing the etiological distribution of 112 patients with systemic AA amyloidosis showed that FMF (52.7 %), chronic inflammatory and neoplastic diseases (35.7 %) were the leading causes of systemic AA amyloidosis, while periodontal disease found in 11.6 % of the patients under study. The prevalence of moderate to severe periodontitis was 47.5 % in FMF patients, 72.5 % in patients with known chronic inflammatory diseases, and 84.7 % in patients with periodontal disease. Serum levels of APRs in amyloidosis patients were reduced significantly following nonsurgical periodontal therapy. They suggested that periodontitis may be an important occult source of chronic inflammation that increases the levels of acute-phase reactants in the patients and hence might affect the development of amyloidosis.

Periodontal disease shares several clinical and etiopathogenic characteristics with systemic AA amyloidosis. First, periodontal disease is a long-standing infectious or inflammatory disease and can cause a dramatic increase in the levels of systemic inflammation and periodontal treatment can result in the reduction in the levels of these markers. The increased serum APRs including SAA cause to the etiopathogenesis of systemic AA amyloidosis. Second, there is a close relationship between the severity of both diseases and serum APR levels. Third, the systemic immune response, genetic and environmental factors also affect the risk of developing periodontitis and systemic AA amyloidosis. Fourth, a limited number of experimental studies have shown that SAA and other APRs were elevated in response to an intravenous challenge with p.gingivalis. Fifth, treatment of periodontal disease reduces serum levels of inflammatory markers and underlying chronic inflammatory disease like systemic AA amyloidosis. Lastly, serum APRs that increase during the periodontal disease, are the cause to etiopathogenesis of systemic AA amyloidosis.

Collectively, these findings support the notion that periodontitis can elicit a potentially harmful systemic inflammatory response and may thus provide a potential risk factor for systemic AA amyloidosis and other diseases of inflammatory origin. Chronic periodontitis may be an additive factor to traditional etiologic factors for systemic AA amyloidosis as well as being primary etiological factor for systemic AA amyloidosis. Periodontal evaluation should be performed as part of a medical assessment.

Although the inflammation hypothesis provides a plausible and attractive explanation for the periodontitis-amyloidosis relationship, further research is needed to define the mechanisms linking the two diseases and how patients with periodontitis should best be managed to reduce their risk factor of systemic AA amyloidosis.

5. Auto-inflammatory syndromes and amyloidosis

The term "autoinflammatory disease" encompases an expanding group of inflammatory disorders defined as Mendelian genetic diseases of the innate immune system. This group is expanding considering the fact that diseases sharing strong similarities with this core group can be defined as auto-inflammatory. Familial Mediterranean fever (FMF) is the most frequent entity within this group of disorders which further consists of hyperimmunoglobulinaemia D and periodoic fever syndrome (HIDS), tumour necrosis factor receptor-associated periodic syndrome (TRAPS), cryopyrin-associated periodic syndrome (CAPS), Aphthous-like oral ulceration has been reported as one manifestation in several of the syndromes, including periodic fever, aphtous-stomatitis, pharyngitis, adenitis ((PFAPA), and pyogenic sterile arthritis, pyoderma gangrenosum acne (PAPA). Chronic jaw recurrent osteomyelitis has been recorded in chronic recurrent multifocal osteomyelitis (Juric, 2004; Girschic et al., 2007). Reactive (AA, secondary) amyloidosis is a severe complication of these diseases (Grateau et al., 2005). This is caused by deposition of fibrils that consist of the proteolytically cleaved acute-phase protein serum amyloid A (SAA). Several genetic and environmental factors modify the risk for systemic AA amyloidosis (van der Hilst et al., 2005; Scully and Hodgson 2008) Aphthous-like ulceration has been reported as one manifestation in some of the auto-inflammatory syndromes. Associations of other aphthous-like ulcers including Behçet's disease, Reiter's syndrome, Crohn's disease, systemic lupus erythematosus, and cyclic neutropenia support an immuno-pathological etiology (Livneh et al., 1996). Genetic, inflammatory and environmental factors predispose individuals to autoinflammtory and periodontal diseases. Periodontitis-induced autoinflammatory response also may play a role in development/severity of some autoinflammatory diseases and systemic AA amyloidosis via IL-1 gene alteration (Scully et al., 2008, Akman et al., 2008; Grateau and Duruöz, 2010). FMF and Behçet's disease are most frequent entities within this group of disorders.

6. Relationship between periodontal parameters and Behçet's disease and systemic AA amyloidosis

Behçet's disease (BD) is a chronic relapsing, systemic vasculitis of unknown etiology. Although several immunological abnormalities have been demonstrated in patients with BD, the exact machanism of the inflammatory changes occuring remains to be elucidated (Sakane et al., 1999; Verity et al., 2003; Everekoğlu, 2005). The most probable hypothesis is that of an immunological driven inflammatory response set off by infectious agents in genetically predisposed individuals, a major pathologic process is vasculitis (Sakane et al., 1997; Alpsoy et al., 1998). Overexpression of proinflammatory cytokines from various cellular sources seem to be responsible for the enhanced inflammatory reaction in BD, and it may be associated with genetic susceptibility (Sakane et al., 1997; Gül, 2001).

In recent years, many studies emphasized the gene-environment interaction in the development of periodontitis and BD (Akman et al., 2008; Shirodaria et al., 2000; Gül 2001). Periodontitis-induced autoinflammatory response may also play a role in the development/severity of BD and periodontitis (Akman et al., 2008; Shirodaria et al., 2000; shimpuku et al., 2003).

Oral microbial flora have long been implicated in the pathogenesis, as BD starts mostly from the oral mucosal surface (Lehner 1997; Mumcu et al., 2004). In a recent study, Mumcu et al., (2006) have shown that oral health-related quality-of-life assessments were impaired in patients with BD and associated with disease activity and treatment modalities. Previous studies demonstrated that periodontal scores were higher in patients with BD than the healthy subject (Nakae et al., 1981; Celenligil-Nazlıel et al., 1999; Mumcu et al., 2004; Akman et al., 2007; Karaçaylı et al., 2009; Arabacı et al.2009). Also, it has been speculated that BD might develop after the periodontitis and advenced periodontal disease may represent a risk factor for severe organ involvement (Akman et al., 2007).

Systemic AA amyloidosis has been important complication in the past, even in childhood onset patients. AA-type amyloid fibrils were found in all case studies (Akpolat et al., 2002). Oral ulcers are usually the first sign and the main classification criteria (97-100%) in BD, causing an unpredictable course with remission and exacerbations. Genetic/environmental factors are implicated on the pathogenesis of amyloidosis. Serum amyloid A (SAA) polymorphism was found to be a risk factor for amyloidosis in BD (Utku et al., 2007). Furthermore, it has been demonstrated that long term periodontal follow-up and education of oral hygiene in patients with BD may help to prevent the development and/or progression of these diseases (Akman et al., 2008; Karaçaylı et al., 2009; Arabacı et al., 2008).

7. Familial Mediterranean fever – Periodontal disease and systemic AA amyloidosis

Familial Mediterranean fever (FMF) is an autosomal recessive inflammatory disease, which occurs worldwide but predominantly affects population from the Eastern Mediterranean Basin (Livneh et al., 2001). FMF is an autoinflammatory disease, characterized by recurrent attacks of fever and serosal inflammation, along with a very intense acute-phase response. The most important complication of FMF is systemic AA amyloidosis (Soher et al., 1967). Secondary amyloidosis also occurs in some FMF patients with chronic inflammatory conditions and chronic infections. The activation pattern of serum amyloid A (SAA) protein in the presence of inflammation was similar to that of CRP. Increased levels of CRP and SAA protein have been reported to be associated with increased FMF (Cengiz et al., 2009; De Beer et al., 1982; Akar et al., 2003), Periodontitis (Cengiz et al., 2009; Craig et al., 2003; D'Aiuto et al., 2005). and systemic AA amyloid (Cengiz et al., 2009; Lachmann et al., 2007) diseases activity and poor outcome in patients.

The genetic causes of amyloidosis have yet to be completely understood. It seems to be associated with M694V homozygous mutations of the FMF gene, MEFV, and with differences in SAA (Ben-Chetrit 2003; Aringer, 2004; Yiğit et al., 2008). Several investigators claimed that (Sidi et al., 2000, Cazeneuve et al., 1999, Mansour et al., 2001; Shohat et al., 1999) the M694V homozygote genotype was associated with the development of amyloidosis, whereas others (El-Shanti et al., 2006; Yalçınkaya et al., 2000) have not confirmed this finding.

It has been reported that APRs are generally elevated during acute attacks of FMF and return to normal upon clinical remission (Ben-Chetrit et al.1998). However, there are articles reporting that in some patients, even in those using colchicine regularly, the levels of APRs remain high in the intervals between acute attacks of FMF (Tunca et al., 1999), but the nature and source of this inflammation is unclear. Although changes in the salivary concentration of secretory immunoglobulin A and phagocytic activity of neutrophils in blood from the gingiva have been reported in patients with FMF (Akapion, 1998), the possibility that periodontal inflammation might contribute to increased APR levels in patients with FMF has not been investigated previously. Periodontitis is a local inflammatory process caused by bacteria and it may be associated with changes in the systemic inflammatory and immune responses (Slade et al., 2003; Craig et al., 2003). In fact, several reports have suggested that effective periodontal therapy may result in a decrease of the systemic markers of inflammation (D'Aiuto et al., 2004; D'Aiuto et al., 2005; Cengiz et al 2009).

Periodontitis and FMF have many potential pathogenic mechanisms in common. Both diseases have complex causes including genetic and gender predisposition, and might share many risk factors, such as age, education, smoking, social status and stress (Page, 1998; Touitou et al., 2007). Moreover, both diseases cause the release of the inflammatory markers. During the inflammatory response, local cells are stimulated to release APRs (Korkmaz et al., 2002; Ben-Chetrit et al., 1998; Tunca et al., 1999; Slade et al., 2003; D'Aiuto et al., 2005). Chlamydia pneumoniae has been found in patients with FMF and periodontitis (Altun et al., 2004; Paju et al., 2007). It is also known that chronic infection or inflammatory disease may cause systemic AA amyloidosis, even without obvious infection or inflammation (Cengiz, 2005; Nasr et al., 2006). Chronic inflammation and periodontal microbial burden may predispose patients with FMF to acute attacks of FMF or may be associated with amyloidosis in ways proposed for other infections, such as C. Pneumonia. Also, in approximately 6 to 11.86 % of cases of systemic AA amyloidosis no underlying disease can be found (Lachmann et al., 2007; Paydaş, 1999).

Recently, a paper published by Cengiz et al., (2009) claimed that the prevalence of moderate to severe periodontitis in FMF patients with amyloidosis (80.6%) was significantly greater than in FMF patients without amyloidosis (38%) and controls (20%). Serum levels of APRs in FMF patients were reduced significantly following nonsurgical periodontal therapy. In this study, it has been shown that periodontitis might be an important source of chronic inflammation or infection in FMF patients with and without amyloidosis.

The results of these studies confirm that periodontitis is highly prevalent in FMF patients, particularly in FMF patients with amyloidosis, and show a significant association between severe periodontitis and increased levels of APRs. Therefore, its diagnosis and management deserve a better interdisciplinary approach. Although most of the evidence regarding the relationship between periodontal disease and those systemic conditions is consistently supportive of this notion, more research is needed. Treating periodontitis might help to alleviate the disease burden in patients with FMF and systemic AA amyloidosis.

8. References

Agrawal, AA., Kapley, A., Yeltiwar, RK., Purohit, HJ. (2006) Assessment of single nucleotide polymorphism at IL-1 A+4845 and IL-1 B+3954 as genetic susceptibility test for chronic periodontitis in Maharashtrian ethnicity. *J Periodontol* 77 (9):1515-1521.

Akopian, GV. (1998) The local immune mechanisms of the involvement of the teeth and periodontium in periodic disease. *Stomatolagiia* (Mosk) 77: 4-7.

Akar, N., Hasipek, M., Akar, E., Ekim, M., Yalcınkaya, F., Çakar, N. (2003) Serum amyloid A1 and tumor necrosis factor-alpha allels in Turkish Familial Mediterranean Fever patients with and without amyloidosis. *Amyloid* 10: 12-16.

Akman, A., Kaçaroğlu, H., Dönmez, L., Bacanlı, A., Alpsoy, E. (2007) Relationship between periodontal findings and Behcet's disease: a controlled study. *J Clin Periodontal* 34: 485-491.

Akman, A., Çiçek-Ekinci, N., Kaçaroğlu, H., Yavuzer, U., Alpsoy, E., Yeğin, O. (2008) Relationship between periodontal findings and specific polymorphisms of interleukin- 1(alfa) and 1 (beta) in Turkish patients with Behçet's disease. *Arch Dermatol Res* 300: 19-26.

Akpolat, T., Akkoyunlu, M., Akpolat, I., Dilek, M., Odabaş, AR., Ozen, S. (2002) Renal Behçet's disease: a cumilative analysis. *Semin Arthritis Rheum* 31: 317-337.

Alpsoy, E., Yılmaz, E., Coskun, M., Savas, A.,Yegin, O. (1998) HLA antigens and linkage disequilibrium patterns in Turkish Behçet's patients. *Journal of Dermatology* 25: 158-162.

Altun, S., Kasapçopur, O., Aslan, M., Karaarslan, S., Koksal, V., et al., (2004) Is there any relationship between Chlamydophila Pneumoniae infection and juvenile idiopathic arthritis? *J Med Microbiol* 53: 787-790.

Arabacı, T., Kara, C., Çiçek, Y. (2009) Relationship between periodontal parameters and Behçet's disease and evaluation of different treatments for oral recurrent aphthous stomatitis. *J Periodontal Res* 44: 718-725.

Aringer, M. (2004) Periodic fever syndrome-a clinical overview. *Acta Med Austriaca* 31: 8-12.

Armitage, GC. (1999) Development of a classification system for periodontal diseases and conditions. *Ann Periodontol* 4: 1–6.

Ben-Chetrit, E. (2003) Familial Mediterranean Fever (FMF) and renal amyloidosis-phenotype-genotype correlation, treatment and prognosis. *J Nephrol* 16: 431–434.

Celenligil-Nazlıel, H., Kansu, E.,Ebersole, J. (1999) Periodontal findings and systemic antibody responses to oral microorganisms in Behcet's disease. *Journal of Periodontology* 70: 1449–1456.

Cengiz, K. (2005) Uncommon etiology in renal amyloidosis. *Acta Clin Belg* 60: 109–113.

Cengiz, Mİ., Bağcı, H., Cengiz, S., Yiğit, S., Cengiz, K. (2009) Periodontal disease in patients with Familial Mediterrenean Fever: from inflammation to amyloidosis. *J Periodontol Res* 44(3): 354-361.

Cengiz, MI., Yayla, N., Cengiz, K., Bağcı, H., Taksın, E. (2010b) Interaction between periodontal disease and sytemic aa amyloidosis: from inflammation to amyloidosis. *J. Periodontol* [accepted, Ahead, of Print].

Cengiz, MI., Wang, HL., Yıldız, L. (2010a) Oral involvement in a case of AA amyloidosis: a case report. *J Med Case Reports*. 4(1): 200–206.

Craig, RG., Kotanko, P., Kamer, AR., Levin, NW. (2007) Periodontal disease-a modifiable source of systemic inflammation for the end-stage renal disease patient an hemodialysis therapy? *Nephrol Dial Transplant* 22: 312–315.

Craig, RG., Yip, JK., So, MK., Boylan, RJ., Socransky, SS., Hoffajee, AD. (2003) Relationship of destructive periodontal disease to the acute-phase response. *J Periodontol* 74: 1007–1016.

D'Aiuto, F., Nibali, L., Parker, M., Suvan, J., Tonetti, MS. (2005) Short-term effects of intensive periodontal therapy on serum inflammatory markers and cholesterol. *J Dent Res* 84: 296–273.

D'Aiuto, F., Parkar, M., Andreou, G., Suvan, J., Brett, PM., Ready, D., Tonetti, MS. (2004) Periodontitis and systemic inflammation: control of the local infection is associated with a reduction in serum inflammatory markers. *J Dent Res* 83: 156–160.

De Beer, FC., Mallya, RK., Fagan, EA., Lanham, JG., Hughes, GR. Pepys MB. (1982) Serum amyloid-A protein concentration in inflammatory diseases and its relationship to the incidence of reactive systemic AA-amyloidosis. *Lancet* 2: 231–234.

Elimova, E., Kisilevski, JB. (2009) Heparan sulfate promotes the aggregation of HBL associated serum amyloid A: evidence of a proamyloidogenic histidine molecular switch. *FASEB J* 23(10): 3436–3448.

El-Shanti, H., Majeed, AH., El-Khateeb, M. (2006) Familial Mediteranean Fever in Arabs. *Lancet* 367: 1016–1024.

Evereklioğlu, C. (2005) Current concepts in the etiology and treatment of Behçet's disease. *Survival Ophthalmology* 50: 297–350.

Falk, RH., Comenzo, RL., Skinner, M. (1997) The systemic amyloidosis. *N Engl J Med* 337: 898–909.

Geerts, SO., Nys, M., De, MP., Charpentier, J., Albert, A., Legrand, V., Rompen, EH. (2002) Systemic release of endotoxin-induced by gentle mastication: association with periodontitis severity. *J Periodontol* 73: 73–78.

Girschick, HJ., Zimmer, C., Klaus, G., Darge, K., Dick, A., Morbach, H. (2007) Chronic recurrent multifocal osteomyelitis: what is it and how should it be treated? *Nat Clin Pract Rheumatol* 3: 733–738.

Gleneer, GG. (1980) Amyloid deposits and amyloidosis: the beta-fibrilloses (second of the two parts). *N Eng J Med* 302: 1333–1343.

Glurich, I., Grossi, S., Albini, B., Ho, A., Shah, R., Zeid, M., et al., (2002) Systemic inflammation in cardiovascular and periodontal disease: comparative study. *Clin Diagn Lab Immunol* 9: 425–432.

Grateau, G., Jeru, I., Rouaghe, S., Cazeneuve, C., Ravet, N., Duguesnoy, P., et al., (2005) Amyloidosis and auto-inflammatory syndromes. *Curr Drug Target Inflamm Allergy.* 4: 57–65.

Grateau, G., Duruöz, MT. (2010) Autoinflammatory Conditions: When to suspect? How to treat? *Best Pract Res Clin Rheumatol* 24(3) 401–411.

Gul, A. (2001) Behcet's disease: an update on the patogenesis. *Clinical and Experimental Rheumatology* 19: 6–12.

Hujoel, PP., White, BA., Garcia, RI., Listgarten, MA. (2001) The dentogingival epithelial surface area revisited. *J Periodontol Res* 36: 48–55.

Inaba, H., Amano, A. (2010) Roles of Oral bacteria in cardiovascular diseases from molecular mechanisms to clinical cases: Implication of periodontal diseases in development of systemic diseases. *J Pharmacol Sci* 113:103–109.

Jurik, AG. (2004) Chronic recurrent multifocal osteomyelitis. *Semin Musculoskelet Radiol* 8: 243–253.

Karaçaylı, U., Mumcu, G., Şimşek, I., Pay, S., Kose, O., Erdem, H., Direskenli, H., Günaydın, Y., Dinç, A. (2009) The close association between dental and periodontal treatments and oral ulcer in Behçet's disease: a prospective clinical study. *J Oral Pathol Med* 38: 410–415.

Kisilevski, R. (1992) Proteoglycans, glycosaminoglycans, amyloid enhancing factor, and amyloid deposition. *J Entern Med* 232:515–516.

Knuuttila, M. Hampaiden kiinnityskudossairaudet [periodontal diseases] in Suominen-Taipale L, Nordblad A, Vehkalahti M, Aromaa a, editors. (2004) Suomalaisten aikuisten suunterveys [Oral health among the adult Finnish Population]. Terveys 2000-tutkimus [Health 2000-health examinationsurvey]. Finland: Helsinki: *Publication of the National Public Health Institute;* P 88–97.

Korkmaz, C., Özdoğan, H., Kasapçobur, O., Yazıcı, H. (2002) Acute phase response in Familial Mediterranean Fever. *Ann Rheum Dis* 61: 79–81.

Lachmann, HJ., Hawkins, PN. (2006) Systemic amyloidosis. *Current Opinion in Pharmacology* 6: 214–220.

Lachmann, HJ., Goodman, HJB., Gallimore, J., Gilbertson, JA., Joshi, J., Pepys, MB., Hawkins, PN. (2005) Characteritic and clinical outcome of 340 patients with systemic AA amyloidosis. In Amyloid and Amyloidosis. Edited by Grateau G, Kyle RA, Skinner M, *CRC Press* 173–175.

Lachman, HJ., Goodman, HJB., Gilbertson, JA., Gallimore, RJ., Sabin, CA., Gillimore, JD., Hawkins, PN. (2007) Natural history and outcome in systemic amyloidosis. *N Engl J Med* 356: 2361–2371.

Lehner, T. (1997) The role of heat shock protein, microbial and autoimmune agents in the aetiology of Behcet's disease. *International Review of Immunology* 14: 21-32.

Li, L., Massas, E., Batista, EL JR., Levine, RA., Amar, S. (2002) Porphyromonas gingivalis infection accelerates the progression of atherosclerosis in a heterozygous apolipoprotein E-deficient murine model. *Circulation* 105: 861-867.

Li, X., Kolltveit, KM., Tronstad, L., Olsen, I. (2000) Systemic diseases caused by oral infection. *Clin Microbiol Rev* 13: 547-558.

Livneh, A., Aksentijevich, I., Langevitz, P. Torosyan, Y., G-Shoham, N., et al., (2001) A single mutated MEFV allele in Israeli Patients suffering from Familial Mediterranean Fever and Behcet's disease (FMF-BD). *Eur J Hum Genet* 9: 191-196.

Malle, E., De Beer, FC. (1996) Human serum amyloid A (SAA) protein: a prominent acute-phase reactant for clinical practice. *Eur J Clin Invest* 26: 427-435.

Mansour, I., Delague, V., Cazeneuve, C., Dode, C., Chouery, E., et al., (2001) Familial Mediterranean Fever in Labanon: Mutation Spectrum, evidence for cases in Maronites, Greek Orthodoxes. Greek Catholics, Syriacs and Chiites and for an assocation between amyloidosis and M694V and M6941 Mutations. *Eur J Hum Genet* 9: 51-55.

Mumcu, G., Ergun, T., Inanc, N., Fresko, I., Atalay, T., Hayran, O.,Direskeneli H. (2004) Oral health is impaired in Behcet's disease and is associated with disease severity. *Rheumatology* 43: 1028-1033.

Mumcu, G., Inanc, N., Ergun, T., Ikiz, K., Gunes, M., Islek, U., Yavuz, S., Sur, H., Atalay, T., Direskeneli, H. (2006) Oral health related quality of life is affected by disease activity in Behcet's disease. *Oral Dis* 12: 145-151.

Nakae, K., Agata, T., Maeda, K., Masuda, K., Hashimoto, T.,Inaba, G. (1981) Behcet's Disease Pathogenic Mechanism and Clinical Future: Case Control Studies on Behcet's Disease, 1st edn. Tokyo: University of Tokyo Press: 41-49.

Nasr, SH., Schwarz, R., D'Agoti, VD., Markowitz, GS. (2006) Paraplegia, proteinuria, and renal failure. *Kidney Int* 69: 412-415.

Offenbacher, S. (1996) Periodontal diseases: pathogenesis. *Ann Periodontol* 1: 821-828.

Page, RC. (1998) The pathobiology of periodontal diseases may affect systemic diseases: inversion of a paradigm. *Ann Periodontal* 3: 108-120.

Paju, S., Sinisalo, J., Pussinen, PJ., Valtonen, V., Nieminen, MS. (2007) Is periodontal infection behind the failure of antibiotics to prevent coronary events? *Atherosclerosis* 193: 193-195.

Paydas, S. (1999) Report on 59 patients with renal amyloidosis. *Int Urol Nephrol* 34(5): 619-631.

Pihlstrom, BL., Michalowicz, BS., Johnson, NW. (2005) Periodontal diseases. *Lancet* 366: 1809-1820.

Pizzo, G., Guiglia, R., Russo, LL., Campisi, G. (2010) Dentistry and internal medicine: from the focal infection theory to the periodontal medicine concept. *European Journal of Internal Medicine* 21: 496-502.

Pras, M., Schubert, M., Zucker-Franklin, D., Rimon, A., Franklin, EC. (1968) The characterisation of soluble amyloid prepared in water. *J Clin Invest* 47: 924-933.

Röcken, C., Shakespeare, A. (2002) Pathology, diagnosis and pathogenesis of AA amyloidosis *Virchows Arch* 440: 111-112.

Sakane, T., Takeno, M., Suzuki, N.,Inaba, G. (1999) Behçet's disease. *New England Journal of Medicine* 341: 1284-1291.

Scannapieco, FA. (1998) Position paper of the American Academy of periodontology: periodontal disease as a potential risk factor for systemic diseases. *J Periodontal* 69: 841-850.

Scully, C., Hodgson, TA. (2008) Recurrent oral ulcers; there is a trap. Oral Surg Oral Med Oral *Pathol Oral Radiol Endod.* 6: 845-852.

Scully, C., Hodgson, T., Lachmann, H. (2008) Auto-inflammatory syndrome and Oral Health. *Oral Diseases* 14: 690-699.

Seymour, GJ., Ford, PJ., Cullinan, MP., Leishman, S., Yamazaki, K. (2007) Relationship between periodontal infections and systemic disease. *Clin Microbiol Infect* 13 (Suppl 4): 3-10.

Shimpuku, H., Nosaka, Y., Kawamura, T., Tachi, Y., Shinohara, M., Ohura, K. (2003) Genetic polymorphisms of the interleukin-1 gene and early marginal bone loss around endosseous dental implants. *Clin Oral Implants Res* 14: 423-429.

Shirodaria, S., Smith, J., McKay, IJ., Kenet, CN., Hughes, FJ. (2000) polymorphism in the IL-1A gene are correlated with levels of interleukin-1 alpha protein in gingival crevicular fluid of teeth with severe periodontal disease. *J Dent Res* 79: 1864-1869.

Sidi, G., Shinar, Y., Livneh, A., Langevitz P., Pras, M., Pras, E. (2000) Protracted febrile myalgia of Familial Mediterranean Fever: mutation analysis and clinical correlations. *Scand J Rheumatol* 29: 174-176.

Slade, GD., Ghezzi, EM., Heiss, G., Beck, JD., Riche, E., Offenbacher, S. (2003) Relationship between periodontal disease and c-reactive protein among adults in the atherosclerosis Risk in Communities study. *Arch Intern Med* 163:1172-1179.

Sohar, E., Gafni, J., Pras, M., Heller, H. (1967) Familial Mediterranean Fever. A survey of 470 cases and review of the literature. *Am J Med* 43: 227-253.

Thoden van Velzen, SK., Abraham-Inpijn, L., Moorer, WR. (1984) Plaque and systemic disease: a reappraisal of the focal infection concept. *J Clin Periodontol* 11: 209-220.

Touitou, I., Sarkisian, T., Medlej-Hashim, H., Tunca, M., Livneh, H., et al., (2007) Country as the primary risk factor for renal amyloidosis in Familial Mediterranean Fever. *Arthritis Rheum* 56: 1706-1712.

Tunca, M., Kırıkali, G., Soyturk. M., Akar, S., Pepys, MB., Hawkins, PN. (1999) Acute Phase response and evolution of Familial Mediterranean Fever. *Lancet* 353:1415.

Utku, U., Dilek, M., Akpolat, I., Bedir, A., Akpolat, T. (2007) SAA1 alpha/alpha alleles in Behçet's disease related amyloidosis. *Clin Rheumatol* 26: 927-929.

Van der Hilst, JCH., Simon, A., Drenth, JPH. (2005) Hereditary periodic fever and reactive amyloidosis. *Clin Exp Med* 5: 87-98.

Verity, DH., Wallace, GR., Vaughan, RW., Stanford, MR. (2003) Behçet's disease: from Hippocrates to the third millennium. *British Journal of Ophthalmology* 87: 1175-1183.

Yalçınkaya, F., Çakar, N., Mısırlıoğlu, M. et al., (2000) Genotype -phenotype correlation in a large group of Turkish patients with Familial Mediterranean Fever: evidence for mutation-independent amyloidosis. *Rheumatology (Oxford)* 39: 67-72.

Yamada, T. (1999) Serum amyloid A (SAA): a concise review of biology, assay methods and clinical usefulness. *Clin Chem Lab Med* 37: 381–388.

Yiğit, S., Bağcı, H., Özkaya, O., Özdamar, K., Cengiz, K., Akpolat, T. (2008) MEFV mutations in patients with Familial Mediterranean Fever in Black Sea region of Turkey: Samsun experience. *J Rheumatol* 35: 106–113.

7

Amyloidosis in the Skin

Toshiyuki Yamamoto
Department of Dermatology, Fukushima Medical University
Japan

1. Introduction

Amyloidosis is induced by deposition of amyloid proteins in various organs. Both systemic and localized type amyloidosis present with a variety of skin manifestations. Based on biochemical and immunological aspects, amyloid proteins are subdivided into several subtypes from different origins. Amyloid fibrils in primary and multiple myeloma-associated systemic amyloidosis are composed of immunoglobulin protein AL (light chain), whereas in secondary systemic amyloidosis, they are composed of a non-immunoglobulin protein (amyloid AA). In primary localized cutaneous amyloidosis, amyloid materials are derived from cytokeratin; however, in nodular primary cutaneous amyloidosis, amyloid is AL type. Dialysis-related amyloidosis is composed of β2-microglobulin.

So far, there are several reviews of skin features associated with amyloidosis [1-3]. Cutaneous amyloidosis is characterized by deposition of amyloid in the skin, which is seen in association with systemic amyloidosis and also restricted to the skin. In case of association with systemic amyloidosis, skin lesions are important as one of the extra-hematologic manifestations, because cutaneous lesions may occasionally be the initial presentation of systemic amyloidosis. Representative lesions include petechiae, purpura, ecchymoses, and eyelid translucent papulonodular lesions. By contrast, amyloidosis limited to the skin is called primary localized cutaneous amyloidosis, which is clinically classified into more common macular, papular, and the rare nodular form. Also, reports of cases showing peculiar forms of cutaneous amyloidosis are seen, depending on the different races. Additionally, amyloid deposition is secondarily seen in association with skin tumors, such as basal cell carcinoma, Bowen's disease, and other benign tumors. In this review, both primary and secondary skin lesions associated with systemic as well as cutaneous amyloidosis are discussed, making a focus on mucocutaneous manifestations.

2. Amyloid materials

Various subtypes of cutaneous amyloid are distinguished. Amyloid deposits are verified by several specific stains such as PAS, thioflavine T fluorescence, Congo red, and Dylon (Fig. 1). Light microscopy reveals amorphous materials extracellularly. Investigation by electron microscopy shows fibrillar materials (Fig. 2).

3. Systemic amyloidosis

Primary systemic amyloidosis (AL amyloidosis) is caused by plasma cell dyscrasia, and develops in 10-20% of patients with multiple myeloma. Various organs are affected such as

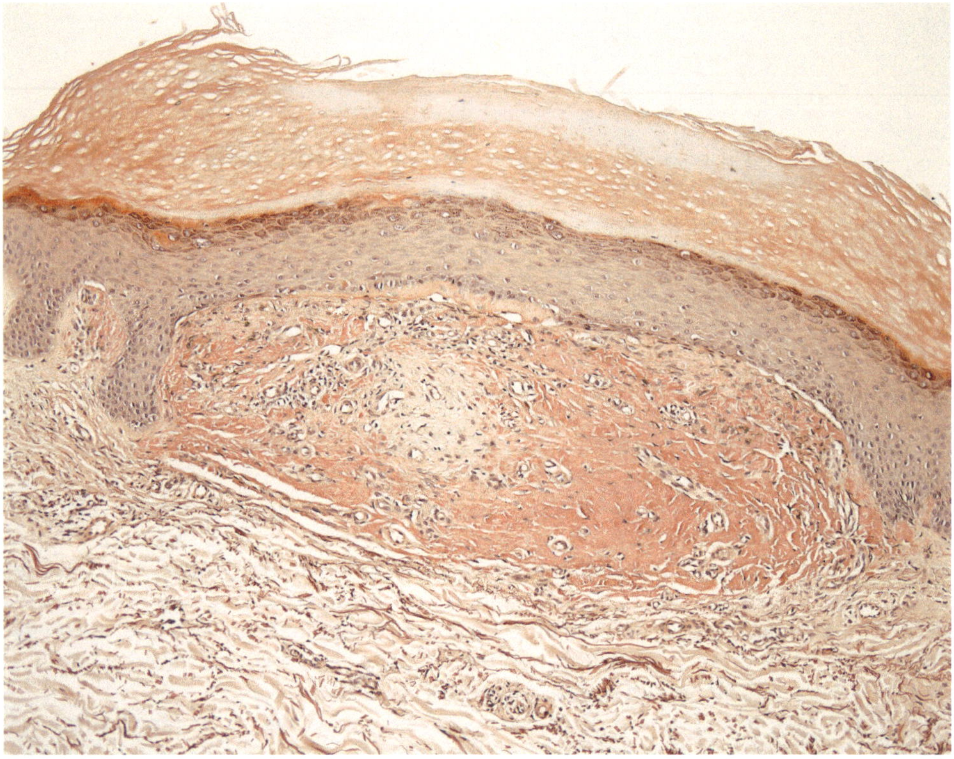

Fig. 1. Massive amyloid deposition with melanophages is seen in the papillary dermis in the lesional skin of lichen amyloidosis (Congo red staining). Hyperkeratosis of the overlying epidermis is also seen

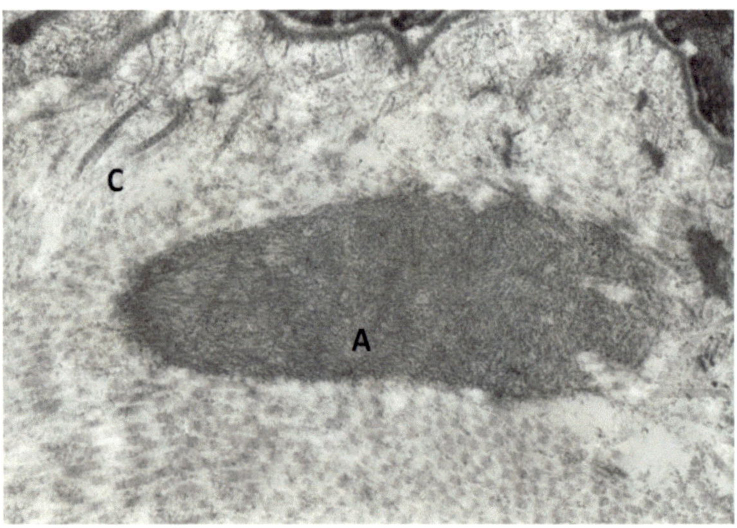

Fig. 2. Electron microscopy shows fibrillar materials consistent with amyloid (A) and normal collagen (C)

renal, cardiac, neuronal, gastrointestinal, hepatic, and splenic involvement. Skin manifestation is seen in approximately 30-40% of patients. Purpura, petechiae, and ecchymoses are induced in the skin as well as mucous membranes. Eyelid purpura is frequently seen (Fig. 3), and purpura are also seen elsewhere in the body. Purpura is caused by minor trauma, slight stimuli, or even spontaneously. Amyloid deposition is seen around the blood vessels, which causes capillary fragility. As periorbital lesions, translucent nodules, xanthomatous plaques, waxy yellowish hemorrhagic lesions are seen (Fig. 4, 5).

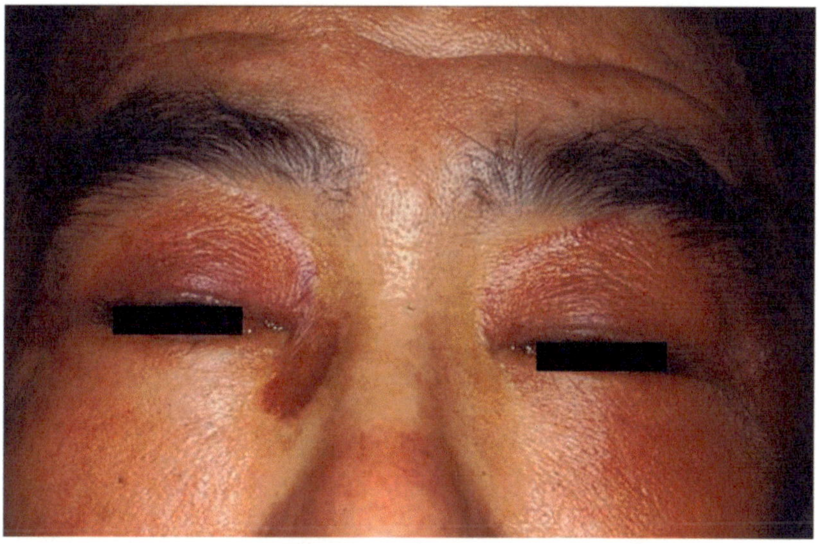

Fig. 3. Purpuric plaques around the bilateral eyelids

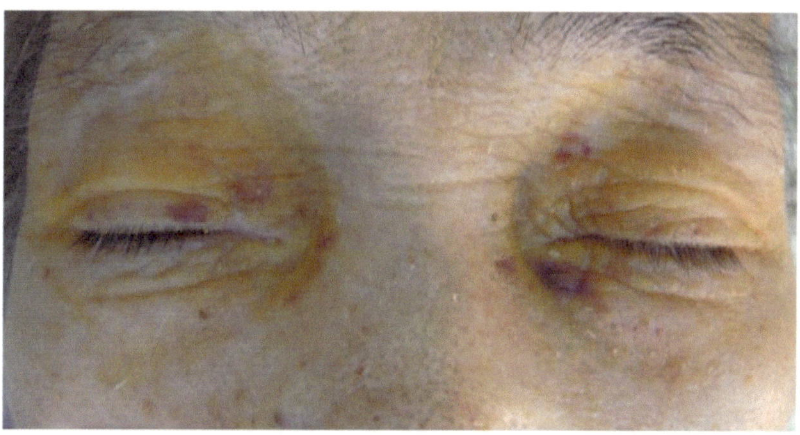

Fig. 4. Periorbital xanthomatous plaques and purpura

Other rare forms of cutaneous amyloidosis associated with systemic amyloidosis include subcutaneous nodules, whitish nodules, bullous lesions, and refractory ulcers [4, 5]. Amyloid deposition is also occasionally seen in the tongue and oral mucosa. Macroglossia is the representative sign (Fig. 6). Nail involvement is due to amyloid deposition in the nail matrix, and can be an initial manifestation of systemic amyloidosis [6]. Nail lesions present

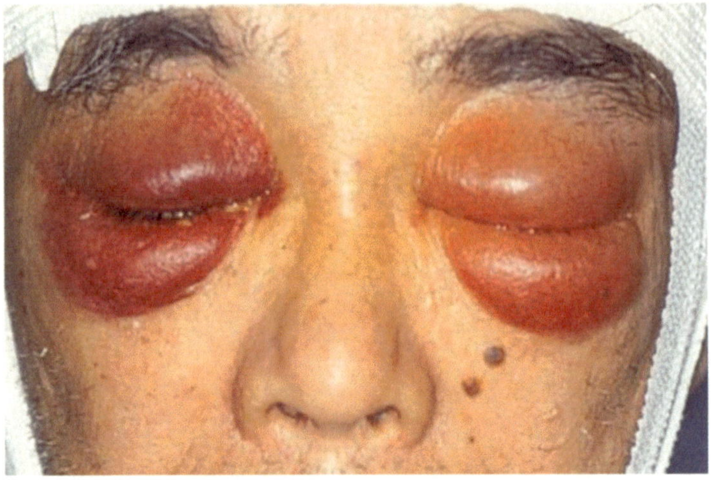

Fig. 5. Waxy, yellowish hemorrhagic lesions

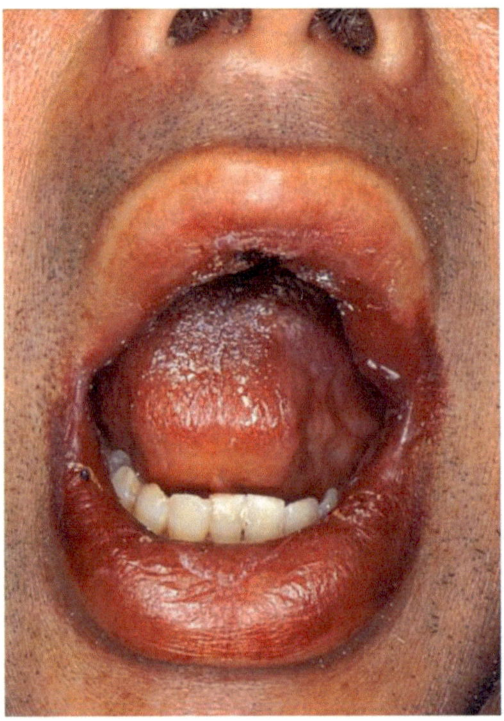

Fig. 6. Macroglossia in a patient with systemic amyloidosis

with dystrophy, thinning, whitening, banding, striations, brittleness, onycholysis, fragility, and even anonychia (Fig. 7). Alopecia may develop when amyloid deposition occurs on the hair matrix. Scleroderma-like manifestations are rarely seen, especially on the fingers, in patients with primary systemic amyloidosis [7-9]. Skin biopsy is important for the diagnosis, because amyloid deposition can be detected even in the skin of normal appearance. Blind aspiration biopsies from the abdominal subcutaneous fat tissues or the rectal submucosa are sometimes useful for the definitive diagnosis for systemic amyloidosis.

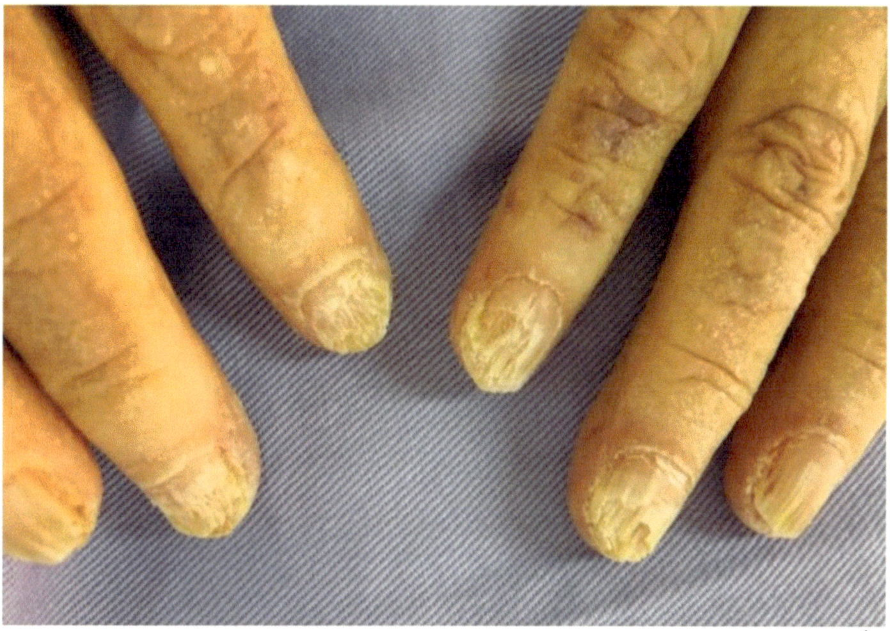

Fig. 7. Fingernails of a patient with systemic amyloidosis showing longitudinal ridging and splitting

4. Localized amyloidosis

Primary localized cutaneous amyloidosis (PLCA) is defined by deposition of amyloid in previously normal skin with no evidence of deposits in internal organs, and classified into more common macular, papular, and the rare nodular form. PLCA may be induced by chronic stimuli or minor trauma [10].

Lichen amyloidosis is frequently seen on the dorsal aspect of the lower legs and forearms, which is characterized by pruritic, firm, hyperkeratotic, reddish-brown papules or nodules (Fig. 8). Main component of amyloid in lichen amyloidosis is considered to be cytokeratin, suggesting that amyloid deposits may be derived from degenerated epithelial cells.

Macular amyloidosis is predominantly localized on the upper back, and characterized by dark pigmented macules with a rippled pattern of pigmentation (Fig. 9). In severe cases, macular amyloidosis involves all over the back (Fig. 10). Lichen amyloidosis and macular amyloidosis are occasionally seen in a single patient, and is known as biphasic forms. Unique features of macular amyloidosis are rarely seen on the upper back or exterior aspects of upper extremities. Lesions are pigmented, discrete spotty papules and not presented hyperkeratotic papules like lichen amyloidosis (Fig. 11). Those lesions are induced by prolonged scraching or rubbing with various objects such as bath sponges, brushes, towels, plant sticks and leaves, which resulted in keratinocyte degenereation. The same clinical entity includes friction amyloidosis, friction melanosis, and towel melanosis [11]. Friction amyloidosis is induced by long-term use of a nylon towel or scrub brush over

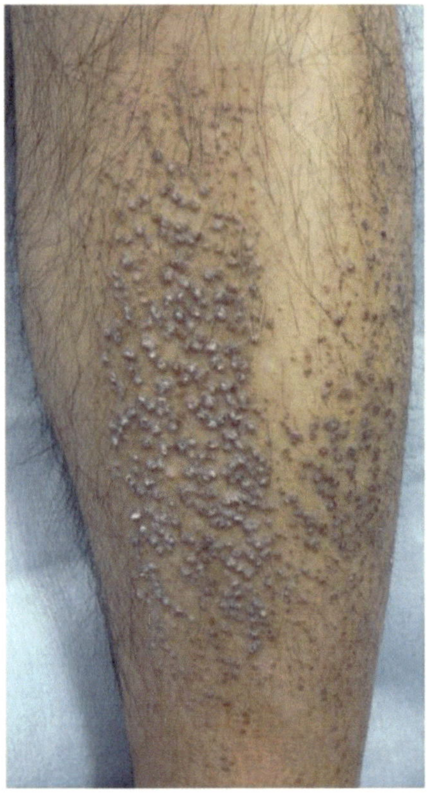

Fig. 8. Lichen amyloidosis on the lower leg

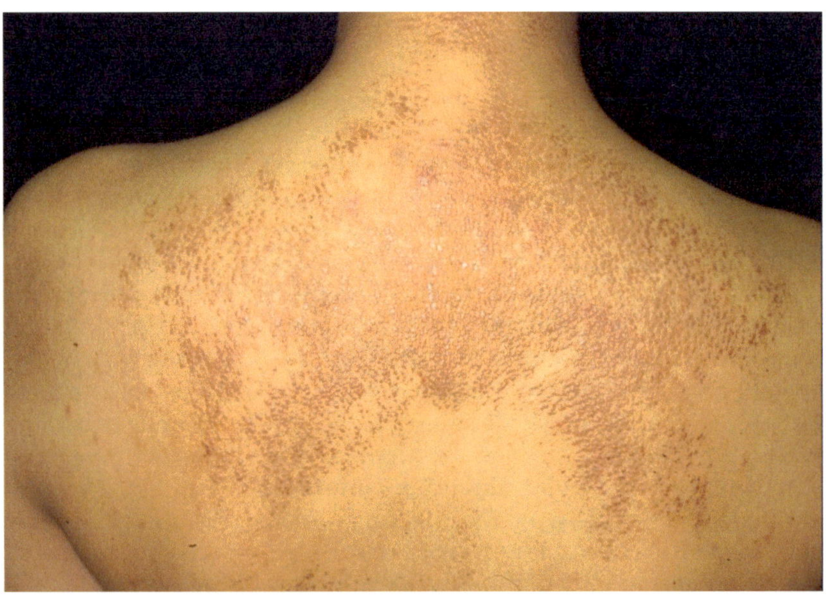

Fig. 9. Macular amyloidosis on the upper back

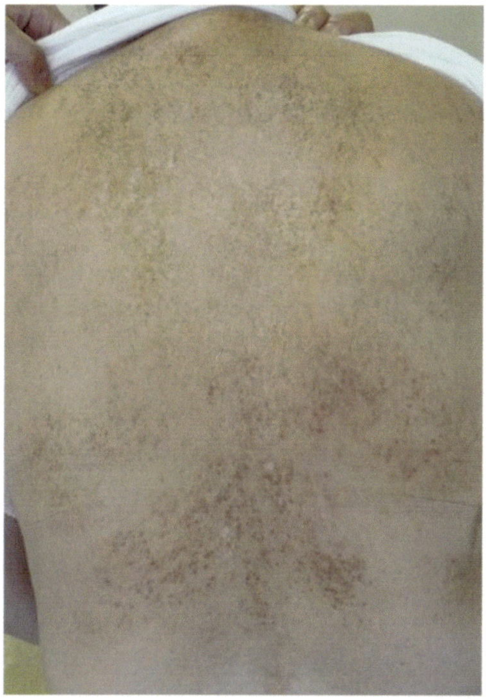

Fig. 10. Widespread primary cutaneous localized amyloidosis (macular form)

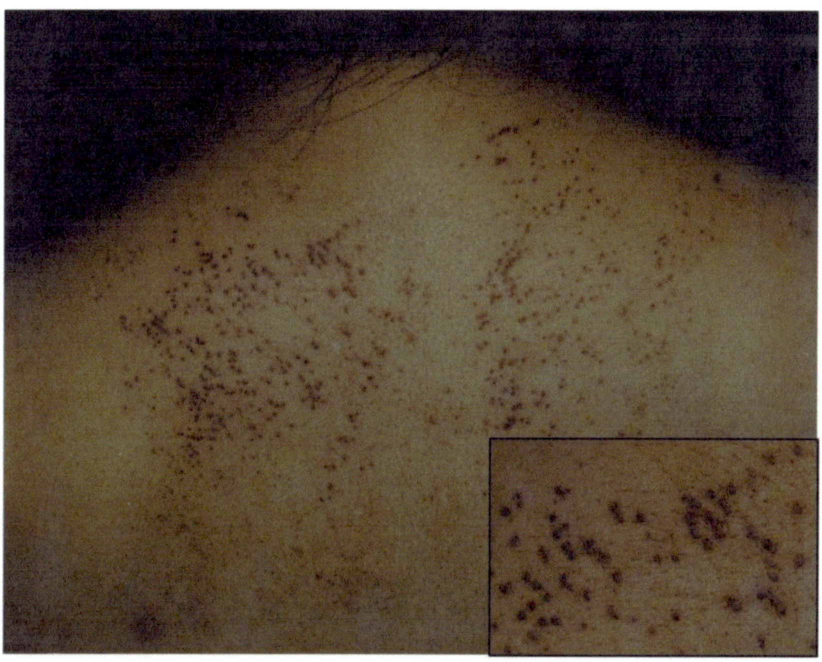

Fig. 11. Pigmented papular form of macular amyloidosis on the upper back (insert: higher magnification)

the bony regions such as the arms, forearms, clavicle, scapula, and neck [12, 13]. Amyloid deposits in the skin may be derived from degenerated epithelial keratinocytes [14], possibly through filamentous degeneration or apoptosis [15]. Histological investigation by amyloid stain show deposition of amorphous materials in the papillary dermis. Amyloid is usually detected unassociated with hair follicles, but rarely recognized around the follicles (Fig. 12).

Nodular amyloidosis presents with a single or multiple nodules on the face, trunk and extremities [16, 17], which sometimes develop following trauma (Fig. 13). Also, periorbital small, waxy nodules are multiply seen. In the nodular type, amyloid is originated from AL protein by local plasma cells, and modified β2-microglobulin is also shown to be a component of amyloid fibrils [18]. Apart from other types, amyloid materials are situated up to in the deep dermis. Plasma cell infiltration is prominent within or peripheral areas of the amyloid materials (Fig. 14). Although patients with nodular amyloidosis may develop systemic amyloidosis after long-term follow-up, recent papers indicate that the ratio is lower than previously reported [16]. In the series of 16 cases of nodular amyloidosis, 2 patients had Sjögren's syndrome, 2 had diabetes mellitus, and 3 had liver disease. In particular, association with Sjögren's syndrome is remarkable [19].

PLCA usually is unassociated with systemic disorders; however, a few cases of HCV-related amyloidosis have been reported [20, 21], one of which was biphasic PLCA [20]. Nodular lesions showing the surface atrophy are described as amyloidosis cutis nodularis atrophicans.

Additionally, other unusual variants of PLCA have been reported depending on genetic, racial, and environmental factors. Those include poikiloderma-like appearance, reticular

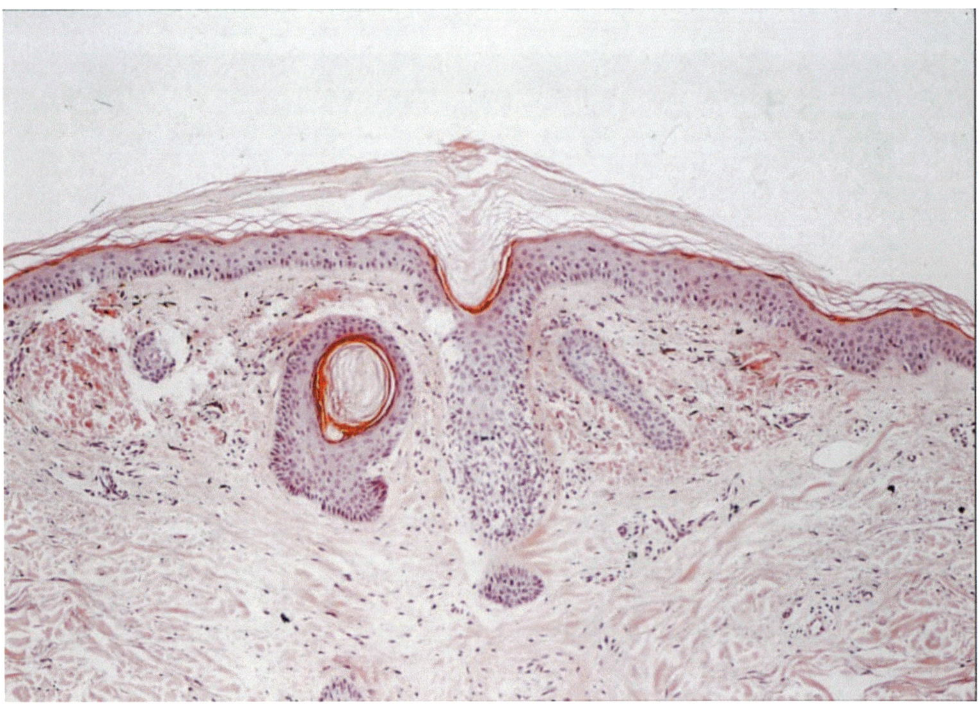

Fig. 12. Amyloid deposition around the hair follicle in the papillary dermis in the lesional skin of macular amyloidosis (Congo red)

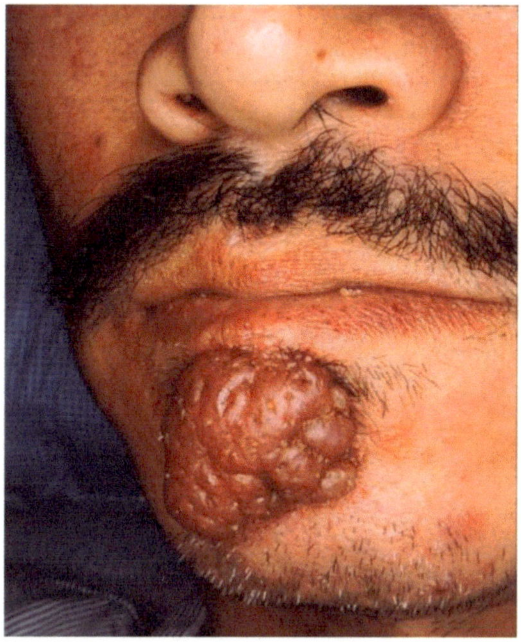

Fig. 13. Nodular amyloidosis on the chin

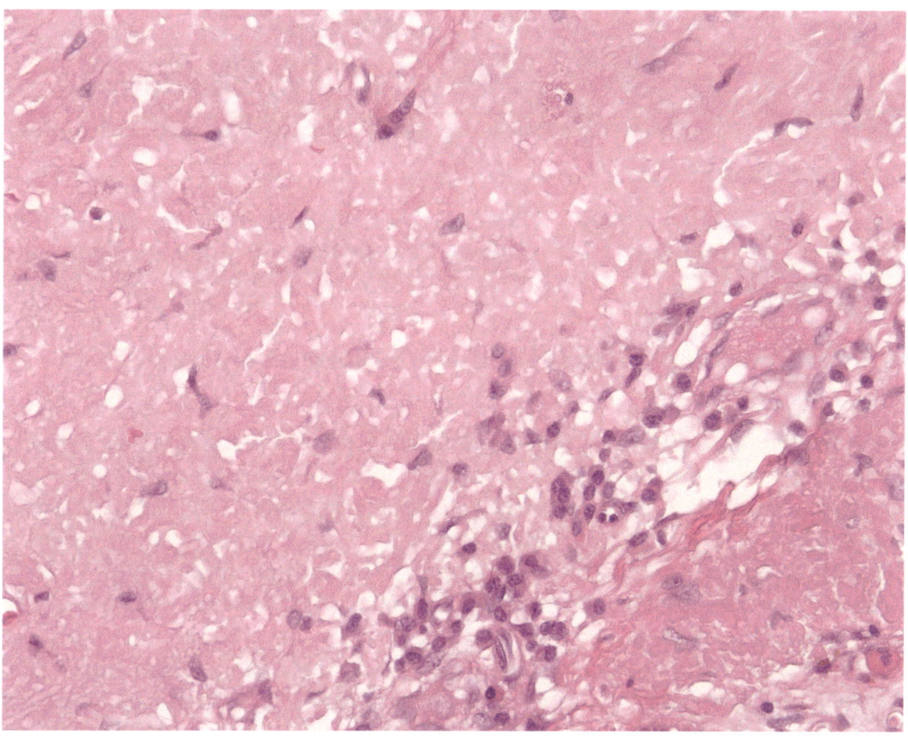

Fig. 14. Plasma cell infiltration in the lesional skin of nodular amyloidosis

form, hypopigmented, widespread diffuse pigmentation, incontinentia pigmenti-like pattern, homogenous pigmented patched, and amyloidosis cutis dyschromia [22-30]. Also, eczematous lesions [31, 32] and bullous lesions mimicking bullous pemphigoid [33] have been reported. Rare sites include ear, nose, and cheek [34-38]. Anosacral cutaneous amyloidosis is frequently seen in Asian elderly people, and hyperkeratotic, pigmented plaques are located on the bilateral outer area of the anus (Fig. 15).

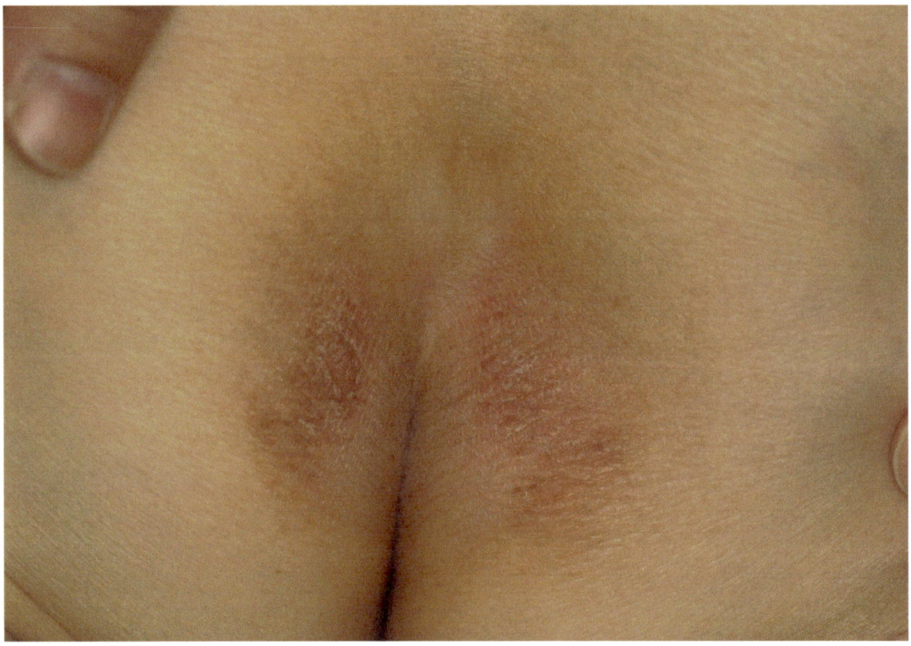

Fig. 15. Anosacral amyloidosis

Therapeutic modalities for cutaneous amyloidosis remain a challenge, although topical application of corticosteroids and dimethylsulfoxide (DMSO), phototherapy, and laser treatment are selected.

5. Secondary amyloidosis associated with various disorders

An association of cutaneous amyloidosis with various disorders (*i.e.* inflammatory disorders, autoimmune disorders, and tumors) has been reported. Amyloid deposition is occasionally seen associated with chronic inflammation, and secondary cutaneous amyloid deposition is sometimes seen in patients with atopic dermatitis [39]. Chronic stimuli by frequent scratching may play a triggering role in amyloid production from keratinocytes. Additionally, secondary amyloid deposition associated with inflammatory disorders, such as psoriasis [40] or disseminated superficial porokeratosis [41] have been reported.

Connective tissue diseases or collagen vascular diseases have been rarely seen, such as systemic sclerosis, lupus erythematosus, Sjögren's syndrome, rheumatoid arthritis, dermatomyositis, Behchet's disease, sclerodermatomyositis, generalized morphea-like scleroderma, sarcoidosis, and so on [42-47]. Association of PLCA with various autoimmune disorders suggests that underlying immune-mediated factors may be implicated [47].

Secondary amyloid deposition is occasionally associated with both benign and malignant skin tumors such as melanocytic naevi, seborrheic keratosis, calcifying epithelioma, dermatofibroma, solar keratosis, Bowen's disease, basal cell carcinoma, trichoepithelioma, and so on [48-56]. Although an epidermal origin of amyloid in secondary cutaneous amyloidosis, particularly in association with skin tumors of epithelial cell origin, is suggested in several conditions, degenerating naevus cells may contribute to the amyloid production [55]. A previous report showed amyloid deposition in Bowen's disease treated with radiotherapy [53]. It is suggested that any insult to the skin leading to degenerative cell changes could result in amyloid deposition.

6. Dialysis-related amyloidosis

In dialysis-related amyloidosis, skin manifestations often present with cutaneous or subcutaneous nodules [57, 58]. Bilateral subcutaneous masses are seen on the buttocks (Fig. 16), which are sometimes painful on sitting. Extensive deposition of β2-microglobulin amyloid is seen in the dermis to subcutis, occasionally associated with local calcification.

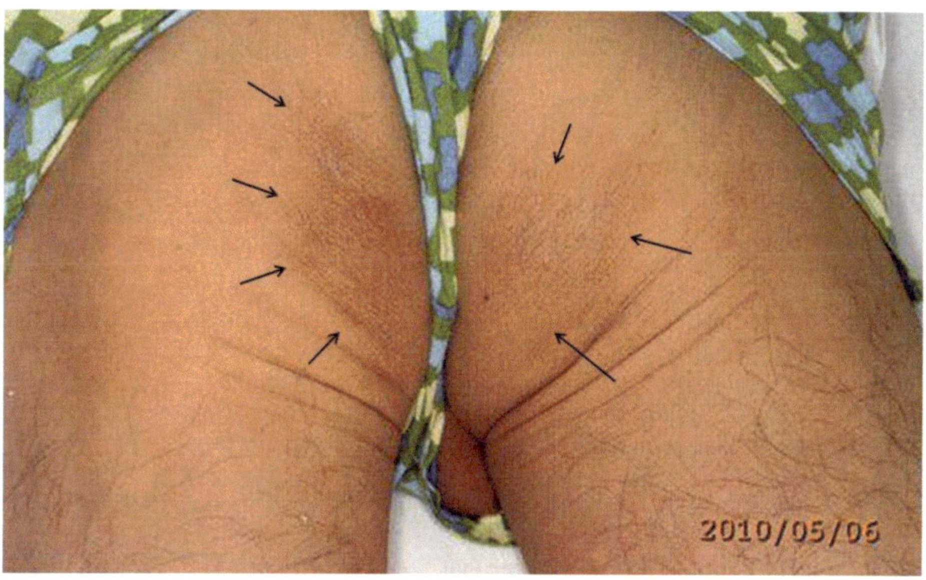

Fig. 16. Dialysis-related amyloidosis on the buttocks

7. References

[1] Steciuk, A., Dompmartin, A., Troussard, X., Verneuil, L., Macro, M., Comoz, F., & Leroy, D. (2002) Cutaneous amyloidosis and possible association with systemic amyloidosis. *International Journal of Dermatology* vol. 41, pp. 127-132.

[2] Silverstein, S.R. (2005) Primary systemic amyloidosis and the dermatologist: where classic skin lesions may provide the clue for early diagnosis. *Dermatology Online Journal* vol. 11, pp. 5.

[3] Schreml, S., Szeimies. R.-M., Vogt, T., Landthaler, M., Schroeder, J., & Babilas, P. (2010) Cutaneous amyloidoses and systemic amyloidoses with cutaneous involvement. *European Journal of Dermatology* vol. 20, pp. 152-160.

[4] Robert, C., Aractingi, S., Prost, C., Verola, O., Blanchet-Bardon, C., Blanc, F., Bagot, M., Dubertret, L., & Fermand, J.P. (1993) Bullous amyloidosis: report of 3 cases and review of the literature. *Medicine* vol. 72, pp. 38-44.
[5] Alhaddab, M., Srolovitz, H., & Rosen, N. (2006) Primary systemic amyloidosis presenting as extensive cutaneous ulceration. *Journal of Cutaneous Medical Surgery* vol. 10, pp. 253-256.
[6] Fujita, Y., Tsuji-Abe, Y., Sato-Matsumura, K.C., Akiyama, M., & Shimizu, H. (2006) Nail dystrophy and blisters as sole manifestations in myeloma-associated amyloidosis. *Journal of American Academy of Dermatology* vol. 54, pp. 712-714.
[7] Lee, D.D., Huang, C.Y., & Wong CK. (1998) Dermatopathologic findings in 20 cases of systemic amyloidosis. *American Journal of Dermatopathology* vol. 20, pp. 438-442.
[8] Cho, S.B., Park, J.S., Kim, H.O., & Chung, K.Y. (2006) Scleroderma-like manifestation in a patient with primary systemic amyloidosis: response to high-dose intravenous immunoglobulin and plasma exchange. *Yonsei Medical Journal* vol. 47, pp. 737-740.
[9] Reyes, C.M., Rudinskaya, A., Kloss, R., Girardi, M., & Lazova, R. (2008) Scleroderma-like illness as a presenting feature of multiple myeloma and amyloidosis. *Journal of Clinical Rheumatology* vol. 14, pp. 161-165.
[10] Lonsdale-Eccles, A.A., Gonda, P., Gilbertson, J.A., & Haworth, A.E. (2009) Localized cutaneous amyloid at an insulin injection site. *Clinical and Experimental Dermatology* vol. 34, pp. e1027-e1028.
[11] Siragusa, M., Ferri, R., Cavallari, V., & Schepis, C. (2001) Friction melanosis, friction amyloidosis, macular amyloidosis, towel melanosis: many names for the same clinical entity. *European Journal of Dermatology* vol. 11, pp. 545-548.
[12] Wong, C.K., & Lin, C.S. (1988) Friction amyloidosis. *International Journal of Dermatology* vol. 27, pp. 302-307.
[13] Venkataram, M.N., Bhushnurmath, S.R., Muirhead, D.E., & Al-Suwaid, A.R. (2001) Friction amyloidosis: a study of 10 cases. *Australasian Journal of Dermatology* vol. 42, pp. 176-179.
[14] Chang, Y.T., Liu, H.N., Wang, W.J., Lee, D.D., & Tsai, S.F. (2004) A study of cytokeratin profiles in localized cutaneous amyloids. *Archives of Dermatological Research* vol. 296, pp. 83-88.
[15] Maeda, H., Ohta, S., Saito, Y., Nameki, H., & Ishikawa, H. (1982) Epidermal origin of the amyloid in localized cutaneous amyloidosis. *British Journal of Dermatology* vol. 106, pp. 345-351.
[16] Moon, A.O., Calamia, K.T., & Walsh, J.S. (2003) Nodular amyloidosis: review and long-term follow-up of 16 cases. *Archives of Dermatology* vol. 139, pp. 1157-1159.
[17] Kalajian, A.H., Waldman, M., & Knable, A.L. (2007) Nodular primary localized cutaneous amyloidosis after trauma: a case report and discussion of the rate of progression to systemic amyloidosis. *Journal of American Academy of Dermatology* vol. 57, pp. S26-S29.
[18] Fujimoto, N., Yajima, M., Ohnishi, Y., Tajima, S., Ishibashi, A., Hata, Y., Enomoto, U., Konohana, I., Wachi, H., & Seyama, Y. (2002) Advanced glycation end product-modified beta2-microglobulin is a component of amyloid fibrils of primary localized cutaneous nodular amyloidosis. *Journal of Investigative Dermatology* vol. 118, pp. 479-484.
[19] Meijer, J.M., Schonland, S.O., Palladini, G., Merlini, G., Hegenbart, U., Ciocca, O., Perfetti, V., Leijsma, M.K., Bootsma, H., & Hazenberg, B.P. (2008) Sjögren's syndrome and localized nodular cutaneous amyloidosis: coincidence or a distinct clinical entity? *Arthritis and Rheumatism* vol. 58, pp. 1992-1999.
[20] Erbagci, Z., Erkilic, S. & Tuncel, A.A. (2005) Diffuse biphasic cutaneous amyloidosis in an HCV-seropositive patient: another extrahepatic manifestation of HCV infection? *International Journal of Clinical Practice* vol. 59, pp. 983-985.

[21] Abe, M., Kawakami, Y., Oyama, N., Nakamura-Wakatsuki, T., & Yamamoto, T. (2010) Cutaneous amyloidosis associated with HCV infection: report of 2 cases. *International Journal of Dermatology* vol. 49, pp. 960-961.
[22] Ho, M.H., & Chong, L.Y. (1998) Poikiloderma-like cutaneous amyloidosis in an ethnic Chinese girl. *Journal of Dermatology* vol. 25, pp. 730-734.
[23] Wang, C.K., & Lee, J.Y.Y. (1996) Macular amyloidosis with widespread diffuse pigmentation. *British Journal of Dermatology* vol. 135, pp. 135-138.
[24] Eng, A.M., Cogen, L., Gunner, R.M., & Blekys, I. (1976) Familial generalized dyschromic amyloidosis cutis. *Journal of Cutaneous Pathology* vol. 3, pp. 102-108.
[25] An, H.T., Han, K.H., & Cho, K.H. (2000) Macular amyloidosis with an incontinentia pigmenti-like pattern. *British Journal of Dermatology* vol. 142, pp. 371-373.
[26] Ahmed, I., Charles-Holmes, R., & Black, M.M. (2001) An unusual presentation of macular amyloidosis. *British Journal of Dermatology* vol. 145, pp. 851-852.
[27] Hung, C.C., Wang, C.M., Hong, H.S., & Kuo, T.T. (2003) Unusual skin manifestation of cutaneous amyloidosis. *Dermatology* vol. 207, pp. 65-67.
[28] Alvarez-Ruiz, S.B., Perez-Gala, S., Aragues, M., Fraga, J., & Garcia-Diez, A. (2007) Unusual clinical presentation of amyloidosis: bilateral stenosis of the external auditory canal, hoarseness and a rapid course of cutaneous lesions. *International Journal of Dermatology* vol. 46, pp. 503-504.
[29] Criado, P.R., Silva, C.S., Vasconcellos, C., Valente, N.Y., & Maito, J.B. (2005) Extensive nodular cutaneous amyloidosis: an unusual presentation. *Journal of European Academy of Dermatology and Venereology* vol. 19, pp. 481-483.
[30] Ho, M.S., Ho, J., & Tan, S.H. (2009) Hypopigmented macular amyloidosis with or without hyperpigmentation. *Clinical and Experimental Dermatology* vol. 34, pp. e547-e551.
[31] Konishi, A., Fukuoka, M., & Nishimura, Y. (2007) Primary localized cutaneous amyloidosis with unusual clinical features in a patient with Sjögren's syndrome. *Journal of Dermatology* vol. 34, pp. 394-396.
[32] Gan, E.Y., & Tey, H.L. (2010) Primary cutaneous nodular amyloidosis initially presenting with eczema. *Singapore Medical Journal* vol. 51, pp. e158-e160.
[33] Asahina, A., Hasegawa, K., Ishiyama, M., Miyagaki, T., Tada, Y., Suzuki, Y., Tanabe, T., & Saito, I. (2010) Bullous amyloidosis mimicking bullous pemphigoid: usefulness of electron microscopic examination. *Acta Dermatology and Venereology* vol. 90, pp. 427-428.
[34] Shimauchi, T., Shin, J.H., & Tokura, Y. (2006) Primary cutaneous amyloidosis of the auricular concha: case report and review of published work. *Journal of Dermatology* vol. 33, pp. 128-131.
[35] Evers, M., Baron, E., Zaim, M.T., & Han, A. (2007) Papules and plaques on the nose: nodular localized primary cutaneous amyloidosis. *Archives of Dermatology* vol. 143, pp. 535-540.
[36] Jhingan, A., Lee, J.S.S., & Kumarasinghe, S.P.W. (2007) Lichen amyloidosis in an unusual location. *Singapore Medical Journal* vol. 48, pp. e165-e167.
[37] Koh, M., Kwok, C.Y., Tan, H.W., & Mancer, J.F. (2008) A rare case of primary cutaneous nodular amyloidosis of the face. *Journal of European Academy of Dermatology and Venereology* vol. 22, pp. 1011-1012.
[38] Neff, A.G., McCuin, J.B., & Mutasim, D.F. (2010) Papular amyloidosis limited to the ears. *Journal of American Academy of Dermatology* vol. 62, pp. 1078-1079.
[39] Lee, D.D., Huang, C.K., Ko, P.C., Chang, Y.T., Sun, W.Z., & Oyang, Y.J. (2011) Association of primary cutaneous amyloidosis with atopic dermatitis: a nationwide population-based study in Taiwan. *British Journal of Dermatology* vol. 164, pp. 148-153.

[40] Wittenberg, G.P., Oursler, J.R., & Peters, M.S. (1995) Secondary amyloidosis complicating psoriasis. *Journal of American Academy of Dermatology* vol. 32, pp. 465-468.
[41] Ginarte, M., Leon, A., & Toribio, J. (2005) Disseminated superficial porokeratosis with amyloid deposits. *European Journal of Dermatology* vol. 15, pp. 298-300.
[42] Yamamoto, T., & Suzuki, Y. (2010) Primary localized cutaneous amyloidosis intermingled with papulopustular lesions in a patient with Behcet's disease. *Rheumatology International* May 15 [Epub ahead]
[43] Orihara, T., Yanase, S., & Furuya, T. (1985) A case of sclerodermatomyositis with cutaneous amyloidosis. *British Journal of Dermatology* vol. 112, pp. 213-219.
[44] Sumi, K., Yamamoto, T., Yokozeki, H., Nishioka, K. (2003) Amyloid deposition associated with generalized morphea-like scleroderma. *European Journal of Dermatology* vol. 13, pp. 509-511.
[45] Kikuchi, N., Sakai, E., Nishibu, A., Otsuka, M., & Yamamoto, T. (2010) Primary localized cutaneous amyloidosis in patients with scleroderma. *Acta Dermatology and Venereology* vol. 90, pp. 326-327.
[46] Taniguchi, Y., Horino, T., & Terada, Y. (2009) Cutaneous amyloidosis associated with amyopathic dermatomyositis. *Journal of Rheumatology* vol. 36, pp. 1088-1089.
[47] Dahdah, M.J., Kurban, M., Kibbi, A.G., & Ghosn, S. (2009) Primary localized cutaneous amyloidosis: a sign of immune dysregulation? International Journal of Dermatology vol. 48, pp. 419-421.
[48] Hashimoto, K., & King, L.E. Jr. (1973) Secondary localized cutaneous amyloidosis associated with actinic keratosis. *Journal of Investigative Dermatology* vol. 61, pp. 293-299.
[49] Peterson, W.C. Jr. (1968) Thioflavine-T reactivity in calcifying epithelioma of Malherbe. *Archives of Dermatology* vol. 97, pp. 340-341.
[50] Aso, M., Hagari, Y., Nakamura, K., Mihara, M., & Shimao, S. (1990) A case of secondary cutaneous amyloidosis: epidermal keratinocytes produce amyloid in the cytoplasm. *Journal of Cutaneous Pathology* vol. 17, pp. 176-181.
[51] Lee, Y.S., & Fong, P.H. (1990) Secondary localized amyloidosis in trichoepithelioma. A light microscopic and ultrastructural study. *American Journal of Dermatopathology* vol. 12, pp. 469-478.
[52] Weedon, D., & Shand, I. (1979) Amyloid in basal cell carcinoma. *British Journal of Dermatology* vol. 11, pp 141-146.
[53] Layton, A.M., Cunliffe, W.J., & Jones, W. (1991) Enhanced amyloid deposition in Bowen's disease treated with radiotherapy. *British Journal of Dermatology* vol. 125, pp. 606-607.
[54] MacDonald, D.M., & Black, M.M. (1980) Secondary localized cutaneous amyloidosis in melanocytic naevi. *British Journal of Dermatology* vol. 103, pp. 553-556.
[55] Hanami, Y., & Yamamoto, T. Secondary amyloid deposition in a melanocytic naevus. *International Journal of Dermatology* (in press).
[56] Quigley, B.C., Ricciuti, J., & Morgan, M.B. (2010) Amyloid light chain deposition associated with dermatofibroma: serendipity or association? *American Journal of Dermatopathology* vol. 32, pp. 298-300.
[57] Shimizu, S., Yasui, C., Yasukawa, K., Nakamura, H., Shimizu, H., & Tsuchiya, K. (2003) Subcutaneous nodules on the buttocks as a manifestation of dialysis-related amyloidosis: a clinicopathological entity? *British Journal of Dermatology* vol. 149, pp. 400-404.
[58] Takayama, K., Satoh, T., Maruyama, R., & Yokozeki, H. (2008) Dialysis-related amyloidosis on the buttocks. *Acta Dermatology and Venereology* vol. 88, pp. 72-73.

Part 2

Localized Amyloidosis

8

Localized Amyloidosis of the Head and Neck

Işıl Adadan Güvenç
Başkent University, İzmir
Turkey

1. Introduction

Amyloidosis is a benign, slowly progressive condition characterized by the presence of extracellular fibrillar proteins in a variety of organs and tissues. It can be categorized as systemic or localized. Head and neck involvement can be seen in both systemic and localized amyloidosis. Systemic amyloidosis results in involvement of many organs, and shortens life expectancy, whereas localized amyloidosis is usually benign (Yiotakis et al., 2009). In this extensive review, the presentation, diagnosis and treatment modalities of localized amyloidosis of the head and neck will be discussed.

2. Localized amyloidosis of the head and neck

Virchow, in 1851, was the first to use the term amyloid because of its starchlike reaction when treated with iodine and sulfuric acid. In 1842, however, Von Rokitansky was the first to identify this material in the liver and spleen. Symmers classified amyloidosis clinically as: primary amyloid (localized or general); secondary amyloid (localized or general); amyloid associated with multiple myeloma; and hereditary or familial amyloid. In systemic or generalized disease, amyloid is deposited in many organ systems and life expectancy is shortened (Kennedy & Patel, 2000). The mean survival of patients with systemic forms is between 5 to 15 months, whereas those with localized forms have an excellent prognosis (Fahrner et al., 2004). Approximately 9% of amyloidosis cases are localized (Kyle & Bayrd, 1975). In localized amyloidosis of the head and neck, deposition of amyloid may be observed in individual organs without any systemic involvement. The progressive accumulation of amyloid deposits interferes with the normal structure of affected tissues resulting eventually in impairment of their function (Yiotakis et al., 2009). Life expectancy is not affected unless an enlarging laryngotracheal lesion goes unattended (Kennedy & Patel, 2000).

Clinically, amyloidosis is divided into two main categories, systemic and localized. Types of systemic amyloidosis are AL, AA, familial and senile amyloidosis.

AL amyloidosis, formerly called, primary amyloidosis is seen in progressive systemic disease, plasma cell dyscrasia/multiple myeloma, and most localized forms of amyloidosis. AL amyloid associated with plasma cell dyscrasia is the most common form of amyloidosis, accounting for 75% of cases in the United States (Penner & Muller, 2006).

AA amyloidosis, formerly called, secondary amyloidosis occurs in association with chronic inflammatory disorders, chronic infections, and accounts for only 5% of all amyloid cases. The amyloid fibril protein is derived from the circulating acute phase protein known as serum amyloid A (Panda et al., 2007). AA amyloidosis shows a predilection for the spleen, liver, kidney, lymph nodes, and adrenals, although no organ system is spared. AA amyloidosis may also occur in association with Hodgkin disease, genitourinary or gastrointestinal malignancies (Penner & Muller, 2006). In systemic amyloidosis, proteinuria with nephrotic syndrome is often the first symptom; other manifestations include peripheral neuropathies, dementia and cognitive dysfunction, and organ enlargement, especially of the liver, kidney, spleen and heart (Sipe & Cohen, 1998). Macroglossia is most frequently noted in the head and neck region. Other nonspecific signs and symptoms such as fatigue, weight loss, orthostatic hypotension, diarrhea, skeletal muscle pseudohypertrophy, skin papules or plaques, arrhythmias, renal failure, congestive heart failure and carpal tunnel syndrome can be seen. Renal failure is the major cause of death in systemic amyloidosis. Sudden death secondary to cardiac arrythmias is also common (Nandapalan et al., 1998). The median survival reported by Kyle and Greipp in 229 cases of systemic amyloidosis was 13 months for patients with amyloidosis only, and 5 months for those with amyloidosis and myeloma (Kyle & Greipp, 1983).

Amyloid Protein	Protein Precursor	Clinical Syndrome
AA	apoSAA	Reactive (secondary) Familial Mediterranean fever Muckle-Wells syndrome
AL	Igλ, Igκ	Idiopathic (primary) Multiple myeloma Local nodular
AH	γ1 heavy chain	Macroglobulinemia
A β_2M	β_2 microglobulin	Chronic hemodialysis arthropathy
A β	β-protein precursor	Alzheimer's disease Down's syndrome Hereditary cerebral angiopathy with bleeding
APrP	Prion protein	Creutzfeldt-Jacob disease Gerstmann-Straussler syndrome Kuru
AIAPP	Amyloid insulin polypeptide	Diabetes mellitus type 2 Insulinoma
AANF	Atrial natriuretic factor	Senile cardiac amyloid
ATTR	Transthyretin	FAP; multiple point mutations Senile systemic cardiac
AGel	Gelsolin	FAP-Finnish
AApoA1	Apolipoprotein A1	FAP-Iowa (Irish)
ACys	Cystatin C	Hereditary cerebral angiopathy with bleeding
AFibA	Fibrinogen A α	Nonneuropathic hereditary amyloid with renal disease
ALys	Lysozyme	Nonneuropathic hereditary amyloid with renal disease

Table 1. Abbreviated classification of amyloid (Sipe & Cohen, 1998)

β2M amyloidosis is associated with patients who are maintained on hemodialysis for more than 7 years. Familial transthyretin-associated (ATTR) patients with normal plasma transthyretin develop senile systemic amyloidosis with predominant cardiac involvement, whereas patients with genetically variant transthyretin develop familial amyloid polyneuropathy (FAP), usually with systemic amyloidosis (Berg et al., 1993; Kennedy & Patel, 2000). Table 1 shows the most common amyloid proteins and associated clinical syndromes (Sipe & Cohen, 1998).

Approximately 9% to 15% of amyloidosis is of the localized type, which usually consists of AL amyloid (Passerotti et al., 2008). In localized idiopathic AL amyloidosis, localized deposition of amyloid is regarded to be the result of local synthesis rather than the deposition of light chains produced elsewhere in the human body (Yiotakis et al., 2009). The benign nature of localized amyloidosis suggests that a localized clone of plasma cells producing an amyloidogenic light chain may represent the pathogenetic mechanism of this disease, which appears to be a form of plasma cell dyscrasia (Berg et al., 1993).

Histologically, amyloid is extracellular deposits of insoluble, homogenous, amorphous, acellular, eosinophilic and proteinaceous material with a well-defined β-pleated sheet ultrastructure (Figure 1). Lymphocytes, plasma cells, and foreign body giant cells may be seen in the surrounding tissue in localized amyloidosis. Infiltration of plasma cells observed near localized amyloid deposits suggests local production of the amyloid precursor protein.

Immunohistochemical and molecular genetic studies have characterized clonal plasma cell populations associated with local amyloid deposits, and have matched the amyloid protein with DNA sequencing of the plasma cell clone (Biewend et al., 2006). These abundant plasma cells are not seen in systemic AL amyloidosis, but rather the circulating light chain proteins are gathered in specific organs. Giant cells frequently accompany localized amyloid deposits. The role of these giant cells is unclear; they may actively participate in amyloid fibril formation by uptake and modification of the precursor protein, or they may be part of a foreign body reaction in an attempt by the body to remove amyloid (O'Halloran & Lusk, 1994; Xu et al., 2005).

Classically, amyloid can be distinguished from other eosinophilic infiltrates via its apple-green birefringence when stained with Congo red and viewed under polarized light (Figure 2). This feature is specific but not sensitive. If the specimen loses its affinity for Congo red after exposure to potassium permanganate, this suggests an AA type amyloid deposit (Pentenero et al., 2006). Immunohistochemistry can differentiate kappa light chains from lambda light chains in AL type amyloidosis as well as excluding AA (inflammation-derived) and ATTR (transthyretin-derived) amyloid chains. Because of deposition of the variable regions of light chains, AL amyloid stains positive with commercially available antibodies only in approximately 40% of cases. Thus, negative immunostaining does not exclude AL amyloid. Isolation of amyloid with biochemical characterization by amino acid sequencing is the best way to confirm the AL type, but this is a very elaborate and time-consuming method and is not useful in normal practice (Bartels et al., 2004). Eventually these studies do not have much influence on patient management, since the number of additional biopsies and the treatment of localized amyloidosis do not differ whether the type of amyloidosis is known or not. Electron microscopy shows that all amyloid subtypes are composed of 7.5–10 nm wide linear, nonbranching tubular protein fibrils loosely arranged in a meshwork (O'Halloran & Lusk, 1994).

It is important to perform detailed investigations at diagnosis to rule out a systemic process. General blood examination (hemoglobin, creatinine, total protein, albumin, bilirubin, alkaline phosphatase), general urine examination (creatinine clearance, proteinuria), ECG, echocardiography, abdominal USG should be undertaken (Bartels et al., 2004). Serum and urine analysis to detect the presence of a monoclonal paraprotein composed of amyloid light chains should also be performed. Serum or urine "Bence Jones proteins" will be found in up to 88% of patients with primary systemic amyloidosis and 100% of patients with multiple myeloma-associated systemic amyloidosis (Fahrner et al., 2004). If electrophoresis fails to demonstrate paraproteins, immunelectrophoresis should be considered (Kyle & Bayrd, 1975). Collagen vascular diseases, tuberculosis, and multiple myeloma (rheumatoid factor, antinuclear antibody, tuberculosis skin test, and chest radiograph) should also be excluded (Friedman et al., 2002). Some authors advocate extensive investigations for patients who present with localized upper aerodigestive tract amyloidosis. Invasive procedures including labial salivary gland (LSG) biopsy, aspiration of abdominal fat, bone marrow biopsy, and rectal biopsy (positive in 84% of the cases) have been suggested as methods to exclude systemic amyloidosis. However, as the diagnostic yield is very low, some authors believe that invasive investigations are not indicated (Green et al., 2000). Fine-needle aspiration of abdominal fat pad (FNAFP) is less invasive compared to tissue biopsies and in a recent report, the estimated sensitivity and specificity of FNAFP was found to be 75% and 92%, respectively. Based on results of follow-up biopsies and compelling clinical findings, others

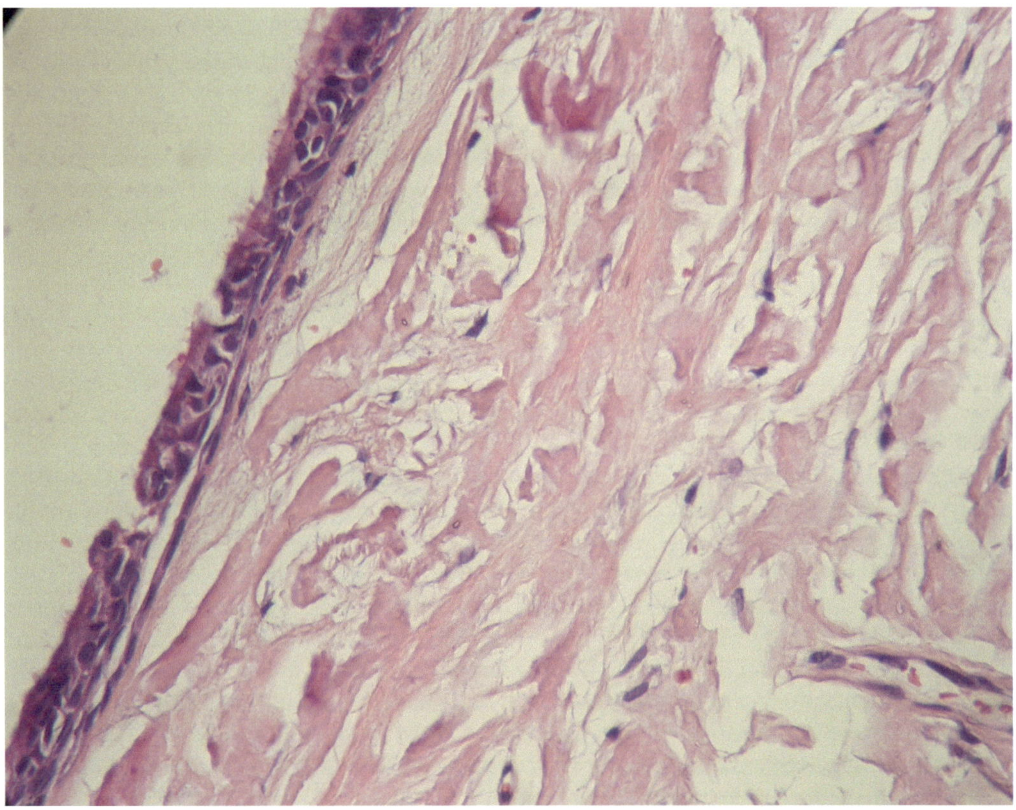

Fig. 1. In an excisional biopsy of localized amyloidosis of nasopharynx, bright pink homogenous, amorphous, acellular, eosinophilic material is seen in the submucosa (hematoxylin eosin, X40) (Özdemir et al., 2010)

have reported specificity of 100% and sensitivity in the range of 58–88%. The overall simplicity and ease of the procedure makes FNAFP the initial technique of choice for the diagnosis of systemic amyloidosis (Ansari-Lari & Ali SZ, 2004). ^{123}I-SAP scintigraphy is another non-invasive test to confirm or rule out occult systemic amyloidosis. However, in a few cases, ^{123}I-SAP scintigraphy can be normal despite systemic amyloidosis with small amyloid deposits. The scintigraphy combined with LSG biopsy gives the clinician valuable information about the local or systemic character of amyloid deposits (Maulin et al. 1997).

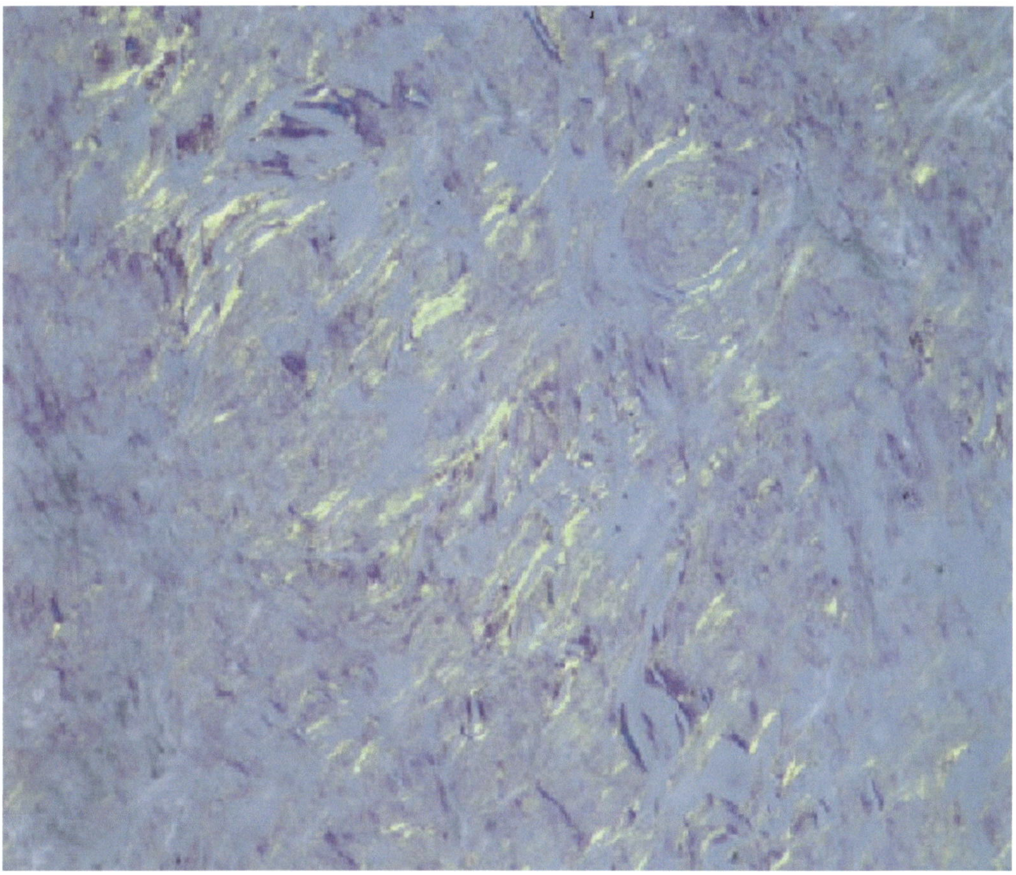

Fig. 2. Apple-green birefringence under polarized light (Congo-red, polarization microscope, ×20) (Akyıldız et al., 2009)

When the diagnosis of localized amyloidosis is finally validated, the risk of further local progression exists, but the risk of systemic progression is low. In fact only three studies have possibly reported localized amyloidosis progressing to systemic disease. Some confusion still exists in the literature, since submucosal progression from laryngeal deposits to the tracheal, bronchial, or gastrointestinal tract is sometimes equated with systemic involvement. In the absence of a systemic involvement or a hematological malignancy, multifocal involvement of the aerodigestive tract should not be considered as systemic dissemination. In this regard, a full endoscopic assessment of the involved tract is necessary in order to clearly determine the number of sites affected by the process, to exclude an associated neoplasm and to anticipate the outcome. Due to the markedly shortened life expectancy in patients with systemic forms of amyloidosis, it is obligatory to differentiate systemic disease from the localized type (Paccalin et al., 2005).

Magnetic resonance imaging (MRI) is the technique of choice to demonstrate the most specific features of amyloidosis. Typically, the amyloid deposits have intermediate T1-weighted signal intensity and low T2-weighted signal intensity, similar to skeletal muscle. This is secondary to the β-pleated structure of the amyloid deposits that occurs as protein fibrils in a parallel sheetlike configuration, similar to the organization of skeletal muscle fibers (Gilad et al., 2007). MRI taken before and after excision, helps in the evaluation and follow-up of the deposits, and can prevent further endoscopic examination (Chin et al., 2004).

Computed tomography (CT) scanning can discriminate between localized and diffuse disease in patients with amyloidosis of the respiratory tract (Chin et al., 2004). On CT scans, amyloid deposits appear as relatively well-defined, submucosal, homogenous masses, usually demonstrating different forms of calcification (Figure 3).

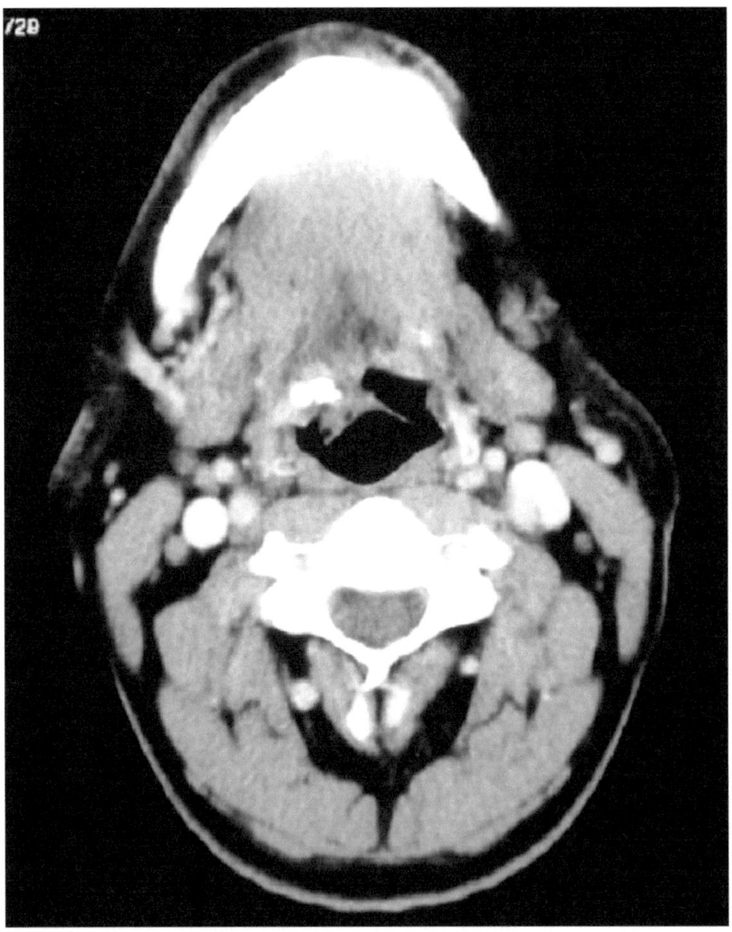

Fig. 3. CT scan of a lesion on the right side of the tongue base. Calcification is seen within the lesion. (Akyıldız et al., 2009)

Although the amyloid itself does not enhance with contrast material administration, peripheral enhancement in the region of the amyloid deposits has been noted. This may be caused by the foreign-body giant cell reaction that is evoked around the amyloid deposits. The lack of enhancement of the amyloid deposits helps to distinguish them from cellular tumors, all of which enhance to varying degrees (Chin et al., 2004).

The low risk of subsequent systemic disease does not mean that localized amyloidosis is always benign. Although most patients remain free of disease, a few others have symptomatic recurrences, sometimes after many symptom-free years. Complications and fatal local progression have been reported despite optimal symptomatic treatment in respiratory tract and laryngeal amyloidosis because of recurrent obstruction, progressive respiratory failure or fatal hemorrhage (Gean-Marton et al., 1991).

Localized amyloidosis in the head and neck is a rare and benign disease. However 90% of the patients with systemic amyloidosis will develop amyloid deposits in the upper aerodigestive tract. Owing to its poor prognosis, the latter condition should be differentiated from primary localized amyloidosis of the head and neck. Localized amyloidosis may involve any site in the head and neck including the orbit, nose, paranasal sinuses, nasopharynx, oropharynx, tonsils, oral cavity, salivary glands, tongue, tracheobronchial tree and larynx (Passerotti et al., 2008; Penner & Muller S, 2006). The larynx is the most common site of involvement and is rarely associated with systemic disease. In contrast, amyloid macroglossia is usually associated with systemic AL amyloidosis, either plasma cell dyscrasia or multiple myeloma. Most other locations in the head and neck are extremely rare with limited cases reported (Penner & Muller S, 2006).

3. Localized laryngeal amyloidosis

Localized laryngeal amyloidosis accounts for 0.2% to 1.5% of benign laryngeal tumors (Ma et al., 2005). The first case of localized laryngeal amyloidosis was documented by Borow in 1873. McAlpine and Fuller, in a review of the literature, found 235 cases of localized amyloidosis of the upper and lower respiratory tracts, and the larynx was involved in 177 cases (75%) (Nandapalan et al., 1998, as cited in McAlpine & Fuller, 1964). Until 1990, only approximately 300 cases of upper airway amyloidosis were reported in the literature. This condition most commonly occurs in the fourth to sixth decades of life, with a male-female predominance of 3:1 (Ma et al., 2005).

The precise etiology and pathogenesis of laryngeal amyloidosis remain unknown. There is no definite established link with smoking, drinking, vocal abuse or recurrent infection (Ma et al., 2005). A large percentage of these patients also have significant reflux esophagitis. Amyloid deposits can result from chronic inflammatory process, and gastroesophageal reflux may be the cause in these cases.

Laryngeal amyloidosis most frequently presents with progressive dysphonia. Other complaints are dysphagia, dyspnea with exertion, choking, occasional aspiration, cough, fullness in the throat or globus sensation and rarely, hemoptysis (Bartels et al., 2004; Kennedy& Patel, 2000; Yiotakis et al., 2009).

The gross appearance usually suggests a mucosally covered mass. The initial diagnosis is thought to represent a malignant neoplasm in most patients. Furthermore, at laryngoscopy and frozen section biopsy, the diagnosis may suggest only granulation tissue or a foreign body type of reaction and it may not be until after the permanent sections are analyzed that amyloidosis is considered (Kennedy& Patel, 2000).

The lesion is usually a firm, nonulcerated yellow, orange or gray submucosal nodule, mass or a pedunculated polypoid lesion. Amyloid deposits are most commonly located in the false vocal cords (55%) and ventricles (36%), less commonly in the subglottis (36%), vocal folds (27%), the aryepiglottic folds (23%) and anterior commissure (14%) (Mitrani & Biler, 1985). It is frequent to have multiple laryngeal sites, or even, that of the aerodigestive tract, and tongue and trachea are the ones most frequently associated with laryngeal amyloidosis and, in such cases, systemic involvement is also more common (Passerotti et al., 2008). A case of laryngocele caused by localized laryngeal amyloidosis has been reported in the literature (Cankaya et al., 2002). Only one case of localized AL-type hypopharyngeal amyloidoma has been reported to date. (Ghekiere et al., 2003). Two other cases of localized amyloidosis of hypopharynx were secondary to multipl myeloma (Chadwick et al, 2002; Hammami et al, 2010)

Four histological patterns of laryngeal amyloidosis have been described. These include amorphous random masses, deposits around blood vessels, deposits in continuity with the basilar membrane of seromucinous glands, and deposits within adipose tissue (Gallivan & Gallivan, 2010).

Laryngeal amyloidosis is usually associated with amyloid protein of the light chain (amyloid L; AL) type. Restricted light chain staining (lambda or kappa) in both plasma cells and the amyloid has been observed in cases of laryngeal amyloidosis. In one series, more than 60% of laryngeal deposits displayed a lambda light chain staining pattern, and 25% a kappa pattern. (Lewis et al., 1992; Ma et al., 2005).

Diagnosis should focus on evaluating the extent of local amyloidosis and on ruling out systemic involvement. Macroscopic examination of the larynx should be performed by indirect videolaryngostroboscopy. A thorough voice analysis is also required.

Radiological examination involves CT and MRI. On CT scans, laryngeal amyloidosis presents with submucosal and homogeneous amyloid deposits which are not associated with the cartilage changes. These deposits are firm lesions that tend to occur in the supraglottic larynx (Figure 4), although all laryngeal sites may be affected (Bartels et al., 2004). CT two-dimensional reconstruction images, along with their axial views, are found to be more helpful than any other scan in mapping the location of the amyloid before surgery as well as in planning the time of the surgery (Kennedy& Patel, 2000). The differential diagnosis includes other submucosal diseases such as laryngeal sarcoidosis, lymphoma and pseudotumor. Submucosal lesions such as paragangliomas and hemangiomas are more localized on CT scans and MR images, and the entire lesion enhances rather than periphery (Bartels et al., 2004). However, even though the radiological studies are helpful, amyloidosis is usually not included in the differential before the material for biopsy is obtained by direct laryngoscopy (Kennedy & Patel, 2000).

Systemic work-up should include a thorough history (including family history), physical examination (enlargement of spleen or liver, cardiac failure, edema), laboratory screening (levels of hemoglobin, serum creatinine, bilirubin, total protein, albumin, alkaline phosphatase, and proteinuria and a search for monoclonal proteins in serum and urine). ECG, echocardiography, and at least one other biopsy of a different site of the body, preferably the rectum or abdominal subcutaneous fat tissue (Bartels et al., 2004). Use of ^{123}I-SAP scintigraphy may be helpful, especially if combined with labial biopsy (Maulin et al., 1997).

Diagnostic work-up should also look for collagen vascular diseases, tuberculosis, and multiple myeloma (rheumatoid factor, antinuclear antibody, tuberculosis skin test, chest

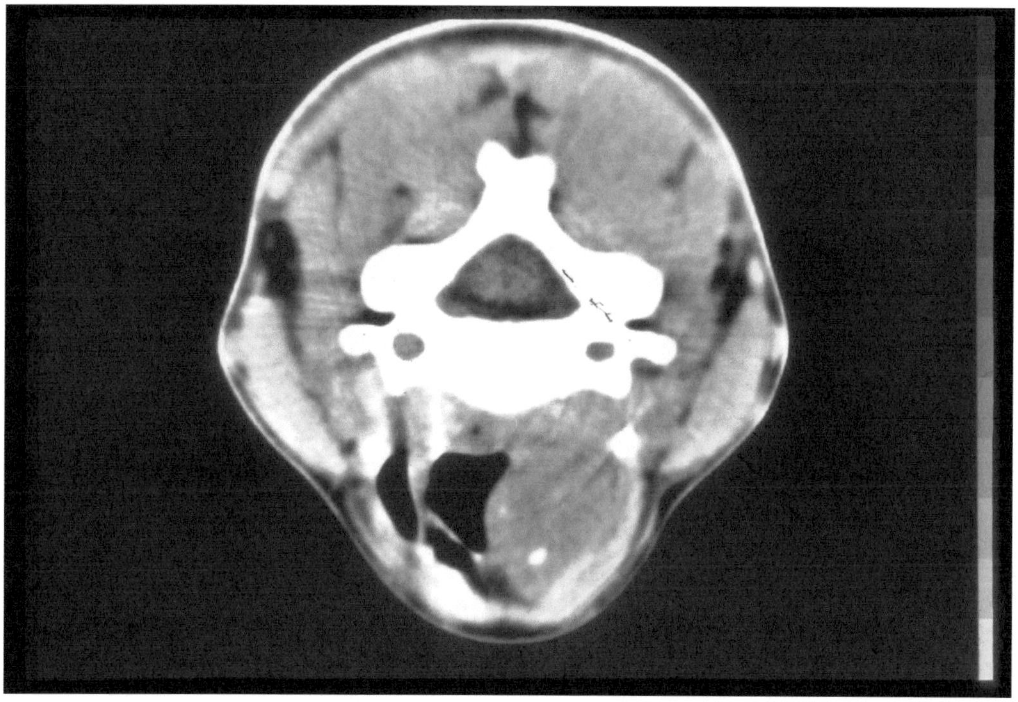

Fig. 4. Amyloidosis localized in supraglottic larynx. In this case thyroid cartilage appeared intact and no nodal involvement was detected (Yiotakis et al., 2009)

radiograph). The differential diagnosis should also include metastatic medullary thyroid cancer, laryngeal sarcoidosis, benign laryngeal polyps, laryngeal malignancies, benign minor salivary gland tumors and chondromas (Friedman et al., 2002)

The larynx is rarely the first location of systemic amyloidosis; however, systemic amyloidosis should never be ruled out from the differential diagnosis because of its potentially poor prognosis. In a case with localized laryngeal amyloidosis, systemic amyloidosis developed after an 8-year period, therefore yearly visits with a follow-up period of at least 10 years is recommended. Yearly monitoring of the presence of monoclonal free light chains in serum and urine may be helpful in detecting progression into systemic AL amyloidosis at an earlier stage of the disease (Bartels et al., 2004).

Laryngeal involvement may be a part of laryngo-tracheobronchial amyloidosis (LTBA) causing airway obstruction, hemoptysis, chronic cough, recurrent respiratory infections, dysphonia and dysphagia. LTBA is usually a primary, localized form of the disease, with deposits of AL amyloid fibrils. This evidence, together with the presence of plasma cells in and around amyloid deposits, may suggest that localized plasma cell dysfunction is responsible for this pathology. The precise etiology of primary localized airway amyloidosis still remains unclear, and the most recent hypothesis about its origin involves derangement of immunoregulation after recurrent or prolonged antigen challenge. Others have speculated that idiopathic production of structurally abnormal immunoglobulins by monoclonal plasma cells may overwhelm the clearing mechanisms leading to deposition of their cleavage products in the airway submucosa.

Classifying patients in a series of 32 LTBA cases showed purely laryngeal involvement in 12.5% of cases, isolated tracheal localization in 3% of cases, laryngo-tracheal amyloidosis (or "proximal airway disease") in 28% of cases, tracheobronchial disease (or "mid and distal airway disease") in 44% of cases, and extensive involvement of the entire laryngotracheobronchial tree in 12.5% of cases. A full endoscopic assessment of the involved tract clearly defines the number of sites affected by the process.

The endoscopic appearance of LTBA lesions can be classified as submucosal plaques and nodules, pseudotumor or tumor-like appearance, circumferential wall thickening. These appearances represent different stages of the same process of amyloid deposition. In fact, it seems to start with the formation of submucosal yellowish plaques, seen nearly everywhere in the tracheobronchial tree. Then lesions grow progressively in a confluent manner leading to a circumferential thickening or pseudotumor appearance. It is believed that these different endoscopic appearances have no prognostic implications, but effect the surgical options. In a pseudotumor mass or a circumferential wall thickening, mechanical resection and/or dilatation coupled with transmucosal Nd:YAG laser treatment with low power and high energy density are recommended. On the other hand, submucosal plaques, particularly when located at the glottic or subglottic levels, should be treated by a mucosa-sparing approach or by CO_2 laser, thus minimizing scar tissue formation and subsequent complications (Piazza et al., 2003).

Localized laryngeal amyloidosis is a slowly progressive disease that should be treated according to the complaints of the patient. The indication for treatment is not determined by the presence of amyloid deposits, but the symptoms these deposits result in, such as dysphonia or dyspnea. Bronchoscopy is important to identify subglottic amyloid deposits and more distal tracheal or bronchial lesions. While the prognosis for laryngeal amyloidosis is usually good, death has rarely been reported. This usually occurs from diffuse tracheobronchial disease with pulmonary failure (Lewis et al., 1992).

The primary treatment described in localized laryngeal amyloidosis is endoscopic surgical removal of deposits that interfere with laryngeal or airway function, although extensive surgical procedures have been performed, depending on the size of the lesions. The location and size of the amyloid deposits should determine the surgical instruments of choice. Biopsy specimens are preferably removed by cold endoscopic excision. The specimens can be examined more minutely if no carbonization is present. Cold endoscopic excision is preferable for the removal of small deposits and those located at critical anatomic sites such as the true vocal cords. In these cases, a standard cordotomy is performed, after which the cheese-like contents can be taken out of the subepithelial space, and then the epithelial flap is glued back. In the same way, coring out subglottic lesions has a lasting and effective result. CO_2 laser or powered instrumentation is usually used in supraglottic deposits. The epithelium is excised with these techniques. This may be the reason why supraglottic lesions tend to recur (Bartels et al., 2004).

Because of the propensity of amyloid to infiltrate blood vessels, cold resection of amyloid lesions may be complicated by bleeding. CO_2 laser excision may be advantageous, but if used in very extensive lesions, there may be scarring. In very large lesions, external approaches, employing laryngofissure for treatment of diffuse subglottic and tracheal amyloidosis have been used. Repeated excision and curettage may be necessary to achieve stabilization of lesions and subsequent decannulation of those patients who are tracheotomy dependent (Gallivan & Gallivan, 2010). Large supraglottic amyloid deposits, can be handled by supraglottic laryngectomy, or, by a more conservative approach, a lateral supraglottic procedure can be used (Kennedy & Patel, 2000). Local or systemic steroids are ineffective in controlling or reversing lesions of amyloidosis.

Gallivan and Gallivan report in their article that at the airway clinic they work with, 8 of 10 patients (3 laryngeal and 7 tracheobronchial recurrent amyloidosis cases) had achieved disease stability with low dose radiation. (Gallivan & Gallivan, 2010). In another recent case report, a case of localized laryngeal amyloidosis involving false vocal cord was treated with surgical debulking and adjuvant external beam radiation to a dose of 45 Gy (Neuner et al., 2010).

There have been several proposed mechanisms by which radiation exerts its effects on amyloid deposits. One theory is that localized radiation therapy has a destructive effect on local abnormal plasma cells, which tend to be low dose radiation sensitive, as has been shown in patients with multiple myeloma and plasmacytomas. However, the amyloid deposits in laryngo-tracheobronchial amyloidosis contain scarce plasma cells, so a radiation effect on plasma cell function or turnover is unlikely to be the only mechanism of action. Other possibilities include a radiation effect on local vascular structures or induction of immune responses against the deposits by causing local inflammation. In addition, there may be other blood, tissue, or pH factors in the local milieu that mediate the response (Neben-Wittich et al., 2007).

Localized laryngeal amyloidosis tends to recur and it usually takes a number of years until the disease is stabilized. A detailed history of current symptoms and local examination of the larynx should be encountered with yearly follow-ups, and local recurrences should be treated as conservative as possible. There has been no report of malignant change in amyloid tumor however one must be aware of the possibility of a subsequent development of systemic amyloidosis (Friedman et al., 2002).

4. Localized nasopharyngeal amyloidosis

Localized amyloidosis occurs most commonly in the head and neck region. Among the sites, larynx is affected most frequently (61%), followed by oropharynx (23%), trachea (9%), and orbit (4%). Only 3% of cases occur in the nasopharynx. Up to 2007 there were only 14 reported cases (Panda et al., 2007). A Pubmed search up to the present revealed 4 more cases including the case we had reported in 2010. (Geller et al., 2010; Özdemir et al., 2010; Passerotti et al., 2008; Zhuang et al., 2015) Table 2 shows a list of all of the reported cases.

The presentation of head and neck amyloidosis varies according to the site of involvement. A patient with nasopharyngeal amyloidosis may present with postnasal discharge, nasal obstruction, recurrent epistaxis (due to vessel wall invasion), dysphagia, foreign body sensation in the throat, voice change, eustachian tube dysfunction and secondary ear problems such as conductive hearing loss due to middle ear effusion. Lesions appear as yellowish, mucosa covered, irregular polypoidal masses (Patel et al., 2002).

On CT scan, amyloid deposits appear as relatively well-defined, submucosal, homogenous masses, usually demonstrating different forms of calcification (Figure 5). The mass exhibits minimal, if any, enhancement after administration of contrast. On MRI, the submucosal location and distinctive hypointensity on T2-weighted images excludes many of the other differential diagnosis. (Gean-Marton et al., 1991) Dynamic MR further defines the vascular changes due to localized amyloid deposition (Asaumi et al., 2001).

Nasopharyngeal amyloidosis is generally a slow growing, benign tumor, but it may be locally aggressive and produce osteolysis and even invade the skull base. CT and MRI are helpful in revealing any bony destruction or intracranial extension (Patel et al., 2002).

Authors	Year	Age/Sex	Site of Involvement	Symptoms
Kramer	1935	-	NF	Nasal obstruction
Johner	1972	-	NF	Nasal obstruction
Simpson	1984	29/F	NF	Postnasal discharge, glue ear
Zack Zonk	1984	14/M	NF	Hearing loss, glue ear
Gean Marton	1991	-	NF (3 cases)	Nasal obstruction, glue ear
Hegarty	1993	-	NF with skull base erosion	Nasal obstruction, postnasal discharge
Panda	1994	82/M	NF	Oral bleeding
Dominguez	1996	13/F	NF and soft palate	Nasal obstruction, oral bleeding
Lim	1999	42/F	NF	Nasal obstruction
Pitkaranta	2000	-	NF	Nasal obstruction
Patel	2002	-	NF	Hearing loss, glue ear
Zhuang	2005	-	NF and cervical LN	Nasal obstruction, cervical mass
Panda	2007	43/M	NF, oropharynx	Nasal obstruction, foreign body sensation of throat
Passerotti	2008	55/F	NF, Tonsil pillar, larynx	Hoarseness, dysphonia, dysphagia
Geller	2010	62/F	NF and nasolacrimal duct	Nasolacrimal duct obstruction
Özdemir	2010	67/F	NF and cervical LN	Nasal obstruction, cervical mass

F: Female, M: Male, NF: Nasopharynx, LN: Lymph node

Table 2. Reported cases of nasopharyngeal amyloidosis

Diagnosis of nasopharyngeal amyloidosis is made with histopathological examination of amyloid deposits in biopsy specimens as mentioned earlier. Systemic involvement should be ruled out. In the absence of a systemic disease, localized nasopharyngeal amyloidosis has an excellent prognosis.

Surgery is reported to be the choice of therapy. Transpalatal approach or nasopharyngeal curettage is preferred (Özdemir et al., 2010). Bleeding due to the loss of vascular integrity caused by amyloid infiltration of the blood vessels may be a major complication during surgery (Patel et al., 2002). Excision of the amyloid deposits should only be considered if they cause morbidity. However if localized amyloidosis do not cause morbidity, conservative treatment with careful observation is suggested (Domínguez et al., 1996).

In the English literature two cases of localized nasopharyngeal amyloidosis associated with lymph node involvement in the neck are reported (Özdemir et al., 2010; Zhuang et al., 2005). This presentation mimics nasopharyngeal carcinoma with neck metastases. In such a case, diagnosis of localized amyloidosis should be confirmed with biopsy of nasopharyngeal mass and fine needle aspiration biopsies of the neck masses. If asymptomatic, the removal of the neck masses showing amyloid deposits is not necessary.

Nasopharyngeal amyloidosis may coexist with carcinoma of nasopharynx. In a series of 434 cases of nasopharyngeal carcinoma, amyloid deposits were found in 12% of the cases (Munichor et al., 2000, as cited in Pratap et al., 1984). In another recent case report of nasopharyngeal carcinoma with cervical metastasis, the blind biopsies obtained from nasopharynx and fine needle aspiration biopsy (FNAB) of the metastatic cervical lymph nodes revealed carcinoma with amyloid deposits. Authors draw attention to the fact that a potential association of these two conditions may be more frequent than expected and diagnosis of carcinoma with amyloidosis can be made with the use of FNAB (Munichor et al., 2000).

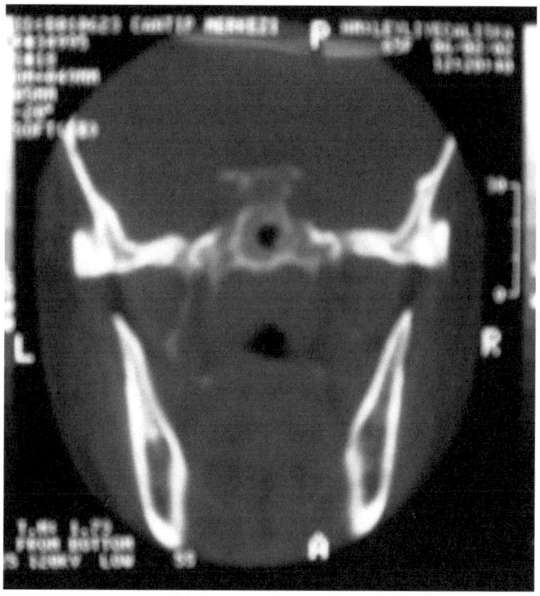

Fig. 5. In the CT scan, the nasopharynx is obliterated by a granular mass with irregular borders. No calcification is seen. Histological examination of the lesion revealed amyloidosis (Özdemir et al., 2010)

Sometimes, amyloid tumors in the nasopharynx can be difficult to treat and recur despite surgical excision. Less recurrence is reported following laser excision of localized amyloidosis (Simpson et al., 1984). Localized nasopharyngeal amyloidosis is a rare disease, for which slow progression and spontaneous regression is expected, therefore it is difficult to predict the outcome. Recurrent masses and extensive lesions involving the head and neck should be handled conservatively (Patel et al., 2002).

5. Localized sinonasal amyloidosis

Primary amyloidosis localized to the nose and/or paranasal sinuses is rare with only 27 reported cases in the English literature (Chin et al., 2004; Mufarrij et al., 1990; Paccalin et al., 2005; Pang et al., 2001; Prasad et al., 2009; Teo et al., 2003; Tsikoudas et al., 2001). Out of these 8 of them are solely localized to the nasal cavity (Pang et al., 2001).

Smooth, soft to firm, non tender, pale waxy gray, yellow or pale pink masses of amyloid deposits are found localized to the inferior concha or other parts of the lateral wall, the septum (Figure 6). The diagnostic nasal endoscopy is helpful in exploring yellowish polypoidal masses extending to the choana, though radiological imaging defines the disease more thoroughly (Prasad et al., 2009). Amyloid deposits are composed of AL, kappa or lambda light chain amyloid. Clinical presentation is often insidious, with symptoms that are slowly progressive over months to years prior to diagnosis. Presenting symptoms are nasal obstruction, nasal discharge, epistaxis and glue ear; facial pain and neuralgia can be seen in amyloidosis of the maxillary antrum (Paccalin et al., 2005; Pang et al., 2001).

The extent of the localized disease is best evaluated by CT and/or MRI scans. In CT scans, calcification seems to be a nonspecific finding. Besides this, in the paranasal sinuses, a "fluffy" appearance is noted in the sinonasal cavity bones adjacent to the amyloid deposits in a case. This could be a result of an osteoblastic reaction incited by the deposition of the proteinaceous amyloid fibrils in the submucosal layers of the sinonasal cavities. Although sinonasal calcifications can also be seen in inspissated secretions, fungal mycetomas, cartilaginous tumors, and olfactory neuroblastomas, the "fluffy" bone changes have not been seen with these diseases (Chin et al., 2004).

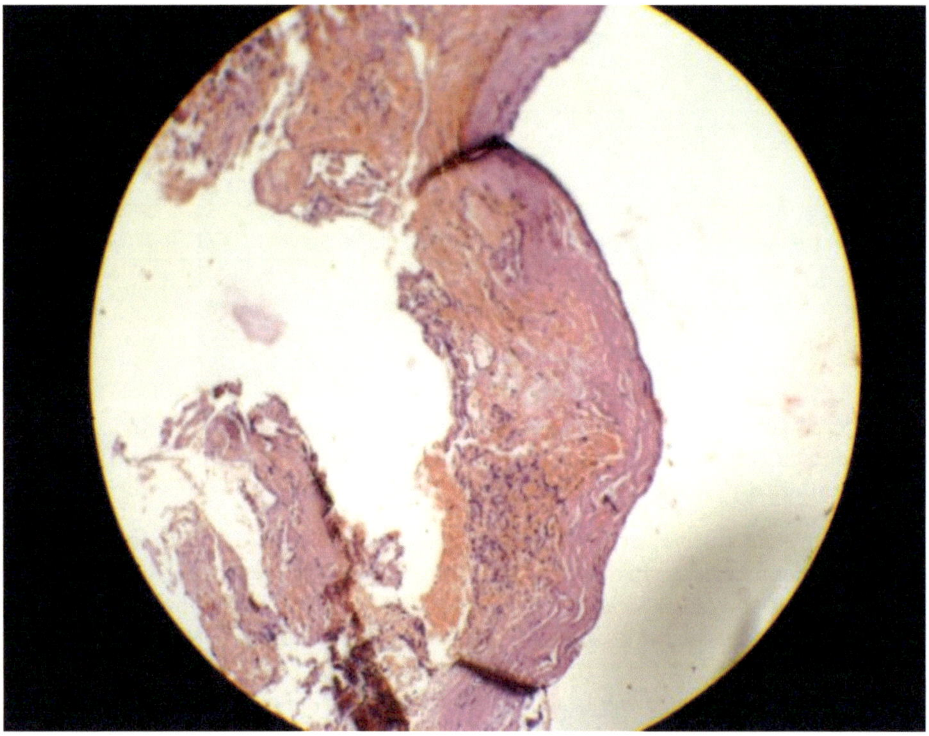

Fig. 6. Amyloid deposits beneath nasal mucosa (hematoxylin eosin) (Prasad et. al., 2009)

Systemic disease should be excluded with appropriate tests. Multifocal involvement is possible therefore endoscopic examination of the entire respiratory tract is indicated including nasopharynx, oropharynx, larynx and tracheobronchial tree. Medical treatment has been unsuccessful and radiotherapy is ineffective and contraindicated in this region. When the disease is symptomatic, conservative surgery is the only option, however recurrences are common (Tsikoudas et al., 2001). Simpson et al. reported that complete excision using the CO_2 laser was satisfactory with no recurrence in a 14-year follow-up period, whereas incomplete excision resulted in recurrence (Simpson et al., 1984).

6. Localized amyloidosis of the oral cavity and oropharynx

Oral amyloidosis often appears with a variety of manifestations, such as multiple soft nodules that appear hemorrhagic or pink to yellow. Amyloidosis presents as a diffuse or a nodular mass mimicking a neoplasm such as granular cell tumors, schwannomas, neurofibromas and mucosal neuromas (Asaumi et al., 2001).

The tongue is the most frequently observed oral subsite, which almost always suggests systemic disease. This can cause a firm or rubbery macroglossia, manifested by increased tongue volume, tongue protrusion beyond the alveolar ridge, speech impairment, and dysphagia (Fahrner et al., 2004). The patients with macroglossia typically demonstrate scalloping of the lateral border of the tongue due to indentations from the teeth (Penner & Muller, 2006). Yellow nodules or raised white lesions occurring predominately along the lateral border are also common (Fahrner et al., 2004). Sometimes petechiae, ecchymoses and hemorrhagic blisters can also be observed. The tongue involvement with numerous smooth surfaced, white-yellow nodules has been reported in cases of long term dialysis related amyloidosis (Pentenero et al., 2006). Amyloid of the tongue is usually secondary to primary amyloidosis with plasma cell dyscrasia, consisting of the monoclonal AL immunoglobulin light-chain amyloid. Additionally, macroglossia occurs in 26% to 83% of patients with multiple myeloma. For generalized macroglossia, besides amyloidosis; tuberculosis, lymphangioma, hypothyroidism, acromegaly, lingual infarction caused by giant-cell arteritis, idiopathic muscular hypertrophy, and Beckwith-Wiedemann syndrome should be considered in the differential diagnosis.

Localized amyloidosis of the tongue is rare and associated with AL type amyloidosis. So far, only thirteen cases have been reported in the English literature. (Biewend et al., 2006; Fahrner et al.,2004; Koren et al., 1998; Penner & Muller, 2006; Simpson et al., 1984), although for four of these cases, a full evaluation for systemic disease was not documented. One of these cases was reported to develop Hodgkin's lymphoma 12 years after the diagnosis of localized amyloidosis (Penner CR & Muller S (2006). Two of the cases presented with glossodynia and glossopyrosis with lesions which were thought to represent median rhomboid glossitis (Koren et al., 1998; Yamoka et al., 1978). One other patient presented with pyrosis of tongue and a well-circumscribed, rubbery, nodular mass in the tongue base (Akyıldız et al, 2009). Others had discrete, firm, pink to yellowish, multiple or solitary nodular lesions on the tongue (Penner & Muller, 2006). For nodular localized lesions, fibroma, lipoma, granular cell tumor, sarcoma, and salivary gland tumors are among the differential. MR images of tongue involvement of amyloidosis appear slightly low on T1-weighted images and slightly high on T2-weighted images compared with T1-T2 images of residual normal tongue (Asaumi et al., 2001).

Localized amyloid of the tonsil is also rare and, to date there have only been thirteen reports in the world literature.(Green et al., 2000; López et al., 1996; Passerotti et al., 2008; Tsuji et al., 2008) Four of these cases also involve other parts of the Waldeyer's ring. (Green et al., 2000; Passerotti et al., 2008) In four reports amyloid was found to affect both tonsils (Green et al., 2000). Immunohistochemical investigations undertaken in some of the reports revealed AL type amyloidosis (López et al., 1996; Tsuji et al., 2008)

Localized amyloidosis of other sites of the oral cavity is extremely rare. Only 5 cases of localized amyloidosis involving palate have been reported to date. (Aono et al., 2009; Pentenero et al., 2006) One of these cases was found to be AA type of amyloidosis while others were AL type. Even though AA type of amyloidosis is usually secondary to chronic inflammatory diseases, the systemic work-up for this case was negative, and the case was considered a primary localized involvement of the palate. The authors hypothesized the role of the denture as a local chronic irritant agent (Pentenero et al., 2006). Lips (Simpson et al., 1984), gingiva (Maulin et al., 1997), lateral pharyngeal wall (Penner & Muller 2006), floor of the mouth (Simpson et al., 1984) are other sites involved in various reports.

Although the presentation seems localized, amyloidosis of head and neck mucosal sites excluding larynx is often secondary to an underlying malignancy. In a series of 12 cases involving the tongue, pharynx, and cervical lymph nodes, 9 (78%) were associated with malignancy or plasma cell dyscrasia. A referral to a hematologist is appropriate when a patient presents with lingual amyloidosis or other head and neck sites to exclude malignancy or systemic disease (Penner & Muller, 2006).

7. Localized amyloidosis of other sites of head and neck

Although the parotid gland has been suggested as a possible site of involvement in systemic amyloidosis, only three cases of localized amyloid tumor involving the parotid gland without systemic involvement has been reported in the literature (Stimson et al., 1988; Nandapalan et al., 1998; Biewend et al., 2006). The immunohistochemical work-up for the first case demonstrated staining for immunoglobulin A, lambda and kappa light chains within the amyloid deposits and in the cytoplasm of the lymphocytes, and plasma cell aggregates (Stimson et al., 1988). The second case presented with enlarging, painless swelling of the right parotid region. FNAB of the mass nondiagnostic, but an MRI scan of the head and neck showed that both parotid glands were involved. A right parotidectomy for histological diagnosis was given, and the patient was asymptomatic in the follow-up (Nandapalan et al., 1998). The third case presented with the involvement of both parotid and submandibular glands. The lesions were excised and no recurrence was observed (Biewend et al., 2006).

As far as salivary structures are concerned, one other case of primary localized amyloidosis of the sublingual gland is reported. This case is also the first case of the oral cavity with primary localized amyloidosis consisting AA protein (Kurokawa et al., 1998).

Many cases of cutaneous amyloidosis have been reported in the literature, but only 4 primary localized cases involving the external auditory canal, and one case involving both external and middle ear were reported. The latter case was diagnosed with the biopsy of the external canal and the CT images of the middle ear were similar to the mass in the external ear canal. The patient was treated with regular cleansing and debridement of the ear canal to prevent irritation, deafness and secondary infection. The authors were reluctant to explore the middle ear, fearing to provoke postoperative dizziness or tinnitus, for this could end the patient's job as a roofer. Fourteen months after diagnosis, the disease remained confined to the involved ear (Gheriani et al., 2007). In the English literature, two other cases of hemodialysis-associated amyloidosis localized to external auditory canal have been reported (Yamazaki et al., 2011). Treatment should include local excision and debridement to prevent irritation, deafness, and secondary infection. Topical steroid therapy can also help limit the local inflammatory process (Gheriani et al., 2007).

To date, eight cases of primary cutaneous amyloidosis involving the auricular concha have been reported (Shimauchi et al., 2006). The nodules which appear pink to brown or red, are typically non-pruritic, slightly friable, but tend not to ulcerate. They may be present on both ears. This entity appears to have been described previously as collagenous papules of the ear. The patients do not have lesions of amyloidosis on other parts of the body and no systemic involvement is seen (Hicks et al., 1988). Skin biopsy provides the definitive diagnosis. An optimal biopsy specimen includes the epidermis, papillary dermis, and reticular dermis. The amyloid in nodular localized cutaneous amyloidosis is located in the reticular dermis and subcutaneous fat, and clearly differentiates nodular localized cutaneous amyloidosis from other forms of amyloidosis. A shave biopsy or other superficial samples may not include enough reticular dermis to complete the diagnosis (Biesbroeck & Kauffman, 2010). Histologically amorphous materials are present in the widened dermal papillae positive for Congo red (Shimauchi et al., 2006). Procedures such as excision, curettage and electrodesiccation as well as laser treatment have provided satisfactory

cosmetic results for nodular localized cutaneous amyloidosis. None of these treatment methods totally eradicates lesions, which can recur (Biesbroeck & Kauffman, 2010).
Nodular localized primary cutaneous amyloidosis of the nose is very rare and five cases have been reported to date (Biewend et al., 2006; Blanc et al., 1985; Evers et al., 2007; Kakani et al., 2001) Nodular amyloidosis can be treated successfully with cold steel excision in combination with carbon dioxide laser. Cases of nodular localized cutaneous amyloidosis of the neck present with multiple subcutaneous neck nodules. A literature review showed five reported cases of subcutaneous nodular amyloidosis. Immunohistochemical analysis in one of these cases showed the amyloid deposits consisting of AL lambda light chains. Twenty-four months follow-up in this case showed minimal disease progression (Nguyen et al., 2001).
Finally, amyloid may infiltrate the thyroid or other endocrine glands, but rarely causes endocrine dysfunction. However, local amyloid deposition in the thyroid gland is noted to have a close association with medullary carcinoma, being present in the stroma of 75% of medullary carcinoma. Therefore, a neck mass revealing amyloid should be investigated to rule out occult medullary carcinoma of the thyroid gland. (Nandapalan et al, 1998).

8. Conclusion

Localized amyloidosis in the head and neck is a benign disease, and should be differentiated from localized involvement of a systemic disease. Upper aerodigestive tract can be involved in 90% of the patients with systemic amyloidosis. Owing to its poor prognosis, the latter condition as well as localized amyloidosis should be recognized by otolaryngologists, and systemic investigations should be encountered in order to differentiate localized from systemic amyloidosis. Localized amyloidosis of head and neck tend to recur, and it usually takes a number of years until the disease is stabilized, therefore conservative management is the rule. If the disease is symptomatic, conservative surgery is essential, and yearly follow-ups are recommended for at least 10 years. Local recurrences should be treated as conservative as possible. Asymptomatic disease usually requires no intervention. In the follow-ups, systemic amyloidosis should never be ruled out from the differential diagnosis. Early monitoring of the presence of monoclonal free light chains in serum and urine might be helpful in detecting progression into systemic amyloidosis at an earlier stage of the disease. Finally, localized amyloidosis of the head and neck is rare, therefore publication of more cases should be encouraged in order to contribute to the literature and develop appropriate strategies for management.

9. References

Akyıldız S, Doğanavsargil B, Göde S & Veral A (2009). Solitary Amyloid Tumor of the Tongue Base. *International Journal of Otolaryngology* Vol: 2009

Ansari-Lari MA & Ali SZ (2004). Fine-needle aspiration of abdominal fat pad for amyloid detection: a clinically useful test? *Diagn Cytopathol.* Mar;30(3), pp. 178-81.

Aono J, Yamagata K & Yoshida H (2009). Local amyloidosis in the hard palate: a case report. *Oral Maxillofac Surg.* Jun;13(2),pp. 119-22.

Asaumi J, Yanagi Y, Hisatomi M, Konouchi H &, Kishi K (2001). CT and MR imaging of localized amyloidosis. *Eur J Radiol.* Aug;39(2),pp. 83-7.

Bartels H, Dikkers FG, Van der Wal JE, Lokhorst HM & Hazenberg BP (2004). Laryngeal amyloidosis: localized versus systemic disease and update on diagnosis and therapy. *Ann Otol Rhinol laryngol.* Sep;113(9),pp. 741-8.

Berg AM, Troxler RF, Grillone G, Kasznica J, Kane K, Cohen AS & Skinner M (1993). Localized amyloidosis of the larynx: evidence for light chain composition. *Ann Otol Rhinol Laryngol.* Nov;102(11), pp. 884-9.

Biesbroeck L & Kauffman CL (2010). Amyloidosis, Nodular Localized Cutaneous, *In: Medscape Reference,* 2011,
Available from: < http://emedicine.medscape.com/article/1102770-workup >

Biewend ML, Menke DM & Calamia KT (2006). The spectrum of localized amyloidosis: a case series of 20 patients and review of the literature. *Amyloid.* Sep;13(3),pp. 135-42.

Blanc F, Triller R, Ferte JF, Itasse H, Schernberg C, Pluot M & Kalis B (1985). Nodular primary localized cutaneous amyloidosis of the tip of the nose. *Ann Dermatol Venereol.*;112(9), pp. 701-2.

Cankaya H, Egeli E, Unal O & Kiris M (2002). Laryngeal amyloidosis: a rare cause of laryngocele. *Clin Imaging.* Mar-Apr;26(2), pp. 86-8.

Chadwick MA, Buckland JR, Mason P, Randall CJ & Theaker J (2002). A rare case of dysphagia: hypopharyngeal amyloidosis masquerading as a post-cricoid tumour. *J Laryngol Otol*;116, pp. 54–56.

Chin SC, Fatterpeckar G, Kao CH, Chen CY & Som PM (2004). Amyloidosis concurrently involving the sinonasal cavities and larynx. *AJNR Am J Neuroradiol.* Apr;25(4), pp. 636-8.

Domínguez S, Wienberg P, Clarós P, Clarós A & Vila J (1996). Primary localized nasopharyngeal amyloidosis. A case report. Int J Pediatr Otorhinolaryngol. Jun;36(1), pp. 61-7.

Evers M, Baron E, Zaim MT & Han A (2007). Papules and plaques on the nose. Nodular localized primary cutaneous amyloidosis. Arch Dermatol. Apr;143(4),pp. 535-40.

Fahrner KS, Black CC & Gosselin BJ (2004). Localized amyloidosis of the tongue: a review. *Am J Otolaryngol.* May-Jun;25(3),pp. 186-9.

Friedman AD, Bhayani R, Memeo L & Kuriloff DB (2002). Localized laryngeal amyloidosis. *Otolaryngol Head Neck Surg.* Nov;127(5)pp. 487-9.

Gallivan GJ & Gallivan HK (2010). Laryngeal amyloidosis causing hoarseness and airway obstruction. *J Voice.* Mar;24(2),pp.235-9. Epub 2008 Dec 25.

Gean-Marton AD, Kirsch CF, Vezina LG & Weber AL (1991). Focal amyloidosis of the head and neck: evaluation with CT and MR imaging. *Radiology.* Nov;181(2),pp. 521-5.

Geller E, Freitag SK & Laver NV (2010). Localized Nasopharyngeal Amyloidosis Causing Bilateral Nasolacrimal Duct Obstruction. *Ophthal Plast Reconstr Surg.* Sep 23. [Epub ahead of print]

Ghekiere O, Desuter G, Weynand B & Coche B (2003). Hypopharyngeal amyloidoma. Am J Radiol 181,pp. 1720–1721.

Gheriani H, Tewary R& O'Sullivan TJ (2007). Amyloidosis of the external auditory canal and middle ear: unusual ear tumor. *Ear Nose Throat J.* Feb;86(2),pp. 92-3,106.

Gilad R, Milillo P & Som PM (2007). Severe diffuse systemic amyloidosis with involvement of the pharynx, larynx, and trachea: CT and MR findings. *AJNR Am J Neuroradiol.* Sep;28(8),pp. 1557-8.

Green KM, Morris DP, Pitt M & Small M (2000). Amyloidosis of Waldeyer's ring and larynx. *J Laryngol Otol.* Apr;114(4):296-8.

Hammami B, Mnejja M, Kallel S, Bouguecha L, Chakroun A, Charfeddine I & Ghorbel A (2010). Hypopharyngeal amyloidosis: A case report. *Eur Ann Otorhinolaryngol Head Neck Dis.* May;127(2),pp. 83-5. Epub 2010 Mar 31.

Hicks BC, Weber PJ, Hashimoto K, Ito K Koreman DM (1988). Primary cutaneous amyloidosis of the auricular concha. J Am Acad Dermatol. Jan;18(1 Pt 1),pp.19-25.

Kakani RS, Goldstein AE, Meisher I & Hoffman C (2001). Nodular amyloidosis: case report and literature review. *Cutan Med Surg.* Mar-Apr;5(2),pp. 101-4. Epub 2001 Mar 2.

Kennedy TL & Patel NM (2000). Surgical management of localized amyloidosis. *Laryngoscope.* Jun;110(6),pp.918-23.
Koren R, Veltman V, Halpern M, Szabo R & Gal R (1998). Localized amyloid tumor of the tongue. A case report and review of the literature. *Rom J Morphol Embryol.* Jan-Dec;44(1-4), pp.179-82.
Kurokawa H, Takuma C, Tokudome S, Yamashita Y & Kajiyama M (1998). Primary localization amyloidosis of the sublingual gland. *Fukuoka Igaku Zasshi.* Jul;89(7),pp. 216-20.
Kyle RA & Bayrd ED (1975).Amyloidosis: Review of 236 cases. *Medicine* 54,pp. 271-299.
Kyle RA & Greipp PR. (1983). Amyloidosis (AL), clinical and laboratory features in 229 cases. *Mayo Clin Proc* 58,pp. 665–683.
Lewis JE, Olsen KD, Kurtin PJ & Kyle RA (1992). Laryngeal amyloidosis: a clinicopathologic and immunohistochemical review. *Otolaryngol Head Neck Surg.* Apr;106(4) pp. 372-7.
López AM, Lorenzo PMJ, López BG & Arnal MF (1996). Giant primary amyloidoma of the tonsil. *J Laryngol Otol.* Jun;110(6), pp. 613-5.
Ma L, Bandarchi B, Sasaki C, Levine S & Choi Y (2005). Primary localized laryngeal amyloidosis: report of 3 cases with long-term follow-up and review of the literature. *Arch Pathol Lab Med.* Feb;129(2),pp. 215-8.
Maulin L, Hachulla E, Deveaux M, Janin A, Wechsler B, Godeau P, Rousset H, Barrier JH, Hatron PY, Devulder B, Huglo D & Marchandise X (1997). 'Localized amyloidosis': 123I-labelled SAP component scintigraphy and labial salivary gland biopsy. *QJM.* Jan;90(1), pp.45-50.
Mitrani M & Biller HF (1985). Laryngeal amyloidosis. *Laryngoscope.* Nov;95(11), pp. 1346-7.
Munichor M, Cohen H, Kerner H, Szvalb S & Iancu TC (2000). Localized amyloidosis in nasopharyngeal carcinoma diagnosed by fine needle aspiration and electron microscopy. A case report. *Acta Cytol.* Jul-Aug;44(4),pp. 673-8.
Mufarrij AA, Busaba NY, Zaytoun GM, Gallo GR & Feiner HD (1990). Primary localized amyloidosis of the nose and paranasal sinuses. A case report with immunohistochemical observations and a review of the literature. *Am J Surg Pathol.* Apr;14(4),pp. 379-83.
Nandapalan V, Jones TM, Morar P, Clark AH & Jones AS (1998). Localized amyloidosis of the parotid gland: a case report and review of the localized amyloidosis of the head and neck. *Head Neck.* Jan;20(1), pp. 73-8.
Neben-Wittich MA, Foote RL & Kalra S (2007). External beam radiation therapy for tracheobronchial amyloidosis. *Chest.* Jul;132(1),pp. 262-7.
Neuner GA, Badros AA, Meyer TK, Nanaji NM & Regine WF (2010). Complete resolution of laryngeal amyloidosis with radiation treatment. *Head Neck.* Nov 10. [Epub ahead of print]
Nguyen TU, Oghalai JS, McGregor DK, Janssen NM & Huston D (2001). Subcutaneous nodular amyloidosis: a case report and review of the literature. *Hum Pathol.* Mar;32(3):346-8.
O'Halloran LR & Lusk RP (1994). Amyloidosis of the larynx in a child. *Ann Otol Rhinol Laryngol;*108,pp. 339-40.
Özdemir İ, Öztürkcan S, Güvenç IA, Özkul Y, Başoğlu S & Etit D (2010). Localized Amyloidosis in the Nasopharynx and Neck: Case Report *Turkiye Klinikleri J Med Sci;* 30(1),pp. 421-4
Paccalin M, Hachulla E, Cazalet C, Tricot L, Carreiro M, Rubi M, Grateau G & Roblot P (2005). Localized amyloidosis: a survey of 35 French cases. *Amyloid.* Dec;12(4), pp. 239-45.
Panda NK, Saravanan K, Purushotaman GP, Gurunathan RK & Mahesha V (2007). Localized amyloidosis masquerading as nasopharyngeal tumor: a review. *Am J Otolaryngol.* May-Jun;28(3),pp. 208-11.

Pang KP, Chee LW & Busmanis I (2001). Amyloidoma of the nose in a pediatric patient: a case report *Am J Otolaryngol.* Mar-Apr;22(2),pp. 138-41.

Passerotti GH, Caniello M, Hachiya A, Santoro PP, Imamura R & Tsuji DH (2008). Multiple-sited amyloidosis in the upper aerodigestive tract: case report and literature review. *Braz J Otorhinolaryngol.* May-Jun;74(3):462-6.

Patel A, Pambuccian S & Maisel R (2002). Nasopharyngeal amyloidosis. *Am J Otolaryngol.* Sep-Oct;23(5),pp. 308-11.

Penner CR & Muller S (2006). Head and neck amyloidosis: a clinicopathologic study of 15 cases. *Oral Oncol.* Apr;42(4),pp. 421-9. Epub 2006 Feb 20.

Pentenero M, Davico Bonino L, Tomasini C, Conrotto D & Gandolfo S (2006). Localized oral amyloidosis of the palate. *Amyloid.* Mar;13(1)pp., 42-6.

Piazza C, Cavaliere S, Foccoli P, Toninelli C, Bolzoni A & Peretti G (2003). Endoscopic management of laryngo-tracheobronchial amyloidosis: a series of 32 patients. Eur Arch Otorhinolaryngol. Aug;260(7),pp. 349-54. Epub 2003 Feb 26.

Prasad D, Somayaji GK, Aroor R & Abdulla MN (2009). Primary nasal amyloidosis. *The Internet Journal of Otorhinolaryngology.* Volume 9 Number 2

Simpson GT 2nd, Strong MS, Skinner M & Cohen AS (1984). Localized amyloidosis of the head and neck and upper
aerodigestive and lower respiratory tracts. Ann Otol Rhinol Laryngol. Jul-Aug;93(4 Pt 1),pp. 374-9.

Sipe JD & Cohen AS (1998). Amyloidosis, In: *Harrison's Principles of International Medicine,* Fauci AS, Braunwald E, Isselbacher KJ, Wilson JD,Martin JB, Kasper DL, Hauser SL, Longo DL pp.1856-60, McGraw-Hill Companies, Inc., ISBN 0-07-115272-5, USA.

Shimauchi T, Shin JH & Tokura Y (2006). Primary cutaneous amyloidosis of the auricular concha: case report and review of published work. J Dermatol. Feb;33(2),pp. 128-31.

Stimson PG, Tortoledo ME, Luna MA & Ordõnez NG (1988). Localized primary amyloid tumor of the parotid gland. *Oral Surg Oral Med Oral Pathol.* Oct;66(4), pp. 466-9.

Teo DT, Lau DP & Sethi DS (2003). Recurrent localized sinonasal amyloidosis: A case report. *Otolaryngology- Head and Neck Surgery.* Aug; 129, pp. 270.

Tsikoudas A, Martin-Hirsch DP & Woodhead CJ (2001). Primary sinonasal amyloidosis. *J Laryngol Otol.* Jan;115(1),pp. 55-6.

Tsuji T, Yamasaki H, Sasho H, Arima N & Tsuda H (2008). Localized amyloidosis in the tonsil. *Rinsho Ketsueki.* Dec;49(12):1628-30.

Xu L, Cai BQ, Zhong X & Zhu YJ (2005). Respiratory manifestations in amyloidosis. *Chin Med J (Engl).* Dec 20;118(24),pp. 2027-33.

Yamaoka Y, Sukuki H, Hatakeyama S, Noda M, Hiraga M & Sekiyama S, (1978). Median rhomboid glossitis associated with amyloid deposition. *Acta Pathologica Japonica* 28,pp.319-323.

Yamazaki K, Sato H, Ishijima K, Abe T & Ishikawa K (2011). A case of hemodialysis-associated amyloidosis localized to the external auditory canal. *Auris Nasus Larynx.* Apr;38(2),pp. 295-9. Epub 2010 Oct 28.

Yiotakis I, Georgolios A, Charalabopoulos A, Hatzipantelis P, Golias C, Charalabopoulos K & Manolopoulos L (2009). Primary localized laryngeal amyloidosis presenting with hoarseness and dysphagia: a case report. *J Med Case Reports.* Sep 16;3,pp. 9049.

Zhuang YL, Tsai TL & Lin CZ (2005). Localized amyloid deposition in the nasopharynx and neck, mimicking nasopharyngeal carcinoma with neck metastasis. *Chin Med Assoc.* Mar;68(3),pp. 142-5.

9

Localized ENT Amyloidosis – Literature Overview

Bouthaina Hammami, Malek Mnejja, Moncef Sellami, Hanene Hadj Taieb, Adel Chakroun, Ilhem Charfeddine and Abdelmonem Ghorbel
Sfax Faculty of Medicine /Habib Bourguiba University Hospital
Tunisia

1. Introduction

Amyloidoses from a group of disorders characterized by extracellular tissue accumulation of amorphous hyaline material. They are categorized in two main forms: systemic and localized (Zhuang YL, 2005). Localized forms involve a single organ, whereas systemic amyloidosis involves multiple organ systems.

Localized forms often involve the head and neck. The aerodigestive tract is a common location, the nasopharynx or soft palate are rarely envaded (Panda NK, 2007) (Pitkäranta A, 2000).

The distinction between localized and systemic disease is important because localized amyloidosis can be managed conservatively with an excellent prognosis, whereas systemic amyloidosis is associated with significant morbidity and mortality (Kyle RA, 1975).

Although the pathogenesis is not completely understood, soluble protein subunits undergo a conformational change to become insoluble and aggregate in an antiparallel β-pleated sheet conformation (Panda NK, 2007). The diagnosis of amyloidosis is made based on Congo red staining on tissue biopsy which leads to apple-green birefringence on polarized microscopy (Patel A, 2002).

Amyloidomas are benign tumorlike lesions consisting of localized deposits of amyloid and are the rarest form in the group of amyloidosis-related lesions (Parmar H, 2010).

Amyloidosis should not be considered as a single clinical entity, but rather as a nonhomogeneous group of diseases characterized by the common presence of a fibrillar structure of linear, aggregated fibers with a cross β-pleated sheet conformation, and evidenced by x-ray diffraction. In primary amyloidosis, a monoclonal population of marrow cells produces either fragments of light chains that may be processed to form amyloid. Secondary amyloidosis is characterized by a defect in the metabolism of the precursor protein (Comenzo RL, 2006).

Our objective is to study the epidemioloclinical characteristics of ENT amyloidosis and the management of those localizations.

2. Study method

Data Sources a systematic literature search of MEDLINE, SCIENCEDIRECT and Web of Science Review Database from 2000 to 2010 was conducted using specific search terms: head and neck amyloidosis, localized amyloidosis, ENT Diseases, hypopharynx, larynx, oral cavity, oropharynx, nasopharynx and sinonasal cavities.

We considered thirty-three articles for our review and including a total of 43 patients.
Exclusion criteria were: systemic amyloidosis, a concomitant history of chronic inflammatory processes, monoclonal gammopathy and myeloma.

3. Epidemiology

Localized amyloidosis is characterized by the same staining properties as systemic amyloidosis but is usually fortuitously diagnosed.
The majority of patients with head and neck amyloidosis have no underlying chronic systemic disease (primary form).
Nasal or nasopharyngeal amyloidosis is a very rare condition with few case reports seen in the English scientific literature. Both sexes may be affected, with a great variation in age of disease onset (8–86 years old). Laryngeal involvement in amyloidosis is rare and accounts for less than 1% of all benign laryngeal tumors. It usually occurs in the 40–60 years age range with a male to female predominance of about 2:1 (Gallivan GJ, 2010).

3.1 Age and sex

The mean age of patients considered in our review was 52,36 years with ages ranging from 10 to 86 years; 21 were male and 22 were female.

3.2 Localization

This literature review identified 33 articles describing a total of 43 cases of localized head and neck amyloidosis, summarized in Table 1.

Localization	Number of cases	Mean age	Male	Female
Larynx	12	47,5	6	6
Nasopharynx	7	55,5	4	3
Tongue	6	58	4	2
Palate	4	66,7	1	3
Trachea	3	52,3	2	1
Hypopharynx	3	55,3	0	3
Sinonasal cavities	2	32,5	0	2
Oropharynx	1	12	0	1
Tonsil	1	71	1	0
Ear	1	47	1	0
Cervical lymph nodes	3	60	2	1

Table 1. Epidemiological characteristics of localized amyloidosis

Localized amyloidosis is an uncommon benign disorder which occurs most commonly in the head and neck region.

Among the sites, larynx is affected most frequently (61%), followed by oropharynx (23%), trachea (9%), and orbit (4%) (Glenner GG, 1980) (Scott PP, 1986). Only 3% of cases occur in the nasopharynx (Glenner GG, 1980) (Scott PP, 1986). In the larynx, the most commonly involved sites are the vestibular fold, followed by the subglotis, ventricle, vocal folds, and aryepiglottic folds.

Chin *et al.* reported a case of localized amyloidosis involving simultaneously the sinonasal cavities and the larynx (Chin SC, 2004).

Localized amyloidosis of the nasal mucosa is extremely rare with few cases reported in the English literature (Pearlman AN, 2010).

Localized amyloidosis of the palate is extremely rare and only five cases have been reported (Aono J, 2009).

Amyloidosis of Waldeyer's ring has been also described (Walker PA, 1996).

The hypopharyngeal involvement is extremely rare: extensive search of the literature retrieved only 3 primitive localized hypopharyngeal amyloidosis (Ghekiere O, 2003) (Bhavani RS, 2010) (Penner CR, 2006).

Amyloidosis in the external auditory canal is extremely rare. Indeed, only 13 cases have been reported worldwide to date (Yamazaki K, 2011).

Only two cases report of localized amyloidosis of the parotid glands were described in the literature (Stimson PG, 1988) (Nandapalan V, 1998).

No case of localized submandibular amyloidosis has been reported.

Kurokawa (Kurokawa H, 1998) reported the first case of primary localized of the sublingual gland.

4. Clinical features

There are currently 3 known forms of amyloidosis.

The first, primary systemic amyloidosis is a systemic condition with no known underlying cause. It is different from the secondary systemic amyloidosis, which occurs with other underlying medical problems, such as tuberculosis and rheumatoid arthritis. And this form also includes patients with multiple myeloma, of which 10% to 20% have associated amyloidosis (Kyle RA, 1975) (Gertz MA, 2005). Renal and cardiac diseases are seen in both primary and secondary systemic forms and are the most frequent causes of death (Kyle RA, 1975). Other symptoms may include hypesthesias, syncope, macroglossia, and carpal tunnel syndrome. The third form of amyloidosis is localized and which occurs without any evidence of systemic involvement or underlying disease.

In a review of 236 cases of amyloidosis, Kyle and Bayrd (Kyle RA, 1975) found that only 22 cases (9%) were localized. None of these patients developed systemic disease in a 10-year follow-up. Similarly, in the University of California, Los Angeles series, localized amyloidosis did not evolve to primary or secondary systemic amyloidosis or multiple myeloma (Kerner MM, 1995).

Localized amyloidosis is a clinical entity with variable presentation, depending on the organs involved.

Clinically, amyloidosis can manifest in several different forms: primary versus secondary, heredofamilial versus acquired, and generalized versus localized.

The most frequent types encountered in clinical practice are the amyloid light chain (AL, primary) and a protein called the AA protein (secondary), both of which might involve multiple organ systems (kidney, heart, and liver). In our literature review we analyzed the articles about localized amyloidosis

Isolated deposition of fibrillar proteins in an organ may result in organ-specific syndromes (e.g. Alzheimer's disease and primary localized amyloidosis of the bladder) (Malek RS, 2002). In the head and neck region, the most common site of amyloid depositions is the larynx, and other sites include the orbit, skin, tongue, salivary glands and cervical lymph nodes (Pribitkin E, 2003).

The presentation of head and neck amyloidosis varies according to the site of involvement. A patient can present with nasal obstruction, epistaxis (due to vessel wall invasion), glue ear, dysphagia, foreign body sensation in the throat, and voice change, but most of the cases of oropharyngeal amyloid are asymptomatic (Mufarrij AA, 1990).

They will appear as yellowish mucosa, covered, and irregular polypoidal lesions (Mufarrij AA, 1990).

4.1 Sino-nasal and nasopharyngeal amyloidosis

The presenting symptoms consist of nasal obstruction, recurrent epistaxis, postnasal drip and ear problems due to eustachian tube obstruction with resultant middle ear effusion (Pang KP, 2001) (Patel A, 2002).

Facial pain can be seen in amyloidosis of the maxillary antrum (MCALPINE JC, 1964).

Occasionally, it may manifest as a clinical picture simulating an apparent malignancy with cervical nodal metastasis (Zhuang YL, 2005).

Generally, the appearance is described as a yellowish or whitish polypoid, firm mass.

Macroscopically, organs infiltrated with amyloid have a characteristic firm, rubbery firm consistency, but may also be nodular-like or irregular, mimicking neoplasm. A waxy, gray or yellowish appearance is also typical (Pribitkin E, 2003).

Geller *et al* (Geller E, 2010) reported the first case of localized nasopharyngeal amyloidosis causing bilateral nasolacrimal duct obstruction.

This localization has usually a slow evolution.

4.2 Larynx

Laryngeal amyloidosis remains a rare entity accounting for about 1% of all benign laryngeal tumors. Within the larynx, a number of sites can be involved including ventricular folds (55%), laryngeal ventricle (36%), subglottic space (36%), vocal folds (27%), aryepiglottic folds (23%) and anterior commissure (14%) (Passerotti GH, 2008).

Clinical manifestations are hoarseness, dyspnea, cough, stridor, and rarely, hemoptysis. (Finn DG, 1982)

The lesion is usually a firm, nonulcerated yellow, orange, or gray submucosal nodule, mass or pedunculated polypoid lesion.

It is rare for vocal fold fixation or cicatricial stenosis to occur unless other predisposing factors are also present (Caldarelli DD, 1979). A cystic lesion (Talbot AR, 1979) or infiltrating tumor of the vocal folds and subglottis, multinodular subglottic, tracheal, mainstem bronchial and pulmonary deposits may occur (Simpson GT 2nd, 1984).

4.3 Tracheobronchial

Respiratory symptoms may vary according to the anatomic deposition of amyloid (Gillmore JD, 1999). Patients with upper tracheal or proximal airway disease develop varying degrees of airway obstruction. They have worse prognosis than those with distal airway involvement (Utz JP, 1996).

Common presenting symptoms are dyspnea, cough, and wheezing. These symptoms are not specific and may mimic different pathologies, such as asthma, chronic bronchitis, and endobronchial tumor. Those with distal tracheal and bronchial disease may have atelectasis, recurrent pneumonias, or bronchiectasis (Thompson PJ, 1983).

4.4 Hypopharynx and upper esophagus

The presenting symptoms consist of progressive dysphagia to both solids and liquids.
Nasofibroscopy and endoscopy found salivary stasis in the pyriform sinus with regular swelling with normal mucosa amyloidosis (Ghekiere O, 2003) (Bhavani RS, 2010).

4.5 Oral cavity

Amyloid involvement of tongue is almost always secondary to systemic amyloidosis and localized involvement is extremely rare (Fahrner KS, 2004).
Oral amyloidosis usually appears as multiple soft nodules, sometimes hemorrhagic, which can cause macroglossia (Asaumi J, 2001). Alternatively the nodular masses may resemble benign tumors such as granular cell tumors, schwannomas, neurofibromas and neuromas (Muto T, 1991).
Yellow nodules or raised white lesions occurring predominately along the lateral border are also common.
Sometimes petechiae, ecchymoses and hemorrhagic blisters can also be observed (van der Waal RI, 2002).
Primary localized amyloidosis of the palate is extremely rare and only a few cases have been reported (Balatsouras DG, 2007) (Stoor P, 2004) (Alvi A, 1999).
This type of lesion tends to spread locally and occasionally may result in bleeding, epistaxis, and middle ear effusion.

4.6 Cervical lymph nodes

Few documented cases of isolated amyloidosis of cervical lymph nodes have been reported (Shi Q, 2000) (Bielsa S, 2005).

4.7 Amyloid goiter

Amyloid goiter is a rare pathology due to massive amyloid infiltration of thyroid tissue, which causes diffuse or localized enlargement of the gland. It can be totally asymptomatic or causes only non-specific symptoms (compression of adjacent structures, tracheal deviation). Thyroid dysfunction (hypothyroidism or hyperthyroidism) is rare (Cavallaro G, 2006).

4.8 Ear

Physical examination demonstrates brownish or red mass that occupied ear canal, eventually blocked the visualization of the tympanic membrane associated with conductive hearing loss in tone audiometry (Yamazaki K, 2011).
It's like an otitis externa that did not respond to local treatment.

5. Diagnosis

Localized amyloid tumors in the head and neck region are an extremely rare manifestation that is not usually associated with either multiple myeloma or systemic amyloidosis (Godbersen GS, 1992).

Amyloidosis is a disease complex resulting in the extracellular deposition of waxy insoluble fibrillar protein material called "amyloid." It was first described by Rokitansky in 1842 (Rokitansky K, 1842). Amyloid consists of relatively insoluble fibrils composed of polypeptide chains arranged in a twisted ß-pleated sheet configuration. This particular protein configuration accounts for its characteristic staining properties and permits identification by light microscopy. It imparts unique chemical properties like resistance to protease digestion and insolubility, which promote continued deposition within organs.
Therefore a biopsy from the head and neck that reveals amyloid necessitates evaluation for systemic involvement either by rectal biopsy (75% positive) or fat aspiration of the anterior abdominal wall (90% positive) (Nandapalan V, 1998). The absence of Congo red staining of biopsy specimens from either of these 2 sites establishes that the amyloidosis is not systemic (Simpson GT 2nd, 1984). Specific organ involvement may also be excluded by laboratory or radiologic studies (Nandapalan V, 1998).
While amyloid can be suspected on routine hematoxylin-eosin sections, special stains are important for definitive diagnosis. With the polarized microscope, amyloid is seen to have a green birefringence when stained with Congo red.
The etiology, treatment, and outcome of systemic amyloidosis are totally different from localized amyloidosis. The mean survival of patients with systemic amyloidosis is between 5 to 15 months, whereas patients with localized amyloidosis have excellent prognosis (Fahrner KS, 2004).
Final diagnosis relied on histopathological analysis of endonasal endoscopic biopsy samples taken under local or general anesthesia (Yakoot A, 2010).
Histopathological examination showed eosinophil areas, staining positively on Congo red (expressing birefringence under polarized light and on thioflavin) (Yakoot A, 2010).
These histologic features indicated a diagnosis of amyloidosis without signs of underlying malignancy (no abnormalities on general check-up).
On Congo red staining, green birefringence is revealed under polarized light, and electron microscopy shows 8–10-nm wide, straight, and unbranching fibrils.

6. Radiology

The computed tomography (CT) provides excellent information on the anatomic location and topography of different laryngeal benign lesions (Aspestrand F, 1989) but cannot be used to differentiate inflammatory masses from benign neoplasms.
Computed tomography scans demonstrate focal amyloidosis as a well-defined, submucosal, homogeneous, hyperdense, soft tissue mass in association with calcifications (Gean-Marton AD, 1991) (Panda NK, 2007) (Pitkäranta A, 2000).
The lesions are described as well-defined homogeneous soft-tissue masses, with no or only a slight degree of contrast enhancement (Godbersen GS, 1992).
Occasionally, areas of localized calcification within the mass are present (Hegarty JL, 1993) (Parmar H, 2010).
Although the amyloidosis does not generally induce osteolysis, one case of nasopharyngeal amyloidosis with sinus extension and bone destruction suggestive of malignancy has been reported (Zhuang YL, 2005).
MRI is considered as the technique of choice for diagnosis, showing characteristic aspects: intermediate T1-weighted signal and T2-weighted hyposignal, as in striated muscle, without modification in fat-suppression sequences (Zhuang YL, 2005). This signal pattern is due to the amyloid protein deposits, which are fibrillar as in striated muscle fiber (Gilad R, 2007).

The laryngeal lesion reveals intensity equal to that of surrounding muscles on T1 and remains isointense or slightly hyperintense on T2. In comparison, chondrosarcoma of the larynx is hypo- to isointense on T1 and hyperintense on T2, which parallels the appearance of mature hyaline cartilage. Therefore, T2 signal-intensity characteristics might help differentiate amyloidoma from chondrosarcoma.
Following administration of a contrast agent, the lesion exhibits slight or no enhancement. A "fluffy" appearance of bones surrounding the lesion has been shown, which is thought to result from an osteoblastic reaction provoked by submucosal deposition of amyloid fibrils (Chin SC, 2004).
MRI studies show a submucosal mass with low signal intensity in both T1- and T2-weighted images, and mild enhancement in postcontrast T1-weighted images. However, Motosugi *et al.* (Motosugi U, 2007) reported a case of localized nasopharyngeal amyloidosis which showed high signal intensity on T2-weighted images and marked early enhancement in the periphery of the mass on dynamic contrast-enhanced MRI. This phenomenon was attributed to plasmacyte infiltration which occasionally occurs with amyloidosis, leading to hypervascularity.
The exact mechanism underlying the signal hypointensity of amyloid in T2-weighted images is unknown. There are 3 possible mechanisms described (Gean-Marton AD, 1991): (1) signal loss results from enhanced T2 decay because of the presence of static or slowly fluctuating internal magnetic fields within adjacent amyloid proteins held in fixed positions within the folded protein; (2) rapid chemical exchange and spin-spin interactions may occur between the amyloid protein and adjacent water molecules; and (3) because the amyloid microenvironment is composed of a heterogeneous micromagnetic mixture of collagen, calcification, and vessels as well as the amyloid fibrils, the T2 hypointensity may result from differences in diamagnetic susceptibility (Gean-Marton AD, 1991).

7. Differential diagnosis

7.1 Systemic amyloidosis

Localized amyloidosis has been described in nearly every organ system. Development of systemic disease following a diagnosis of localized amyloidosis was rare, occurring in 2% of cases. One-quarter of patients with primary systemic amyloidosis presents with clinical involvement of only one organ, but investigation leads to the recognition of widespread involvement (Merlini G, 2003).

7.2 Larynx

In the larynx, the amyloid deposits are submucosal and homogeneous and are not associated with the cartilage changes.
They are firm lesions that tend to occur in the supraglottic larynx, although all laryngeal sites may be affected.
The differential diagnosis includes other submucosal diseases such as laryngeal sarcoidosis, lymphoma, and pseudotumor.

7.3 Tracheobronchial

Wegener's granulomatosis, laryngotracheobronchial papillomatosis, idiopathic laryngotracheal stenosis, sarcoidosis, or tracheobronchitis with ulcerative colitis may radiologically mimic tracheobronchial amyloidosis.

7.4 Tongue

There is a wide differential diagnosis that should be considered in patients presenting with macroglossia or nodular tongue lesions.

For generalized macroglossia, amyloid, tuberculosis, lymphangioma, hypothyroidism, acromegaly, lingual infarction caused by giant-cell arteritis, idiopathic muscular hypertrophy, and Beckwith-Wiedemann syndrome should be considered.

For nodular lesions, fibroma, lipoma, granular cell tumor, sarcoma, lingual thyroid. and salivary gland tumors would be among the differential.

7.5 Palate

The differential diagnosis includes candidiasis, vascular lesions and Kaposi's sarcoma.

7.6 Amyloid goiter

Microscopic infiltration of the thyroid gland by amyloid is an uncommon but well recognized phenomenon and significant enlargement of the thyroid due to deposition of amyloid is rarely seen. This condition has to be distinguished from other types of goiters and at times from malignancy.

Amyloid goiter may be diagnosed by cytopuncture (Kapadia HC, 2001), although there is a problem of differential diagnosis with medullary carcinoma, where amyloid deposit is also found in 50% to 80% of cases.

However, cytopuncture excludes other thyroid cancers, notably anaplastic cancer and lymphoma.

Anatomopathology enables positive diagnosis in case of amyloid deposit detected in the form of an amorphous substance showing yellow-green double refraction under polarized light on Congo red staining.

7.7 Sino-nasal and nasopharyngeal amyloidosis

The differential diagnosis for lesion within the maxillary antrum includes malignant conditions such as squamous cell carcinoma, lymphoma, metastatic disease, plasmacytoma, melanoma, neuroblastoma, paraganglionoma and haemangiopericytoma, benign lesions including hamartoma, and local fungal infections such as mucormycosis and aspergilloma (Birchall D, 1997).

Although amyloidoma of the nose is rare, it should be considered as part of the differential diagnosis of a nasal mass presenting with nasal obstruction and epistaxis, even in pediatric patients. The approach should include a scan to exclude a possible vascular tumor, the as the appearance may be fleshy.

Because of its infrequent occurrence, nasopharyngeal amyloidosis is rarely considered in the differential diagnosis of nasopharyngeal tumor (Panda NK, 2007). Initial endoscopic examination in the present case was rather suggestive of adipose tumor.

8. Treatment

In systemic disease, high-dose chemotherapy followed by stem cell reconstitution seems to provide the most effective treatment (Gertz MA, 2005).

The localized amyloidosis has excellent prognosis and never evolves towards systemic forms (Pitkäranta A, 2000). Hence, it may be treated with surgical excision (Stoor P, 2004) , especially to reduce local soft palate mass (Zhuang YL, 2005) (Pitkäranta A, 2000).

Certain reports consider surgery for nasopharyngeal forms to be merely palliative (Stoor P, 2004). In case of recurrence, surgical revision may be recommenced, depending on symptomatology.
For localized amyloidosis, symptomatic removal is required. But, close follow-up is necessary because the recurrence rate reported is as high as 50%.

8.1 Sinonasal cavities and nasopharynx

For localized amyloidosis of the nasopharynx, surgical resection is usually chosen as the treatment modality for symptomatic relief. However, the extent of surgical excision has changed from radical excision to a more conservative approach.
The rationale behind this alteration is that a conservative surgical approach may be associated with a slower rate of recurrence (Lesserman JA FD, 1995). Unfortunately, failure to prevent recurrence by means of surgical excision has been found in the majority of case reports. Simpson *et al.* (Simpson GT 2nd, 1984) have suggested a reduction in the recurrence rate following laser resection.
Emerging treatment approaches employing agents that disrupt fibril formation, destabilize amyloid deposits, or interfere with interaction between amyloidogenic proteins and accessory molecules have shown promising results in animal models, and clinical applications are underway (Lachmann HJ, 2003).
The surgical treatment must be done in case of airway obstruction, bleeding, and other severe symptoms.
Radiotherapy may be a treatment option in nasal and nasopharyngeal amyloidosis.
Symptoms may be improved with steroid treatment (Pearlman AN, 2010).

8.2 Larynx

It is important to treat laryngeal amyloidosis because untreated cases can progress to vocal fold fixation, severe dysphonia, and airway obstruction. Alternatively, "expectant" management with no intervention may be indicated in certain carefully selected cases, owing to the slow progression of the disease over many years (Avitia S, 2007).
In isolated laryngeal amyloidosis, treatment is primarily endoscopic surgical removal of masses that interfere with laryngeal or airway function. The likelihood of recurrent or residual disease is significant (Talbot AR, 1979).
Because of the propensity of amyloid to infiltrate blood vessels, cold resection of amyloid lesions may be complicated by bleeding. Although CO2 laser excision may be advantageous, if used in very extensive lesions, there may be scarring (Talbot AR, 1979) (Simpson GT 2nd, 1984).
In very large lesions, external approaches, employing laryngofissure for treatment of diffuse subglottic and tracheal amyloidosis have been used. Repeated excision and curettage may be necessary to achieve stabilization of lesions and subsequent decannulation of those patients who are tracheotomy dependent.
Local or systemic steroids are ineffective in controlling or reversing lesions of amyloidosis (Finn DG, 1982).
Bartels *et al* (Bartels H, 2004) found five patients over a period of 13 years who had localized laryngeal amyloidosis and free light chains were found in one patient. Amyloid interfering with laryngeal or airway function was excised during microlaryngoscopy. Cold endoscopic excision for glottic deposits and CO2 laser for supraglottic lesions provided best results. Four patients developed recurrent disease.

Localization	Number of cases	Surgery	Phonosurgery or laser treatment	IMRT	External beam radiation (45 Gy)	Tracheostomy	Tympanostomy tube	Steroid	Supervision
Larynx	12	0	9	2	1				
Nasopharynx	7	4					1		2
Tongue	6	3	1						2
Palate	4	1							3
Trachea	3						1		2
Hypopharynx	3	1							
Sinonasal cavities	2	1						1	
Oropharynx	1								1
Tonsil	1								
Ear	1								
Cervical lymph nodes	3								

IMRT: Intensity Modulated Radiotherapy

Table 2. Distribution by the therapeutic procedure

Dedo and Izdebski (Dedo HH, 2004) reported 10 consecutive laryngeal amyloid patients in whom amyloid was found on the undersurface of both vocal folds in two and submucosally in unilateral or bilateral vestibular folds in eight cases. Direct microlaryngoscopy with CO2

laser excision was done on one side at a time to try to prevent anterior commissure scarring. Followup after the first operation was 6 months to 16 years, with an average of 6.5 years. Four vestibular fold patients required re-excision on the same side after the first operation. Because full resection is difficult, Neuner GA (Neuner GA, 2010) recommends a combination of surgery and radiation therapy to cure localized amyloidosis of the larynx.
Other treatments options that have been described include corticosteroids, radiotherapy, and agents like colchicine and melphalan. However, these modalities have yielded variable results (Avitia S, 2007).

8.3 Trachea

The management is dependent on symptoms. Treatment options are bronchoscopic approaches, surgery, radiation, and observation. Therapy may not be required for asymptomatic patients. Cases with proximal airway obstruction are difficult to manage.
Bronchoscopic methods are mechanical debulking, endobronchial laser ablation, and stent or balloon dilatation in selected patients with stenosis. These methods are preferable and safer than surgery. However, such methods may be ineffective and repeated procedures may be required (Gillmore JD, 1999) (O'Regan A, 2000). Bleeding is a common complication of these procedures.
Sometimes external beam radiation or surgical resection is necessary (Neben-Wittich MA, 2007).

8.4 Oral cavity

The definitive treatment of localized amyloidosis was cited to be surgery. Surgery alone may be 100% curative (Fahrner KS, 2004).

8.5 Cervical lymph node

There is no specific treatment for this uncommon entity (Bielsa S, 2005). The cervical lymph nodes dissection may be done (Shi Q, 2000).

8.6 Amyloid goiter

Fine-needle aspiration biopsy can be performed to exclude malignant lesions. In order to diagnose amyloid goiter, definitively thyroidectomy is often necessary. Surgical intervention is indicated either for aesthetic purposes or to relieve the pressure symptoms (Villa F, 2008).

9. Conclusion

Amyloidosis is a rare disease with multifactorial pathogenesis.
Localized amyloidosis affecting the head and neck region is an uncommon and benign process, which has almost no clinical consequences. Once the diagnosis has been made, an extensive workup for systemic amyloidosis should be undertaken. This should include abdominal fat biopsy or rectal biopsy.

10. References

Alvi A, Goldstein MN. (1999). Amyloidosis of the palate. *Otolaryngol Head Neck Sur*, 120, 2, (1999), pp. 287.

Aono J, Yamagata K & Yoshida H. (2009). Local amyloidosis in the hard palate: a case report. *Oral Maxillofac Surg,* 13, 2, (2009), pp. 119-22.
Asaumi J, Yanagi Y & Hisatomi M. (2001). CT and MR imaging of localized amyloidosis. *Eur J Radiol.*, 39, 2, (2001), pp. 83-7.
Aspestrand F, Kolbenstvedt A & Boysen M. (1989). CT findings in benign expansions of the larynx. *J Comput Assist Tomogr,* 13, 2, (1989), pp. 222-5.
Avitia S, Hamilton JS & Osborne RF. (2007). Surgical rehabilitation for primary laryngeal amyloidosis. *Ear Nose Throat J,* 86, 4, (2007), pp. 206- 208.
Balatsouras DG, Eliopoulos P & Assimakopoulos D. (2007). Primary local amyloidosis of the palate. *Otolaryngol Head Neck Surg,* 137, 2, (2007), pp 348-9.
Bartels H, Dikkers FG & van der Wal JE. (2004). Laryngeal amyloidosis: localized versus systemic disease and update on diagnosis and therapy. *Ann Otol Rhinol Laryngol,* 113, 9, (2004), pp. 741-8.
Bhavani RS, Lakhtakia S & Sekaran A. (2010). Amyloidosis presenting as postcricoid esophageal stricture. *Gastrointest Endosc,* 71, 1, (2010), pp. 180-1, discussion 181.
Bielsa S, Jover A & Porcel JM. (2005). Isolated lymph node amyloidosis. *Eur J Intern Med,* 16, 8, (2005), pp. 619.
Birchall D, Fields JM & Poon CL. (1997). Case report: focal amyloidosis of the maxillary antrum: plain film, CT and MR appearances. *Clin Radiol.* 52, 5, (1997), pp.392-4.
Caldarelli DD, Friedberg SA & Harris AA. (1979). Medical and surgical aspects of the granulomatous diseases of the larynx. *Otolaryngol Clin North Am,* 12, 4, (1979) pp. 767-81.
Cavallaro G, Polistena A & Fornari F. (2006). A case of primitive amyloid goiter. *G Chir,* 27, 8-9, (2006), pp. 315-7.
Chin SC, Fatterpeckar G & Kao CH. (2004). Amyloidosis concurrently involving the sinonasal cavities and larynx. *AJNR Am J Neuroradiol,* 25, 4, (2004), pp. 636-8.
Comenzo RL. (2006). Amyloidosis. *Curr Treat Options Oncol,* 7, 3, (2006), 225-36.
Dedo HH, Izdebski K. (2004). Laryngeal amyloidosis in 10 patients. *Laryngoscope,* 114, 10, (2004), pp. 1742-6.
Fahrner KS, Black CC & Gosselin BJ. (2004). Localized amyloidosis of the tongue: a review. *Am J Otolaryngol,* 25, 3, (2004), pp. 186-9.
Finn DG, Farmer JC Jr. (1982). Management of amyloidosis of the larynx and trachea. *Arch Otolaryngol,* 108, 1, (1982), pp. 54-6.
Gallivan GJ, Gallivan HK. (2010). Laryngeal amyloidosis causing hoarseness and airway obstruction. *J Voice,* 24, 2, (2010), pp. 235-9.
Gean-Marton AD, Kirsch CF & Vezina LG. (1991). Focal amyloidosis of the head and neck: evaluation with CT and MR imaging. *Radiology,* 81, 2, (1991), pp. 521-5.
Geller E, Freitag SK & Laver NV. (2010). Localized Nasopharyngeal Amyloidosis Causing Bilateral Nasolacrimal Duct Obstruction, *Ophthal Plast Reconstr Surg,* [Epub ahead of print].
Gertz MA, Lacy MQ & Dispenzieri A. (2005). Amyloidosis: diagnosis and management. *Clin Lymphoma Myeloma,* 6, 3, (2005), pp. 208-19.
Ghekiere O, Desuter G & Weynand B. (2003). Hypopharyngeal amyloidoma. *AJR Am J Roentgenol* 2003, 181, 6, (2003), pp. 1720-1.
Gilad R, Milillo P & Som PM. (2007). Severe diffuse systemic amyloidosis with involvement of the pharynx, larynx, and trachea: CT and MR findings. *AJNR Am J Neuroradiol,* 28, 8, (2007) pp. 1557-8.
Gillmore JD, Hawkins PN. (1999). Amyloidosis and the respiratory tract. *Thorax,* 54, 5, (1999) pp. 444-51.

Glenner GG. (1980). Amyloid deposits and amyloidosis: the beta-fibrilloses (second of two parts). *N Engl J Med,* 302, 24, (1980), pp. 1333-43.

Godbersen GS, Leh JF & Hansmann ML. (1992). Organ-limited laryngeal amyloid deposits: clinical, morphological, and immunohistochemical results of five cases. *Ann Otol Rhinol Laryngol,* 101, 9, (1992), pp. 770-5.

Hegarty JL, Rao VM. (1993). Amyloidoma of the nasopharynx: CT and MR findings. *AJNR Am J Neuroradiol* , 14, 1, (1993), pp. 215-8.

Kapadia HC, Desai RI & Desai IM. (2001). Amyloid goiter--a case report. *Indian J Pathol Microbiol,* 44, 2, (2001), pp. 147-8.

Kerner MM, Wang MB & Angier G. (1995). Amyloidosis of the head and neck. A clinicopathologic study of the UCLA experience, 1955-1991. *Arch Otolaryngol Head Neck Surg,* 121, 7, (1995), pp. 778-82.

Kurokawa H, Takuma C & Tokudome S. (1998). Primary localization amyloidosis of the sublingual gland. *Fukuoka Igaku Zasshi,* 89, 7, (1998), pp. 216-20.

Kyle RA, Bayrd ED. (1975). Amyloidosis: review of 236 cases. *Medicine (Baltimore),* 54, 4, (1975), pp. 271-99.

Lachmann HJ, Hawkins PN. (2003). Novel pharmacological strategies in amyloidosis. *Nephron Clin Pract,* 94, 4, (2003), pp. c85-8.

Lesserman JA FD. (1995). Endoscopic treatment of amyloidosis of the nasopharynx. *Am J Rhinol,* 9, (1995), pp. 43–7.

Lewis JE, Olsen KD & Kurtin PJ. (1992). Laryngeal amyloidosis: a clinicopathologic and immunohistochemical review. *Otolaryngol Head Neck Surg,* 106, 4, (1992), pp. 372-7.

Malek RS, Wahner-Roedler DL & Gertz MA. (2002). Primary localized amyloidosis of the bladder: experience with dimethyl sulfoxide therapy. *J Urol,* 168, 3, (2002), pp. 1018-20.

Mcalpine JC, Fuller AP. (1964). Localized Laryngeal Amyloidosis, A Report Of A Case With A Review Of The Literature. *J Laryngol Otol,* 78, (1964), pp. 296-314.

Merlini G, Bellotti V. (2003). Molecular mechanisms of amyloidosis. *N Engl J Med,* 349, 6, (2003), pp. 583-96.

Motosugi U, Ichikawa T & Araki T. (2007). Localized nasopharyngeal amyloidosis with remarkable early enhancement on dynamic contrast-enhanced MR imaging. *Eur Radiol,* 17, 3, (2007), pp. 852-3.

Mufarrij AA, Busaba NY & Zaytoun GM. (1990). Primary localized amyloidosis of the nose and paranasal sinuses. A case report with immunohistochemical observations and a review of the literature. *Am J Surg Pathol,* 14, 4, (1990), pp. 379-83.

Muto T, Sato K & Lutcavage GJ. (1991). Multiple nodules of the lip, cheeks, and tongue. *J Oral Maxillofac Surg.* 49, 9, (1991), pp. 1003-6.

Nandapalan V, Jones TM & Morar P. (1998). Localized amyloidosis of the parotid gland: a case report and review of the localized amyloidosis of the head and neck. *Head Neck,* 20, 1, (1998), pp. 73-8.

Neben-Wittich MA, Foote RL & Kalra S. (2007). External beam radiation therapy for tracheobronchial amyloidosis. *Chest,* 132, 1, (2007), pp.262-7.

Neuner GA, Badros AA & Meyer TK. (2010). Complete resolution of laryngeal amyloidosis with radiation treatment. *Head Neck,* (2010), [Epub ahead of print].

O'Regan A, Fenlon HM & Beamis JF Jr. (2000). Tracheobronchial amyloidosis. The Boston University experience from 1984 to 1999. *Medicine (Baltimore),* 79, 2, (2000) pp. 69-79.

Panda NK, Saravanan K & Purushotaman GP. (2007). Localized amyloidosis masquerading as nasopharyngeal tumor: a review. *Am J Otolaryngol,* 28, 3, (2007), pp. 208-11.

Pang KP, Chee LW & Busmanis I. (2001). Amyloidoma of the nose in a pediatric patient: a case report. *Am J Otolaryngol,* 22, 2, (2001), pp. 138-41.

Parmar H, Rath T & Castillo M. (2010). Imaging of focal amyloid depositions in the head, neck, and spine: amyloidoma. *AJNR Am J Neuroradiol,* 31, 7, (2010), pp. 1165-70.

Passerotti GH, Caniello M & Hachiya A. (2008). Multiple-sited amyloidosis in the upper aerodigestive tract: case report and literature review. *Braz J Otorhinolaryngol,* 74, 3, (2008), pp.462-6.

Patel A, Pambuccian S & Maisel R. (2002). Nasopharyngeal amyloidosis. *Am J Otolaryngol.* 23, 5, (2002), pp. 308-11.

Pearlman AN, Jeffe JS & Zynger DL. (2010). Localized amyloidosis of the nasal and paranasal mucosa: a rare pathology. *Am J Otolaryngol,* 31, 2, (2010) pp. 130-1.

Penner CR, Muller S. 2006. Head and neck amyloidosis: a clinicopathologic study of 15 cases. *Oral Oncol,* 42,4, (2006), pp.421-9.

Pitkäranta A, Malmberg H. (2000). Localized amyloid tumor of the nasopharynx. *Otolaryngol Head Neck Surg,* 122, 2, (2000) pp. 309-10.

Pribitkin E, Friedman O & O'Hara B. (2003). Amyloidosis of the upper aerodigestive tract. *Laryngoscope,* 113, 12, (2003), pp. 2095-101.

Rokitansky K. (1842). Handbuch der Pathologischen Anatomie. *Vienna, Austria: Braunmuller and Seide,* 311, (1842) pp. 384–424.

Scott PP, Scott WW Jr & Siegelman SS. (1986). Amyloidosis: an overview. *Semin Roentgenol,* 21, 2, (1986), pp. 103-12.

Shi Q, Fan K & Chen H. (2000). Localized amyloidosis of cervical lymph nodes. *Chin Med J,* 113, 2, (2000), pp.184-5.

Simpson GT 2nd, Strong MS & Skinner M. (1984). Localized amyloidosis of the head and neck and upper aerodigestive and lower respiratory tracts. *Ann Otol Rhinol Laryngol.* 93, (4 Pt 1), (1984), pp. 374-9.

Stimson PG, Tortoledo ME & Luna MA. (1988). Localized primary amyloid tumor of the parotid gland. *Oral Surg Oral Med Oral Pathol,* 66, 4, (1988), pp. 466-9.

Stoor P, Suuronen R & Lindqvist C. (2004). Local primary (AL) amyloidosis in the palate. A case report. *Int J Oral Maxillofac Surg,* 33, 4, (2004), pp. 402-3.

Talbot AR . (1979). Laryngeal amyloidosis. *Otolaryngol Clin North Am,* 12, 4, (1979), pp. 767-81.

Thompson PJ, Citron KM. (1983). Amyloid and the lower respiratory tract. *Thorax,* 38, 2, (1983), pp. 84-7.

Utz JP, Swensen SJ & Gertz MA. (1996). Pulmonary amyloidosis. The Mayo Clinic experience from 1980 to 1993. *Ann Intern Med,* 15, 124, 4, (1996), pp.407-13.

Van Der Waal RI, Van De Scheur MR & Huijgens PC. (2002). Amyloidosis of the tongue as a paraneoplastic marker of plasma cell dyscrasia. *Oral Surg Oral Med Oral Pathol Oral Radiol Endod,* 94, 4, (2002), pp. 444-7.

Villa F, Dionigi G & Tanda ML. (2008). Amyloid goiter. *Int J Surg,* 6, Suppl 1, (2008), pp. S16-8.

Walker PA, Courey MS & Ossoff RH. (1996). Staged endoscopic treatment of laryngeal amyloidosis. *Otolaryngol Head Neck Surg,* 114, 6, (1996), pp. 801-5.

Yakoot A, Giusiano S & Sanjuan M. (2010). An unusual cause of serous otitis media. *Eur Ann Otorhinolaryngol Head Neck Dis,* 127, 4, (2010), pp. 156-8.

Yamazaki K, Sato H & Ishijima K. (2011). A case of hemodialysis-associated amyloidosis localized to the external auditory canal. *Auris Nasus Larynx,* pp. 295-9. Epub 2010 Oct 28.

Zhuang YL, Tsai TL & Lin CZ. (2005). Localized amyloid deposition in the nasopharynx and neck, mimicking nasopharyngeal carcinoma with neck metastasis. *J Chin Med Assoc.*68, 3, (2005), pp. 142-5.

10

Oral Localized Amyloidosis

Kenji Yamagata and Hiroki Bukawa
Oral and Maxillofacial Surgery, Clinical sciences, Graduate School of Comprehensive Human Science, University of Tsukuba
Japan

1. Introduction

Amyloidosis is characterized by the proteinaceous fibrillar material amyloid, which is formed by extracellular accumulations of the insoluble protein fibril. This rare disease results from a sequence of changes in protein folding (Sipe et al., 2010) and occurs in response to various cell dyscrasias or inflammatory conditions. Amyloid stained with hematoxylin and eosin appears as a homogeneous, eosinophilic amorphous substance; when stained with Congo red, it demonstrates green birefringence in polarized light. The amyloid deposits can be localized or systemic, and can be large enough to impair normal tissue function.

Localized amyloidosis is relatively mild in contrast to the large-organ involvement seen in the systemic disease. Localized amyloidosis has been described in almost every organ system. Some patients have a progressive form of amyloidosis that is difficult to manage and is associated with severe morbidity. However, how the systemic disease evolves remains unclear. In a survey of 35 patients with local amyloidosis, Paccalin et al. did not find any risk of developing a systemic disease from local amyloid deposits. They suggested that immunolabeling studies be routinely performed. Moreover, since the evolution of the local disease can be life-threatening, these authors recommended that patients be referred to specialists for further evaluation. Management requires close follow-up to exclude recurrence and to determine appropriate treatment of the symptoms (Paccalin et al., 2005).

Localized amyloidosis affecting the head and neck is uncommon and usually benign. The sites most commonly involved are the larynx, subglottis, and thyroid (Nandapalan et al., 1998; Pentenero et al., 2006). Amyloidosis of the oral cavity is less frequent, and usually appears as multiple soft nodules accompanied by yellow, red, blue, or purple coloring in the mucous membrane. Oral amyloidosis is quite uncommon and occurs mostly as localized amyloidosis (Pentenero et al., 2006; Pribitkin et al., 2003), although when present in the most frequent site, the tongue, it may be linked to the systemic disease. In this chapter we focus on the clinical features, diagnosis, management, and prognosis of amyloidosis arising in the oral cavity.

2. Classification and types of amyloidosis

The Nomenclature Committee of the International Society of Amyloidosis met in conjunction with the XII International Symposium on Amyloidosis in 2010 to recommend amyloid fibril protein nomenclature and to consider newly identified amyloid fibril proteins for inclusion in the nomenclature list (Sipe et al., 2010). Amyloidosis is classified as primary or secondary, based on the nature of the precursor plasma proteins that form the fibril deposits (Khan and Falk, 2001). The pathogenesis is multifactorial. Nonetheless, the final pathway, in which amyloid fibrils are formed in the extracellular matrix, is identical in all forms of the disease. All amyloid deposits have a common fibrillar structure, consisting of linear, aggregated fibrils with an approximate diameter of 7.5-10 nm and a cross β–pleated sheet conformation, as evidenced by x-ray diffraction (Steciuk et al., 2002).

Three major amyloid types have been defined. The amyloid light chain (AL) form is seen in primary and idiopathic amyloidosis when there is no associated disease, but it has also been associated with plasma cell dyscrasia and multiple myeloma. The immunoglobulin light chain variable region is the main component of AL deposits. These patients commonly produce urinary free monoclonal light chains of the K or λ isotype, referred to as Bence Jones proteins. In a small percentage of AL amyloidosis cases, bone marrow plasma cells show clonal dominance of a light chain isotype. (Falk et al., 1997). Unlike multiple myeloma and monoclonal gammopathies, in which K chains are more frequent, in AL amyloidosis the ratio of K to λ light chains is 1:3 (Khan and Falk, 2001).

The amyloid A (AA) form of amyloidosis is seen in patients with secondary, acquired, or reactive amyloidosis, and is associated with chronic disease. AA deposits consist of fragments of at least 5 different molecular forms (Kluve-Beckerman et al., 1988) and are commonly seen in patients with rheumatoid arthritis or inflammatory bowel disease (Husby, 1985). The acute phase protein formed is serum amyloid A, which is produced under the regulation of cytokines that include tumor necrosis factor α3. The amino acid sequence in the AA protein is highly conserved, in contrast to the high variability of the amino acid sequence in the AL protein (Skinner, 1992).

Another type of secondary amyloidosis may occur in patients undergoing dialysis. In these patients, β2 microglobulin, which is part of the Class I major histocompatibility complex antigen, fails to cross the dialysis membrane, resulting in amyloid fibril formation (Danesh and Ho, 2001). These fibrils may be deposited in joints, (resulting in arthritis), periarticular tissue (resulting in carpal tunnel syndrome), and in bones (resulting in cysts) (Khan and Falk, 2001).

The third major type of amyloidosis is familial transthyretin-associated amyloidosis (ATTR) (Stoor et al., 2004). ATTR derives from a group of autosomal-dominant diseases in which, beginning in midlife, a mutant protein forms amyloid fibrils. In this case, the aberrant protein is transthyretin, a thyroxine transport protein that is capable of binding retinol. Other hereditary forms of amyloidosis involve mutations in other serum proteins such as apolipoprotein A1, fibrinogen, and gelsolin (Khan and Falk, 2001).

Oral localized amyloidosis has not been associated with either multiple myeloma or systemic amyloidosis, and does not usually progress to a systemic disease. In 13 cases of reported oral localized amyloidosis, 4 were AL, 2 were AA, and no type was described for the remaining 7 (Table 1). None of these cases appeared to have systemic involvement. However, when amyloidosis of the oral mucosa is diagnosed, further investigation is mandatory, both to evaluate the function of the organs most frequently involved in systemic amyloidosis, such as the liver, kidney, and heart, and to exclude an underlying plasma cell dyscrasia.

3. Clinical features and diagnosis of oral localized amyloidosis

3.1 Epidemiology

Although amyloidosis is rare, with an incidence of 12 cases per million population per year, this figure is no less than the incidence of several more widely recognized conditions, including chronic myeloid leukemia and Guillain-Barré syndrome. While the incidence of familial amyloidosis is unknown, it represents 10% to 20% of AL amyloidosis cases seen in referral centers (Falk et al., 1997).

Oral involvement, while identical in all forms of amyloidosis, has been reported in 40% of patients with AL amyloidosis (Mardinger et al., 1999; Reinish et al., 1994) but appears to be less frequent in patients with AA amyloidosis (Mardinger et al., 1999). Oral localized amyloidosis is quite uncommon (Pentenero et al., 2006; Pribitkin et al., 2003). To our knowledge, only 13 cases of oral localized amyloidosis have been reported (Table 1).

Case No	Authors	Age	Sex	Location	Symptom	Type	Treatment
1	Takeda et al (1987)	58	M	Floor of mouth	ND	ND	ND
2	Haraguchi et al (1997)	62	F	Tongue	Tongue discomfort	AA	Surgery
3	Koren et al (1998)	33	M	Tongue	Tongue pain	ND	ND
4	Alvi et al (1999)	65	M	Soft palate	Bleeding	ND	None
5	Asaumi et al (2001)	84	F	Tongue, lower lip, buccal mucosa	Swelling	ND	ND
6	Stoor et al (2004)	80	M	Hard palate	None	AL	Surgery
7	Pentenero et al (2006)	68	F	Hard palate	None	AA	None
8	Balatsouras et al (2007)	45	F	Soft palate	Fullness of ear-nasopharynx	ND	None
9	Henly et al (2007)	63	F	Hard palate	Palatal sore	AL	None
10	Aono et al (2008)	74	F	Hard palate	Painless nodule	AL	None
11	Angiero et al (2010)	36	M	Tongue	None	ND	ND
12	Angiero et al (2010)	63	F	Tongue	Swelling	ND	ND
13	Angiero et al (2010)	57	M	Tongue	Macroglossia	AL	ND

ND: not described

Table 1. Reported cases of localized amyloidosis arising in the oral cavity

3.2 Clinical features and symptoms

In systemic amyloidosis, systemic AL amyloidosis has the widest spectrum of tissue and organ involvement. The most frequent initial symptoms are fatigue and weight loss, but the diagnosis is usually not made until signs and symptoms are linked to a particular organ (Falk et al., 1997). The kidney and heart are the organs most commonly involved, either alone or in combination. Renal amyloidosis may manifest as proteinuria, which may be clinically evident as mild renal dysfunction. Normal serum creatinine and blood urea nitrogen concentrations may mask massive proteinuria, which may be accompanied by profound edema and hypoalbuminemia (Stoopler et al., 2003). Cardiac complications of amyloidosis are most likely to manifest as rapid-onset and progressive congestive heart failure. Electrocardiographic results may be normal, or may demonstrate a pattern of myocardiac infarction in the absence of coronary artery disease (Falk et al., 1997). Echocardiography may reveal a thickened ventricle and an ejection fraction in the low normal or mildly reduced range (Falk et al., 1987). Autonomic and sensory neuropathy are relatively common (Falk et al., 1997). Hepatomegaly is commonly seen in patients with AL amyloidosis, but splenomegaly is rare. Macroglossia, which is characterized by enlargement and stiffening of the tongue, is a frequent finding. If muscle weakness is present, amyloid deposits may be present elsewhere, resulting in the "shoulder-pad sign," nail dystrophy, or, in rare cases, alopecia (Falk et al., 1997).

The characteristic features of oral localized amyloidosis usually resemble those of benign tumors (Muto et al., 1991; Pentenero et al., 2006). The location in the oral cavity seems to have diagnostic importance, as amyloidosis of the tongue has been suggested as a clinical sign associated with blood dyscrasia or a dialysis-related lesion, while none of the reported cases affecting the palate seem to have systemic involvement (Alvi and Goldstein, 1999; Balatsouras et al., 2007; Pentenero et al., 2006; Pribitkin et al., 2003; Stoor et al., 2004). Oral amyloidosis usually appears as multiple soft nodules accompanied by yellow, red, blue, purple, or mixed colors in the mucous membrane (Pentenero et al., 2006, Aono et al., 2009). The symptoms reported in known cases of oral localized amyloidosis include bleeding, painless nodules, palatal sores, swelling, and macroglossia (Table 1). Differentiating amyloidosis from a tumor is clinically difficult and requires a biopsy of the lesion.

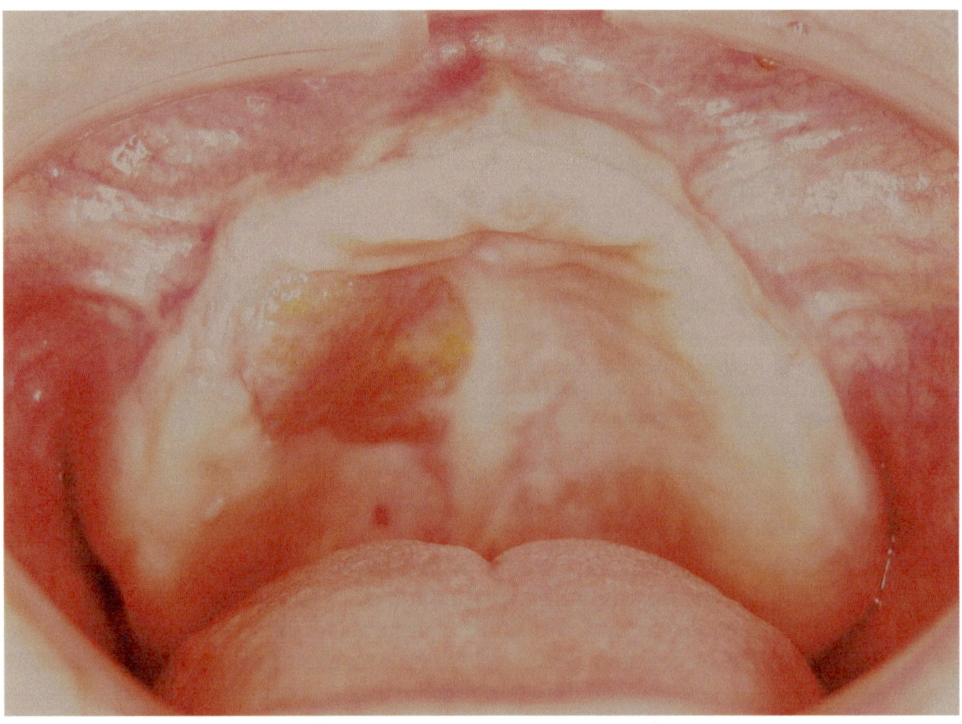

Fig. 1. Examination of the oral cavity. Oral cavity showing a yellow and red papilliform mass on the right side of the palate. The mass was painless and elastic to the touch

3.3 Diagnosis and pathological features

To establish a diagnosis of amyloidosis, clinical suspicions require histological confirmation. Although affected organs such as kidneys are often biopsied, more risky procedures can be avoided by simple subcutaneous aspiration of abdominal fat using a wide-bore needle and syringe (Duston et al., 1987; Libbey et al., 1983). This has an advantage over other widely used methods, such as rectal biopsy, in that it is less invasive but at least as effective. Most oral amyloidosis cases are easily biopsied with local anesthesia.

A tissue biopsy is used to establish a definitive diagnosis. When examined by light microscopy, amyloid stained with hematoxylin and eosin appears as a homogeneous eosinophilic, amorphous substance. When stained with Congo red and observed under polarized light, it shows an apple-green birefringence (Gertz et al., 2005). If the tissue sample yields a positive result, the type of amyloidosis must next be determined (Figure 2).

Since AL is the most common type of amyloidosis, serum or urine immunofixation electrophoresis is used to search for a clonal disorder. If the result is negative, immunohistochemical staining of a bone marrow specimen should be performed to search for Κ or λ light chains. The specific type of amyloid fibril can also be identified by light or electron microscopy with labeled antibodies using immunogold staining; this has been useful for identifying mixed forms of amyloidosis. In the absence of plasma cell dyscrasia, a variant transthyretin should be sought by isoelectric focusing of the serum, which will separate variant from wild-type transthyretin (Khan and Falk, 2001). Genetic testing should be performed if a variant transthyretin is found, since the specific mutation affects prognosis and management. AA amyloidosis is suspected in patients with a chronic inflammatory condition when AL and ATTR amyloidosis have been excluded. The diagnosis is confirmed by immunohistochemical staining for the AA protein.

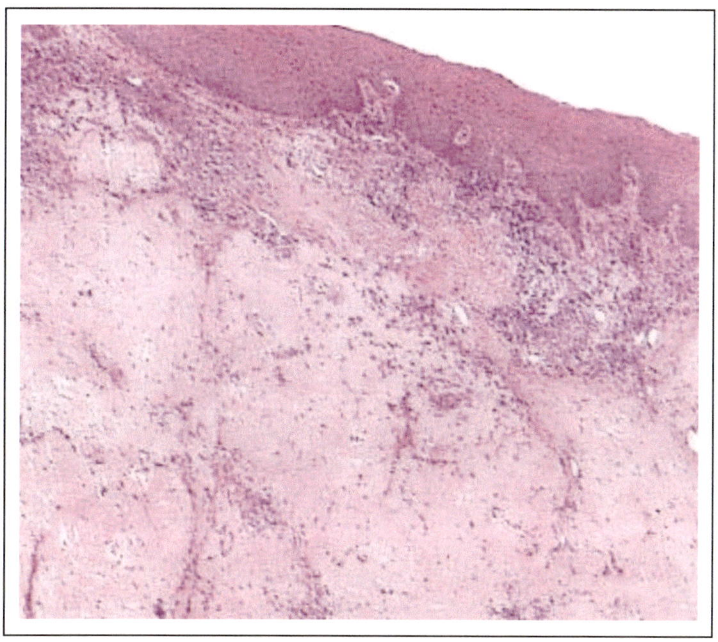

(a)

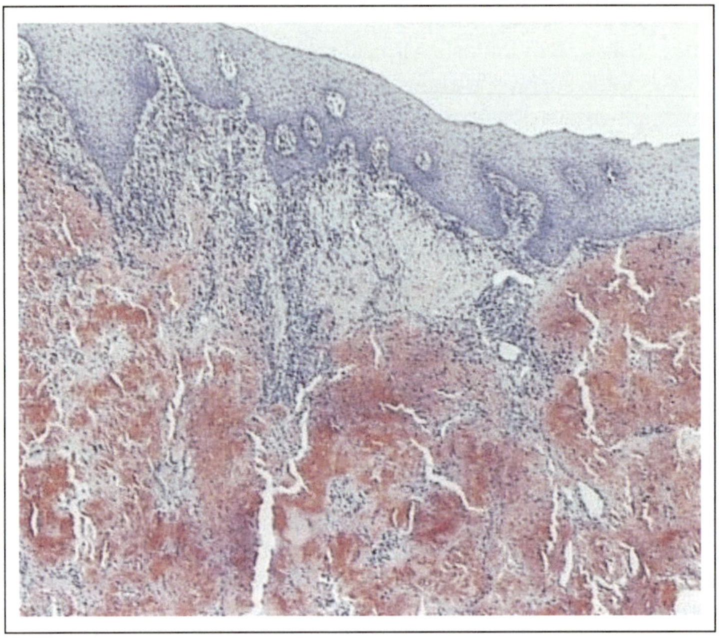

(b)

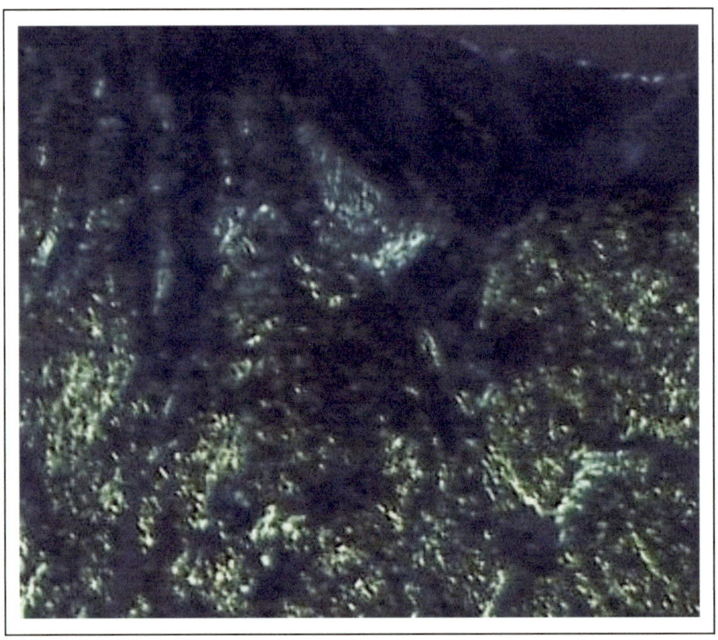

(c)

Fig. 2. (a) Hematoxylin and eosin staining showing an eosinophilic amorphous material in the connective tissue beneath the intact epithelium. (b) Congo red staining showing a red homogenous material under light microscopy. (c) The same area showing apple green birefringence under polarized light. (a–c) Magnification: original ×100

Noninvasive diagnostic tests include ^{123}I serum amyloid P scintigraphy to locate systemic amyloid deposits (Burke et al., 1990) and Tc-99m phosphate radionuclide imaging to demonstrate amyloid deposits in the skin and muscle, including the tongue (Hawkins et al., 1990). In one report, CT scans of amyloid tissue showed soft-tissue masses with no significant enhancement or only slight enhancement (Asaumi et al., 2001). It has also been reported that CT scanning can discriminate between localized and diffuse disease in patients with amyloidosis of the respiratory tract (Gillmore and Hawkins, 1999; Shah et al., 2002). Amyloidosis signals on MR images closely resemble those of skeletal muscle. Moreover, dynamic MR images may be helpful in evaluating localized amyloidosis, because it reveals characteristic features of such lesions (Asaumi et al., 2001). MR images have been shown to be useful in evaluating deposits before and after excision attempts, and could prevent the need for further endoscopic examination (Chin et al., 2004; Ichioka et al., 2004).

4. Typical localized oral amyloidosis

4.1 Tongue amyloidosis

The tongue is the most frequent site of oral amyloidosis. It may be diffusely enlarged due to macroglossia or nodular deposits, or it may be clinically unaffected (Salisbury and Jacoway, 1983; van der Wal et al., 1984). When deposits are extensive, macroglossia may develop; the tongue loses its elasticity and may be firm, dry, hard, fissured, ulcerated, hemorrhagic, and occasionally red and painful. The tongue becomes stiff, interfering with speech, chewing, and swallowing. Surgical management may be required if airway obstruction is anticipated (Mardinger et al., 1999).

Macroglossia is less common in AA than in AL amyloidosis (Mardinger et al., 1999). It is difficult to correlate a particular tongue lesion with a type of amyloid deposit. As lesions frequently recur, requiring repeated excisions, surgical intervention should be considered only in extreme cases of macroglossia with possible airway obstruction (Mardinger et al., 1999; Reinish et al., 1994). Clinicians note that tongue biopsy must include muscle tissue to be of diagnostic value. A biopsy of the tongue is recommended if the presence of amyloidosis is suspected, whether or not the patient is experiencing symptoms. However, other researchers have noted that tongue biopsy is diagnostic in only 60% of cases (Nandapalan et al., 1998). Deep incisional biopsies increase the risk of damaging the tongue's neurovascular supply, and can be painful. This area may also be prone to delayed healing and scarring due to mechanical irritation of the biopsy site (Stoopler et al., 2003). Although most tongue amyloidosis is secondary, five cases of localized tongue amyloidosis have been reported (Angiero et al., 2010; Haraguchi et al., 1997; Koren et al., 1998). One case was determined to be AL amyloidosis, another was AA, and the amyloidosis type was not described in the remaining cases. Reported symptoms included tongue swelling, macroglossia, and tongue pain (Table 1).

4.2 Palatal amyloidosis

Localized amyloidosis of the palate is extremely rare; only six cases have been reported (Alvi and Goldstein, 1999; Balatsouras et al., 2007; Gertz et al., 2005; Muto et al., 1991). Oral localized amyloidosis has not been generally associated with either multiple myeloma or systemic amyloidosis (Alvi and Goldstein, 1999; Balatsouras et al., 2007; Pentenero et al., 2006; Pribitkin et al., 2003; Stoor et al., 2004), and does not usually progress to systemic disease (Stoor et al., 2004). None of the reported cases affecting the palate appeared to have systemic involvement. Of the six patients with localized amyloidosis of the palate, three were diagnosed with AL amyloidosis and one with AA; the type was not reported for the other two patients. While some patients did not experience symptoms, others noted painless nodules, bleeding, and other symptoms. Five patients were not treated for the amyloidosis, and one was treated with surgery (Table 1).

Amyloid deposits have been found in other areas of the oral cavity and maxillofacial complex; however, not all of these areas can be biopsied. Localized amyloidosis has been reported in the nasal septum and maxillary sinus, and an unusual case involving the parotid gland was documented (Nandapalan et al., 1998). These sites are difficult to biopsy because of the mechanical complexities involved. Delgado and Mosqueda (Delgado and Mosqueda, 1989) found amyloidosis in the labial minor salivary glands, which are possible to biopsy (Stoopler et al., 2003).

5. Managing oral localized amyloidosis

In systemic amyloidosis, treatment is directed both toward the affected organ and the specific amyloidosis type. Nephritic involvement may necessitate diuretics and dialysis. Cardiac involvement may also require diuretics. Calcium channel blockers may exacerbate amyloid heart disease (Gertz et al., 1985) and should also be avoided because of their negative isotropism (Khan and Falk, 2001). Digoxin is contraindicated in cardiac amyloidosis, because it binds to amyloid fibrils and may be toxic at therapeutic levels (Khan and Falk, 2001). Previously reported therapies include conventional melphalan and predonisone therapy, dexamethasone-based regimens, thalidomide, stem cell transplantation, and investigational therapies (Gertz et al., 2005). The prognosis for patients with AL amyloidosis depends on the extent of organ involvement. Generally, a patient's prognosis is poor if the condition is left untreated, with a median survival of 1 to 2 years (Kyle and Gertz, 1995).

An optimal therapeutic strategy for amyloidosis would be designed to dissolve amyloid deposits or to prevent their accumulation. Patients with localized amyloidosis generally do not require systemic therapy, and management can be supportive or localized. Surgical intervention may be required when airway obstruction is a concern (Mardinger et al., 1999). Excision can be considered, but lesions often persist or recur (Paccalin et al., 2005). Thalidomide has been shown to be effective in treating refractory multiple myeloma, and is now being considered for treating AL amyloidosis (Singhal et al., 1999). Etarnacept, a tumor necrosis factor receptor antagonist, has shown some early success in treating symptoms of cardiac amyloidosis (Khan and Falk, 2001). The definitive therapy for ATTR amyloidosis is liver transplantation, because of the organ's transthyretin production.

For localized forms of amyloidosis, adjuvant therapies such as chemotherapy and steroids have not been shown to be beneficial. Surgical intervention is usual, but laser treatment may be used if surgical intervention is problematic. Alternatively, the patient may simply be kept under observation (Pentenero et al., 2006; Viggor et al., 2009). While management of oral localized amyloidosis is not commonly needed, local surgical or laser excision can improve functional impairment (Pentenero et al., 2006). Only two of the 13 known cases of oral localized amyloidosis were treated with surgery (Table 1).

6. Prognosis of oral localized amyloidosis

The prognosis of amyloidosis depends on the specific type and the organs involved. If AL amyloidosis is left untreated, the prognosis of a patient with cardiac involvement is poor, with a median survival of 1 to 2 years (Kyle and Gertz, 1995). Patients with ATTR amyloidosis may survive up to 15 years after diagnosis, but survival varies with the specific mutation and the time of diagnosis—the younger the age of presentation, the worse the outcome. The prognosis of patients with AA amyloidosis is affected by the underlying condition.

The prognosis of patients with oral localized amyloidosis is uncertain because of the rarity of the disease. Careful follow-up is advised to monitor its progression. Although rare cases of progressive amyloidosis have been reported (Bartels et al., 2004), there is no documentation to suggest that localized amyloidosis can progress to a systemic involvement (Nandapalan et al., 1998). Although local surgical or laser excision can be used to eliminate functional impairment, recurrences have been observed (Pentenero et al., 2006). The low risk of further generalized disease does not mean that localized amyloidosis is benign; it can be clinically silent or have significant consequences.

7. Conclusion

Oral localized amyloidosis is uncommon and has characteristics resembling those of benign tumors. It usually appears as multiple soft nodules accompanied by yellow, red, blue, or purple coloring in the mucous membrane. Differentiating amyloidosis from a tumor is clinically difficult and requires a biopsy of the lesion. Amyloidosis management is not commonly needed, but local surgical or laser excision can be useful for eliminating functional impairment even though the lesions may recur. The prognosis for patients with localized amyloidosis is uncertain because of the rarity of the disease, and careful follow-up is advised to monitor its progression.

8. References

Alvi A, and Goldstein MN. (1999). Amyloidosis of the palate. *Otolaryngol Head Neck Surg*, Vol. 120, No. 2, (February 1999), pp. 287, ISSN 0194-5998

Angiero F, Seramondi R, Magistro S, Crippa R, Benedicenti S, Rizzardi C, and Cattoretti G. (2010). Amyloid deposition in the tongue: clinical and histopathological profile. *Anticancer Res*, Vol. 30, No. 7, (August 2010), pp. 3009-3014, ISSN 1791-7530

Aono J, Yamagata K, and Yoshida H. (2009). Local amyloidosis in the hard palate: a case report. *Oral Maxillofac Surg*, Vol. 13, No. 2, (May 2009), pp. 119-122, ISSN 1865-1550

Asaumi J, Yanagi Y, Hisatomi M, Konouchi H, and Kishi K. (2001). CT and MR imaging of localized amyloidosis. *Eur J Radiol*, Vol. 39, No. 2, (August 2001), pp. 83-87, ISSN 0720-048X

Balatsouras DG, Eliopoulos P, Assimakopoulos D, and Korres S. (2007). Primary local amyloidosis of the palate. *Otolaryngol Head Neck Surg*, Vol. 137, No. 2, (August 2007), pp. 348-349, ISSN 0194-5998

Bartels H, Dikkers FG, van der Wal JE, Lokhorst HM, and Hazenberg BP. (2004). Laryngeal amyloidosis: localized versus systemic disease and update on diagnosis and therapy. *Ann Otol Rhinol Laryngol*, Vol. 113, No. 9, (September 2004), pp. 741-748, 0003-4894

Burke TS, Tatum JL, and Fratkin MJ. (1990). Accumulation of Tc-99m MDP in amyloidosis involving the tongue. *Clin Nucl Med*, Vol. 15, No. 2, (February 1990), pp. 107-109, ISSN 0363-9762

Chin SC, Fatterpeckar G, Kao CH, Chen CY, and Som PM. (2004). Amyloidosis concurrently involving the sinonasal cavities and larynx. *AJNR Am J Neuroradiol*, Vol. 25, No. 4, (April 2004), pp. 636-638, ISSN 0195-6108

Danesh F, and Ho LT. (2001). Dialysis-related amyloidosis: history and clinical manifestations. *Semin Dial*, Vol. 14, No. 2, (March 2001), pp. 80-85, ISSN 0894-0959

Delgado WA, and Mosqueda A. (1989). A highly sensitive method for diagnosis of secondary amyloidosis by labial salivary gland biopsy. *J Oral Pathol Med*, Vol. 18, No. 5, (May 1989), pp. 310-314, ISSN 0904-2512

Duston MA, Skinner M, Shirahama T, and Cohen AS. (1987). Diagnosis of amyloidosis by abdominal fat aspiration. Analysis of four years' experience. *Am J Med*, Vol. 82, No. 3, (March 1987), pp. 412-414, ISSN 0002-9343

Falk RH, Comenzo RL, and Skinner M. (1997). The systemic amyloidoses. *N Engl J Med*, Vol. 337, No. 13, (September 1997), pp. 898-909, ISSN 0028-4793

Falk RH, Plehn JF, Deering T, Schick EC, Jr., Boinay P, Rubinow A, Skinner M, and Cohen AS. (1987). Sensitivity and specificity of the echocardiographic features of cardiac amyloidosis. *Am J Cardiol*, Vol. 59, No. 5, (February 1987), pp. 418-422, ISSN 0002-9149

Gejyo F, Yamada T, Odani S, Nakagawa Y, Arakawa M, Kunitomo T, Kataoka H, Suzuki M, Hirasawa Y, Shirahama T, and et al. (1985). A new form of amyloid protein associated with chronic hemodialysis was identified as beta 2-microglobulin. *Biochem Biophys Res Commun*, Vol. 129, No. 3, (June 1985), pp. 701-706, ISSN 0006-291X

Gertz MA, Falk RH, Skinner M, Cohen AS, and Kyle RA. (1985). Worsening of congestive heart failure in amyloid heart disease treated by calcium channel-blocking agents. *Am J Cardiol*, Vol. 55, No. 13, (June 1985), pp. 1645, ISSN 0002-9149

Gertz MA, Lacy MQ, Dispenzieri A, and Hayman SR. (2005). Amyloidosis: diagnosis and management. *Clin Lymphoma Myeloma*, Vol. 6, No. 3, (December 2005), pp. 208-219, ISSN 1557-9190

Gillmore JD, and Hawkins PN. (1999). Amyloidosis and the respiratory tract. *Thorax*, Vol. 54, No. 5, (April 1999), pp. 444-451, ISSN 0040-6376

Haraguchi H, Ohashi K, Yamada M, Hasegawa M, Maeda S, and Komatsuzaki A. (1997). Primary localized nodular tongue amyloidosis associated with Sjogren's syndrome. *ORL J Otorhinolaryngol Relat Spec*, Vol. 59, No. 1, (January 1997), pp. 60-63, ISSN 0301-1569

Hawkins PN, Lavender JP, and Pepys MB. (1990). Evaluation of systemic amyloidosis by scintigraphy with 123I-labeled serum amyloid P component. *N Engl J Med*, Vol. 323, No. 8, (August 1990), pp. 508-513, ISSN 0028-4793

Husby G. (1985). Amyloidosis and rheumatoid arthritis. *Clin Exp Rheumatol*, Vol. 3, No. 2, (April 1985), pp. 173-180, ISSN 0392-856X

Ichioka K, Utsunomiya N, Ueda N, Matsui Y, Yoshimura K, and Terai A. (2004). Primary localized amyloidosis of urethra: magnetic resonance imaging findings. *Urology*, Vol. 64, No. 2, (August 2004), pp. 376-378, ISSN 1527-9995

Khan MF, and Falk RH. (2001). Amyloidosis. *Postgrad Med J*, Vol. 77, No. 913, (October 2001), pp. 686-693, ISSN 0032-5473

Kluve-Beckerman B, Dwulet FE, and Benson MD. (1988). Human serum amyloid A. Three hepatic mRNAs and the corresponding proteins in one person. *J Clin Invest*, Vol. 82, No. 5, (November 1988), pp. 1670-1675, ISSN 0021-9738

Koren R, Veltman V, Halpern M, Szabo R, and Gal R. (1998). Localized amyloid tumor of the tongue. A case report and review of the literature. *Rom J Morphol Embryol*, Vol. 44, No. 1-4, (February 2005), pp. 179-182, ISSN 1220-0522

Kyle RA, and Gertz MA. (1995). Primary systemic amyloidosis: clinical and laboratory features in 474 cases. *Semin Hematol*, Vol. 32, No. 1, (January 1995), pp. 45-59, ISSN 0037-1963

Libbey CA, Skinner M, and Cohen AS. (1983). Use of abdominal fat tissue aspirate in the diagnosis of systemic amyloidosis. *Arch Intern Med*, Vol. 143, No. 8, (August 1983), pp. 1549-1552, ISSN 0003-9926

Mardinger O, Rotenberg L, Chaushu G, and Taicher S. (1999). Surgical management of macroglossia due to primary amyloidosis. *Int J Oral Maxillofac Surg*, Vol. 28, No. 2, (April 1999), pp. 129-131, ISSN 0901-5027

Muto T, Sato K, and Lutcavage GJ. (1991). Multiple nodules of the lip, cheeks, and tongue. *J Oral Maxillofac Surg*, Vol. 49, No. 9, (September 1991), pp. 1003-1006, ISSN 0278-2391

Nandapalan V, Jones TM, Morar P, Clark AH, and Jones AS. (1998). Localized amyloidosis of the parotid gland: a case report and review of the localized amyloidosis of the head and neck. *Head Neck*, Vol. 20, No. 1, (February 1998), pp. 73-78, ISSN 1043-3074

Paccalin M, Hachulla E, Cazalet C, Tricot L, Carreiro M, Rubi M, Grateau G, and Roblot P. (2005). Localized amyloidosis: a survey of 35 French cases. *Amyloid*, Vol. 12, No. 4, (January 2006), pp. 239-245, ISSN 1350-6129

Pentenero M, Davico Bonino L, Tomasini C, Conrotto D, and Gandolfo S. (2006). Localized oral amyloidosis of the palate. *Amyloid*, Vol. 13, No. 1, (May 2006), pp. 42-46, ISSN 1350-6129

Pribitkin E, Friedman O, O'Hara B, Cunnane MF, Levi D, Rosen M, Keane WM, and Sataloff RT. (2003). Amyloidosis of the upper aerodigestive tract. *Laryngoscope*, Vol. 113, No. 12, (December 2003), pp. 2095-2101, ISSN 0023-852X

Reinish EI, Raviv M, Srolovitz H, and Gornitsky M. (1994). Tongue, primary amyloidosis, and multiple myeloma. *Oral Surg Oral Med Oral Pathol*, Vol. 77, No. 2, (February 1994), pp. 121-125, ISSN 0030-4220

Salisbury PL, 3rd, and Jacoway JR. (1983). Oral amyloidosis: a late complication of multiple myeloma. *Oral Surg Oral Med Oral Pathol*, Vol. 56, No. 1, (July 1983), pp. 48-50, ISSN 0030-4220

Shah PL, Gillmore JD, Copley SJ, Collins JV, Wells AU, du Bois RM, Hawkins PN, and Nicholson AG. (2002). The importance of complete screening for amyloid fibril type and systemic disease in patients with amyloidosis in the respiratory tract. *Sarcoidosis Vasc Diffuse Lung Dis*, Vol. 19, No. 2, (July 2002), pp. 134-142, ISSN 1124-0490

Singhal S, Mehta J, Desikan R, Ayers D, Roberson P, Eddlemon P, Munshi N, Anaissie E, Wilson C, Dhodapkar M, Zeddis J, and Barlogie B. (1999). Antitumor activity of thalidomide in refractory multiple myeloma. *N Engl J Med*, Vol. 341, No. 21, (November 1999), pp. 1565-1571, ISSN 0028-4793

Sipe JD, Benson MD, Buxbaum JN, Ikeda S, Merlini G, Saraiva MJ, and Westermark P. (2010). Amyloid fibril protein nomenclature: 2010 recommendations from the nomenclature committee of the International Society of Amyloidosis. *Amyloid*, Vol. 17, No. 3-4, (November 2010), pp. 101-104, ISSN 1744-2818

Skinner M. (1992). Protein AA/SAA. *J Intern Med*, Vol. 232, No. 6, (December 1992), pp. 513-514, ISSN 0954-6820

Steciuk A, Dompmartin A, Troussard X, Verneuil L, Macro M, Comoz F, and Leroy D. (2002). Cutaneous amyloidosis and possible association with systemic amyloidosis. *Int J Dermatol*, Vol. 41, No. 3, (May 2002), pp. 127-132, ISSN 0011-9059

Stoopler ET, Sollecito TP, and Chen SY. (2003). Amyloid deposition in the oral cavity: a retrospective study and review of the literature. *Oral Surg Oral Med Oral Pathol Oral Radiol Endod*, Vol. 95, No. 6, (June 2003), pp. 674-680, ISSN 1079-2104

Stoor P, Suuronen R, Lindqvist C, Hietanen J, and Laine P. (2004). Local primary (AL) amyloidosis in the palate. A case report. *Int J Oral Maxillofac Surg*, Vol. 33, No. 4, (May 2004), pp. 402-403, ISSN 0901-5027

van der Wal N, Henzen-Logmans S, van der Kwast WA, and van der Waal I. (1984). Amyloidosis of the tongue: a clinical and postmortem study. *J Oral Pathol*, Vol. 13, No. 6, (December 1984), pp. 632-639, ISSN 0300-9777

Viggor SF, Frezzini C, Farthing PM, Freeman CO, Yeoman CM, and Thornhill MH. (2009). Amyloidosis: an unusual case of persistent oral ulceration. *Oral Surg Oral Med Oral Pathol Oral Radiol Endod*, Vol. 108, No. 5, (September 2009), pp. e46-50, ISSN 1528-395X

Part 3

Novel Aspects in Therapy

11

Tocilizumab for the Treatment of AA Amyloidosis

Toshio Tanaka, Keisuke Hagihara, Yoshihiro Hishitani and Atsushi Ogata
Department of Respiratory Medicine, Allergy and Rheumatic Diseases, Osaka University Graduate School of Medicine, Osaka, Japan

1. Introduction

Amyloid A (AA) amyloidosis is a serious complication of chronic inflammatory, infectious and neoplastic diseases (Merlin & Bellotti, 2003). Insoluble amyloid fibril deposition resulting from the extracellular aggregation of proteolytic fragments of serum amyloid A (SAA), an acute-phase reactant protein, causes progressive deterioration in various organs (Obici et al., 2009; Perfetto et al., 2010). Moreover, long-term overproduction of the SAA protein is a key component of the resultant pathogenetic cascade (Pettersson et al., 2008). Recent fundamental analyses of SAA gene activation have revealed that proinflammatory cytokines such as IL-1β, TNFα and IL-6 are key players in SAA synthesis, leading to speculation that biological modifiers to block the activity of these cytokines may function as novel therapeutic drugs for AA amyloidosis. Some reports have dealt with the beneficial clinical effects of the IL-1 receptor antagonist, TNF inhibitors, and IL-6 receptor antibody (ab) on AA amyloidosis. In this chapter, we present evidence that tocilizumab, a humanized anti-interleukin-6 receptor ab, is a powerful inhibitor of SAA production and has the potential of becoming a first-line drug for AA amyloidosis.

2. Molecular mechanism of transcriptional activation of SAA1 gene

2.1 IL-6 plays a critical role in the synergistic induction of SAA1 gene by proinflammatory cytokines

SAA, which is mainly produced in the liver, is a precursor protein of amyloid A fibril in AA amyloidosis (Uhlar & Whitehead, 1999). The human SAA family consists of SAA1, SAA2, and SAA4. When the first two, also known as acute phase SAAs, are induced, they increase dramatically up to 1000 times during inflammation (Emery & Luqmani, 1993). The vast majority of human AA protein isolated from amyloid deposits are derived from SAA1 (Yamada et al., 1996).

The SAA2 gene is reportedly regulated by nuclear factor kB (NF-kB) and CAAT enhancer-binding protein β (C/EBPβ) in response to synergistic stimulation by IL-1β and IL-6 (Betts et al., 1993), although the exact induction mechanism of the SAA1 gene by proinflammatory cytokines remains unknown. An SAA isoform real time quantitative RT-PCR assay using the hepatic cell line HepG2 revealed that the combination of IL-6 and IL-1β or of IL-6 and TNFα, but not of IL-1β and TNFα displayed synergistic induction of SAA1 gene mRNA expression

(Hagihara et al., 2004). As shown in Fig. 1, anti-IL-6 receptor ab markedly diminished the synergistic induction of SAA mRNA by the triple stimulation of IL-6, IL-1β, and TNFα, which indicates that IL-6 plays a critical role in the synergistic induction of the SAA1 gene by proinflammatory cytokines.

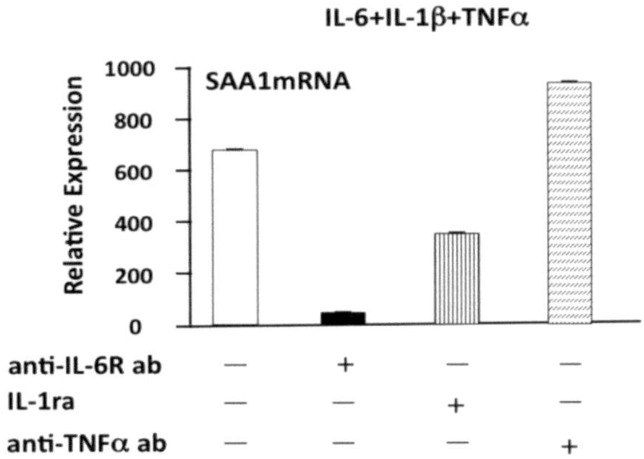

Fig. 1. Inhibitory effects of anti-IL-6R ab (25 μg/ml), IL-1 receptor antagonist (ra) (100 ng/ml), and anti-TNFα ab (4 μg/ml) on the synergistic induction of SAA1 generated by triple stimulation of IL-6, IL-1β, and TNFα. Each specific reagent was incubated with HepG2 cells for 30 min prior to cytokine stimulation. SAA1 mRNA in HepG2 cells was measured by means of real-time quantitative RT-PCR at 6 h after cytokine stimulation. Values shown represent the means + SD of duplicate measurements

Next, we studied the signal transduction pathway leading to the activation of the SAA1 gene. IL-6 was shown to have two main signal transduction pathways, the MAPK and Jak-STAT pathways (Akira, 1997). The Jak2 inhibitor AG490 reduced the synergistic induction of SAA1 to 30%, indicating that the Jak-STAT pathway plays an important role in the synergistic induction of the SAA gene (Hagihara et al., 2004). It was further shown that STAT3 binds to a γ-interferon activation sequence (GAS) like sequence (-TTNNNGAA) and that the C-reactive protein (CRP) gene, a major acute phase protein activated by IL-6, in fact has a STAT3 response element (RE) (-TTCCCGAA) in its promoter (D. Zhang et al., 1996; Nishikawa et al., 2008), while there is no STAT3 RE in the human SAA1 promoter (Uhlar & Whitehead, 1999). We therefore investigated what role STAT3 plays in human SAA1 promoter activity.

2.2 STAT3 is essential for the synergistic induction of human SAA1 genes via the NF-kB RE containing region after complex formation with NF-kB p65

To examine the effect of STAT3 on SAA1 promoter activity, pEF-BOS dominant negative STAT3 Y705F (dn STAT3) or pEF-BOS wild type STAT3 (wt STAT3) were co-transfected with the pGL3-SAA1 promoter luciferase construct (-796/+24) (pGL3-SAA1) into HepG2 cells (Hagihara et al., 2005). dn STAT3 eliminated the transcriptional activity of pGL3-SAA1 even after stimulation with IL-1β+IL-6, while wt STAT3 enhanced the transcriptional activity of pGL3-SAA1 three times more than was attained with IL-6 or IL-1β+IL-6 stimulation.

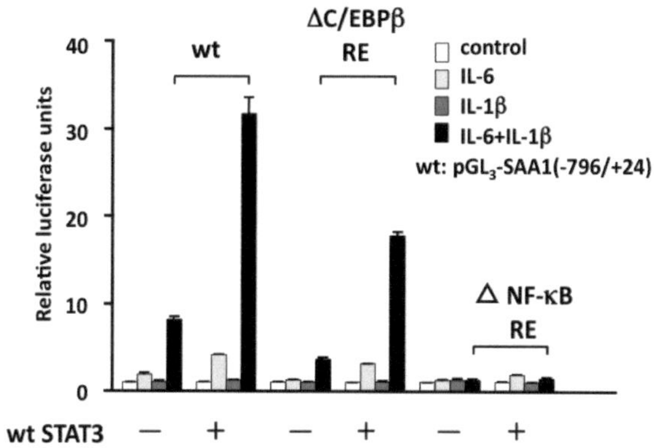

Fig. 2. STAT3 cannot augment the transcriptional activity of SAA1 without NF-kB RE. Wt STAT3 (0.5 μg) was co-transfected with 0.5 μg of pGL3-SAA1 (-796/+24) and pGL3-SAA1 DC/EBPβ RE, pGL3-SAA1 DNF-kB RE. Cytokine stimulation was performed with IL-6 (10 ng/ml) and/or IL-1β (0.1 ng/ml) for 3 h. The relative luciferase activity is expressed as means + SD of triplicate cultures and transfections

As shown in Fig. 2, the co-expression of wt STAT3 enhanced the transcriptional activity of pGL3-SAA1 and pGL3-SAA1 DC/EBPβ RE almost three-fold, but did not augment the transcriptional activity of pGL3-SAA1 DNF-kB RE. These results suggest that STAT3 is involved in the transcriptional activity of SAA, most likely through interacting with NF-kB RE. In the case of rat γ fibrinogen, the CTGGGAATCCC sequence was found to be responsive for transactivation by both STAT3 and NF-kB (Zhang & Fuller, 2000). We postulated that STAT3 might form a complex with NF-kB and contribute to the transcriptional augmentation of the human SAA1 gene. To examine our hypothesis, we performed IP-Western blotting of STAT3 and NF-kB. Fig. 3 clearly shows that STAT3 is associated with NF-kB p65 following IL-1β+IL-6 treatment but that no specific band of NF-kB p50 was detected.

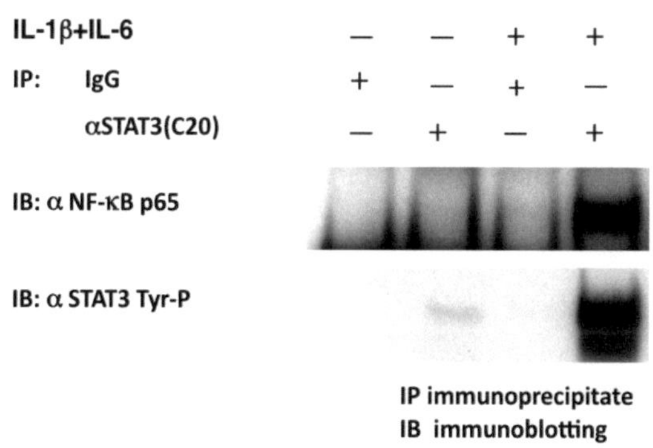

Fig. 3. Endogeneous STAT3 interacts with NF-kB p65 following IL-1β+6 treatment. Nuclear extracts of HepG2 cells stimulated with IL-1β and IL-6 were immunoprecipitated with the anti-STAT3 antibody. Western blots of immunoprecipitates with anti-NF-kB p65 or anti-STAT3 antibodies were performed

These findings indicate that crosstalk between STAT3 and NF-kB p65 contributes to the transcriptional augmentation of SAA1 by IL-1β+IL-6 stimulation.

2.3 STAT3 acts on the SAA1 promoter by means of a newly discovered cis-acting mechanism

STAT3 is reportedly associated with p300 (Nakashima et al., 1999), which raises the possibility that heteromeric complex formation of STAT3, NF-kB p65 and p300 is involved in the transcriptional activity of the human SAA1 gene. To examine this hypothesis, we performed a chromatin immunoprecipitation (ChIP) assay using chromatin isolated from HepG2 cells. STAT3 and p300 were apparently recruited to the SAA1 promoter region (–226 /+24) in response to IL-6 or IL-1β+IL-6 and weakly recruited by IL-1β (Fig. 4), while NF-kB p65 was recruited by IL-1β or IL-1β+IL-6 and slightly recruited by IL-6. These results demonstrate that STAT3 forms a transcriptional complex with NF-kB p65 and p300 on the SAA1 promoter region. Moreover, we found that co-expression of p300 wt in pCMVβ with wt STAT3 dramatically enhanced the luciferase activity in a dose-dependent manner. These findings indicate that STAT3 interacts with p300 in the transcriptional activity of the human SAA1 gene. However, the question remained how STAT3 could bind to the promoter region of the SAA1 gene because there is no typical STAT3 RE. It is likely that STAT3 either binds indirectly to the promoter region of the SAA1 gene, or obtains binding affinity for an unknown DNA sequence in a complex with NF-kB p65. To answer this question, we performed DNA affinity chromatography using a wt SAA1 probe (–196/-73). Nuclear extracts specifically interacting with a biotinylated wt SAA1 probe (–196/-73) were collected with the aid of streptavidin Dynabeads and a magnet, and transcriptional factors were analyzed by Western blotting.

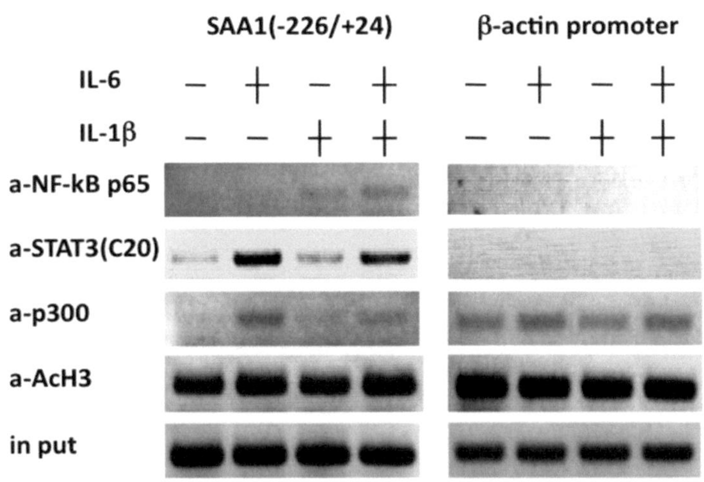

Fig. 4. Chromatin immunoprecipitation assays demonstrate recruitment pattern of STAT3, NF-κB p65, and p300 on the SAA1 promoter (-226/+24) from HepG2 cells treated with IL-6 (10 ng/ml) and/or IL-1β (0.1 ng/ml) for 30 min. Anti-AcH3 antibody was used as a positive control for this assay

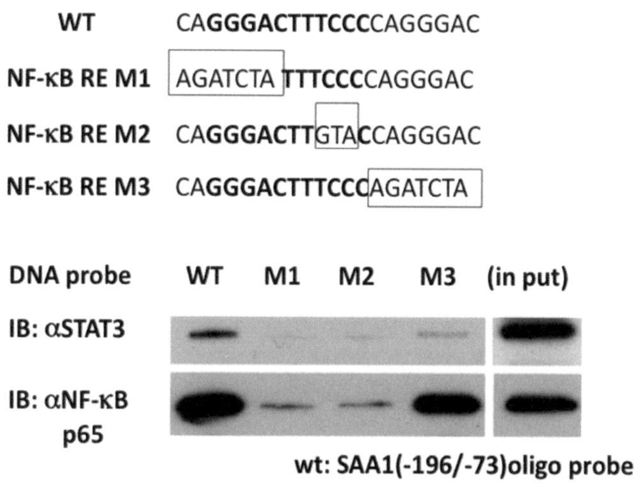

Fig. 5. DNA affinity chromatography shows that STAT3 can act on the SAA1 promoter after binding to NF-kB p65. The nuclear extracts (200 μg) from HepG2 cells after cytokine stimulation were mixed with 1 μg of biotinylated DNA probe, and 50 μl of streptavidin-Dynabeads was added to and mixed in with the samples and collected with a magnet. The trapped proteins were then analyzed by Western blotting. The SAA1 (-196/-73) mt NF-κB RE M1 and M2 probe lost its ability to interact with both STAT3 and NFκB p65, while the SAA1 (-196/-73) mt NFκB RE M3 probe maintained its binding affinity for NF-κB p65 but not STAT3

NF-kB p65 and STAT3 were both pulled down by the wt SAA1 probe from the nuclear extracts of HepG2 cells after IL-1β+IL-6 stimulation. In the case of rat γ fibrinogen, the CTGGGAATCCC sequence was identified as responsible for transactivation by both STAT3 and NF-kB (Zhang & Fuller, 2000). It was also reported that TCC was necessary for NF-kB binding and the CTGGGAA sequence for STAT3 binding because of the loss of transcriptional activity in an AGATCTATCCC mutant. To investigate whether STAT3 could bind to the CAGGGAC sequence of NF-kB RE on the SAA1 promoter region, we created two mutated constructs, the SAA1 NF-kB RE M1 probe (AGATCTATTTCCC) and the M2 probe (CAGGGACTTGTAC). We expected that STAT3 would bind to NF-kB RE M2, but not to NF-kB RE M1. However, neither NF-kB p65 nor STAT3 was detected by the two probes, indicating that the interaction between STAT3 and NF-kB p65 is essential for activation of the binding affinity of STAT3 to the wt SAA1 probe (Fig. 5). We assumed that the formation of the heteromeric complex of STAT3 and NF-kB p65 might confer STAT3 binding affinity to the SAA1 promoter region. On the basis of our results and those obtained with rat γ fibrinogen, we focused our attention on the 3'-site of NF-kB RE (CAGGGACTTTCCCCAGGGAC) as a candidate STAT3 binding site, because sequences contiguous to NF-kB RE could have influenced the binding affinity of STAT3. For vertification of our assumption, we created a SAA1 mt NF-kB RE M3 probe (CAGGGACTTTCCCAGATCTA). As expected, specific bands of STAT3 from the nuclear extracts of HepG2 cells after IL-1β+6 stimulation were markedly reduced by the SAA1 mt NF-kB RE M3 probe compared to the effect obtained with the wt SAA1 probe, although specific bands of NF-kB p65 found to be almost as intact as in the wild type (Fig. 5). These results thus supported our assumption that binding affinity of STAT3 for the human SAA1 promoter region is the result of the formation of a heteromeric complex comprising STAT3 and NF-kB p65. Taken together, our findings demonstrate that STAT3 acts on the human SAA1 promoter via a newly discovered cis-acting mechanism, that is, the formation of a heteromeric complex containing STAT3, NF-kB 65 and p300, resulting in a schematic model which can explain the synergistic induction of human SAA1 gene by IL-1β+IL-6 stimulation (Fig. 6).

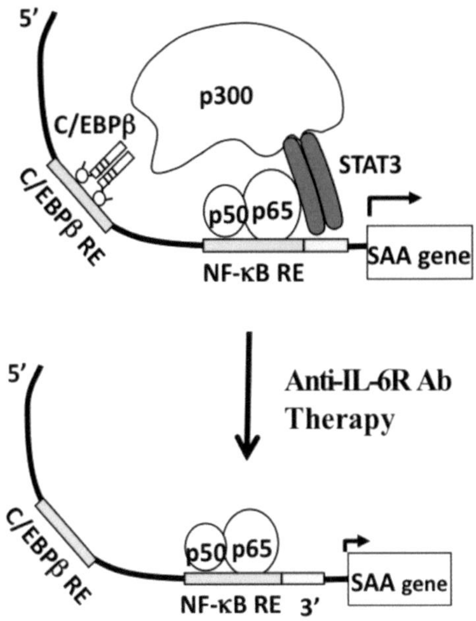

Fig. 6. A model of transcriptional regulation of the SAA1 gene. Cytokine stimulation caused the formation around NF-kB RE of a heteromeric complex with STAT3 and NF-kB p65. STAT3, which is assumed to interact with the 3'-site of NF-kB RE, recruited the co-activator p300, which then coordinated the interaction of NF-kB p65, STAT3, and C/EBPβ thus resulting in the augmentation of transcriptional activity of the human SAA1 gene. Anti-IL-6R ab therapy inhibited the activation of STAT3 and C/EBPβ, and eliminated the formation of the transcriptional complex on the SAA1 promoter

Our results further lead to the conclusion that the serum SAA1 level is affected by the intensity of the interaction between STAT3 and NF-kB p65. At the same time this schematic model explains the effect of anti-cytokine therapy on the transactivation of SAA1. Anti-TNFα or anti-IL-1β therapy can reduce but not completely eliminate the NF-kB signaling pathway, because this pathway is also activated by other cytokines or stimulants to activate toll like receptors (Li & Verma, 2002). As a consequence, the transcriptional complex on the SAA1 promoter is thought to remain after anti-TNFα or anti-IL-1β therapy. On the other hand, IL-6 blocking therapy can inhibit the activation of STAT3 and C/EBPβ, and prevent the formation of the transcriptional complex on the SAA1 promoter (Fig. 6). This model therefore shows that SAA1 gene activation depends on IL-6 more than on other proinflammatory cytokines such as IL-1β and TNFα, thus suggesting that IL-6 blockade is superior to the IL-1 or TNF blockade for the suppression of SAA synthesis.

3. The inhibitory effect of tocilizumab and other biologics on serum levels of SAA

Tocilizumab is a humanized anti-IL-6 receptor monoclonal ab of the IgG1 class that is generated by grafting the complementarity determining regions of a mouse anti-human IL-6 receptor ab onto human IgG1. Tocilizumab blocks IL-6-mediated signal transduction through inhibition of IL-6 binding to transmembrane and soluble IL-6 receptor. So far, tocilizumab has been approved for the treatment of moderate to severe rheumatoid arthritis (RA) in more than 90 countries and of juvenile idiopathic arthritis and Castleman's disease in Japan and may be effective for other autoimmune, inflammatory and neoplastic diseases (Tanaka et al., 2010; Tanaka et al., 2011). For RA, the recommended posology in Japan and the EU is 8 mg/kg once every 4 weeks. In clinical terms, if the serum tocilizumab concentration is maintained at more than 1 μg/ml, CRP remains negative (Nishimoto et al., 2008). The concentration of CRP is therefore a hallmark for determining whether tocilizumab completely blocks IL-6 activity in vivo.

The goal of therapy for AA amyloidosis is treatment of the underlying disorder (Perfetto et al., 2010). Treatment that suppresses the inflammatory activity reduces circulating levels of the SAA protein, but since AA amyloidosis occurs as a complication of chronic inflammatory diseases treated with conventional regimen(s), it is clear that the current treatment of the underlying disorder is not adequate for the prevention of AA amyloidosis development. Another therapeutic strategy therefore needs to be developed. A sustained high concentration of SAA has been found to correlate with a rapid progression of renal amyloid diseases and a low concentration (below 10 mg/L) with a more favorable outcome (Gillmore et al., 2001). Chronic suppression of SAA levels thus leads to a notable regression or stabilization of amyloid load (Lachmann et al., 2007). This makes a strategy to suppress SAA production a rational approach for the treatment of AA amyloidosis and biologics including IL-1 receptor antagonist, TNF blockers and IL-6 receptor ab can be expected to serve as novel therapeutic drugs for AA amyloidosis.

Clinical studies of how tocilizumab affects RA and Castleman's disease have demonstrated its strikingly suppressive effect on serum concentrations of SAA. In an open label trial, 3 doses of tocilizumab (2, 4 or 8 mg/kg) biweekly for 6 weeks were administered to 15 patients with active RA (Nishimoto et al., 2003). In 12 of the patients whose serum tocilizumab level was detectable during the treatment period, SAA was completely normalized after 6 weeks. A multicenter, double-blind, placebo-controlled trial of tocilizumab for RA patients showed that the injection of tocilizumab at 8 mg/kg every 4 weeks resulted in a reduction of the mean concentration of SAA from 365 to 75 mg/L after 3 months (Nishimoto et al., 2004). In a multicenter double-blind, randomized, placebo-controlled, parallel group Phase III OPTION study, patients with RA were randomized to receive tocilizumab (4 or 8 mg/kg) or placebo intravenously every 4 weeks while MTX was continued at stable pre-study doses (10-25 mg/week) for 24 weeks (Smolen et al, 2008). The mean levels of SAA of the group treated with 8 mg/kg, with 4 mg/kg and the placebo-administered group were reduced from 70.4 mg/L to 6.1 mg/L, 69.2 mg/L to 26 mg/L and 64.4 mg/L to 62 mg/L, respectively. For patients with Castleman's disease, tocilizumab treatment at 8 mg/kg every 2 weeks caused a prompt reduction of SAA in 5 patients (Nishimoto et al., 2000) and a striking reduction of SAA in 27 patients at week 60 (Nishimoto et al., 2005).

As for TNF inhibitors, Elliott et al. first demonstrated the suppressive effect of infliximab on SAA levels in patients with RA (Elliott et al., 1993). Twenty patients with active RA were treated with 20 mg/kg of infliximab in an open phase I/II trial lasting 8 weeks and SAA concentrations were reduced from 245 mg/L to 58 mg/L after 1 week and to 80 mg/L after 2 weeks. In a later study, Charles et al. examined the effect of infliximab on 24 RA patients (Charles et al., 1999). After 24 weeks, SAA levels in patients treated with infliximab showed a significant reduction from 378 mg/L to 56 mg/L. Perry et al. reported on the changes in SAA levels during treatment with etanercept of 9 patients with AA amyloidosis complicated by inflammatory arthritis (Perry et al., 2008). In 7 out of 9 patients the median SAA level during ETA treatment was lower than levels before therapy, and in 5 patients, the median post treatment level dropped to below 11 mg/L. Further, the effect of etanercept on SAA in 92 patients with ankylosing spondylitis (AS) reportedly reduced the median pre-treatment level of 4.8 mg/L to 0.9 after 1 month and to 0.8 3 months later (Van Eijk et al., 2009). Similarly, anti-TNF treatment (either with 25 mg of etanercept twice a week or 50 mg once a week, or 5 mg/kg of infliximab every 6 weeks) of 155 AS patients led to a reduction of medial levels of SAA from 7.5 mg/L to 0.7 mg/L after 1 month and to 0.8 mg/L after 3 months (De Vries et al., 2009).

The marked suppressive effect of the IL-1 receptor antagonist, anakinra on serum SAA concentration was demonstrated for an autoinflammatory disease, Muckle-Wells syndrome (Hawkins et al., 2004). The family suffering from this disease was treated with anakinra 100 mg/day subcutaneously. The SAA levels of the mother, son and daughter decreased from 146, 264 and 193 mg/L to 1.3, 2.2 and 1.8 mg/L, respectively. Similarly, anakinra treatment reduced the SAA concentration from a median of 174 mg/L to 8 mg/L in 18 patients with neonatal-onset multisystem inflammatory diseases (Goldbach-Mansky et al., 2006), from a mean level of 133 mg/L to 5 mg/L in 15 patients with autoinflammatory disease associated with CIAS-1/NALP3 mutations (Leslie et al., 2006) and from a mean level of 645 mg/L to 3.4 mg/L in 5 patients with tumor necrosis factor-associated periodic syndrome (TRAPS) (Gattorno et al., 2008). Anakinra thus appears to be highly effective for the suppression of SAA levels in patients with autoinflammatory diseases but there have been no reports on whether anakinra can also inhibit serum concentrations of SAA in patients with inflammatory arthritides.

We compared the inhibitory effects of tocilizumab with TNF inhibitors including infliximab, etanercept and adalimumab, on serum SAAs in RA patients. The results are shown in Fig. 7. Mean SAA levels of patients treated with tocilizumab or anti-TNFs decreased from 194 mg/L to 27 mg/L or from 185 mg/L to 53 mg/L, respectively. In most of the patients who received tocilizumab, SAA immediately dropped to below 10 mg/L except for two patients. Since CRP levels of these two patients were also high, the failure of SAA normalization was due to the low concentration of tocilizumab. In another 25 patients, the mean concentration of SAA was reduced from 186 mg/L to 8.0 mg/L, indicating that, if the concentration of tocilizumab can be consistently maintained at more than 1 μg/ml by changing the infusion interval or dose, the SAA concentration can be expected to remain normalized.

These observations therefore indicate that biologics, including TNF inhibitors, IL-1 receptor antagonist and anti-IL-6 receptor ab are effective for the suppression of serum levels of SAA, while tocilizumab appears to be more effective than TNF inhibitors for the suppression of SAA.

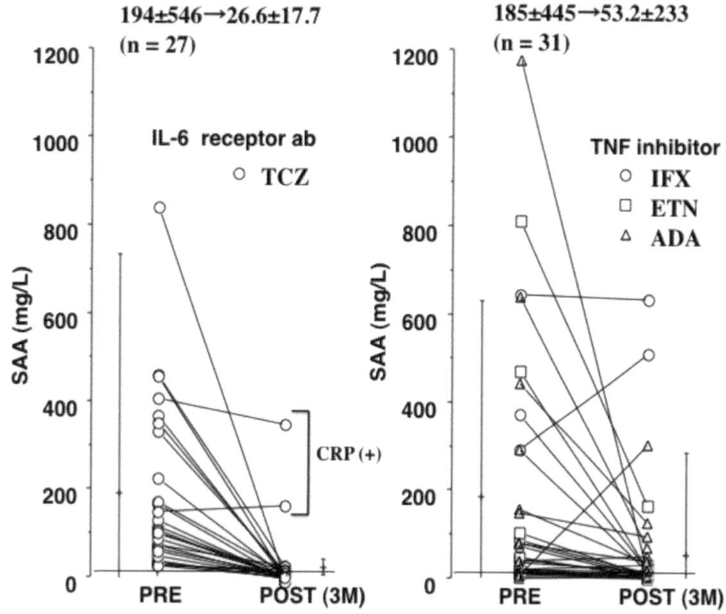

Fig. 7. The serum levels of SAA from patients with RA were more markedly suppressed by tocilizumab than by TNF inhibitors. SAA was measured before and at 3 months after biologics were administered. Twenty-seven patients were treated with tocilizumab (TCZ) and 31 patients anti-TNFs comprising infliximab (IFX), etanercept (ETN) or adalimumab (ADA). There was no significant difference between the baseline SAA of the two groups (p=0.09, Wilcoxon test). The median SAA in the tocilizumab treatment group was reduced from 114.5 mg/L to 6.5 mg/L, and in the anti-TNF treatment group from 72 mg/L to 16 mg/L. Three months after treatment, however, there was a significant difference in SAA between the two groups (p=0.017, Wilcoxon test)

4. The clinical effect of tocilizumab and other biologics on AA amyloidosis

The chronic suppression of SAA levels by anti-proinflammatory agents may lead to clinical amelioration of symptoms, prevention of progressive organ deterioration or recover from the damage, caused by amyloid A deposits. In fact, several studies have reported on the efficacy of biologics for the treatment of AA amyloidosis. In 2002, Elkayam et al. first reported that renal amyloidosis secondary to RA responded well to treatment with infliximab with the pre-therapy SAA level of 29 mg/L decreasing to 4.5 mg/L after 14 weeks. (Elkayam et al., 2002). In addition, rapid and complete clinical and laboratory remission of the nephrotic syndrome was observed within weeks, as well as stabilization of amyloid deposits confirmed by ^{123}I-labeled serum amyloid P (SAP) scintigraphy after 1 year. In 2003, Ortiz-Santamaria et al. reported the effect of infliximab on six patients with AA amyloidosis (complicated by RA in five cases and AS in one case), whose CRP levels improved compared with baseline values (Ortiz-Santamaria et al., 2003). Although three patients were withdrawn from the therapy in the first 2 months, reduced serum creatinine and proteinuria levels were observed in two of the remaining three patients. Gottenberg et al. reported that 15 patients with AA amyloidosis and renal involvement were treated with

TNF inhibitors (10 patients received infliximab, 4 received etanercept, and 1 underwent both types of treatment) (Gottenberg et al., 2003). Frequency of diarrhea was markedly reduced in 2 of the 3 patients with digestive tract amyloidosis, while amyloidosis progressed in 7 patients and was stabilized in 5 patients. Verschueren et al. described a patient with AA amyloidosis secondary to juvenile spondyloarthropathy treated with 3 mg/kg of infliximab (Verschueren et al., 2003). After six months, CRP returned to normal in conjunction with a reduction in proteinuria and after nine months urine analysis showed normal findings and protein excretion had been reduced. However, a renal biopsy after seven months of treatment detected equal amounts of amyloid fibrils in the mesangium, the subendothelial, and subepithelial space. In 2004, Ravindran et al. published a report of a case of RA with secondary Sjögren's syndrome, complicated by AA amyloidosis and nephrotic syndrome, which was treated with etanercept for 2 years (Ravindran et al., 2004). A significant reduction in proteinuria as well as a sustained stabilization of renal function were observed. In addition, a regression of AA amyloid, as quantified by ^{123}I-labeled SAP scintigraphy was established. As described elsewhere, etanercept treatment of patients with AA amyloidosis produced a decrease in SAA, but there were no significant changes in serum creatinine or proteinuria (Perry et al., 2008). In 2009, Kuroda et al. reported the effect of TNF inhibitors on 14 patients with AA amyloidosis associated with RA (Kuroda et al., 2009). For the 4 patients treated with infliximab and 10 patients with etanercept, creatinine clearance improved in 4 patients, did not change in 5 patients, and deteriorated in 3 patients. Urinary protein excretion significantly decreased in 3 patients, remained the same in 6, and increased in 3. The gastroduodenal biopsy from 9 patients showed significant reductions in amyloid deposits and these were no longer detectable in 2 patients. In 2010 it was reported that etanercept treatment of 14 RA patients with AA amyloidosis resulted in the AA amyloidosis improvement and stabilization of AA amyloidosis after 89 weeks (Nakamura et al., 2010). Further, proteinuria decreased from 2.24 to 0.57 g/day and SAA fell from 250 to 26 mg/L, while diarrhea secondary to gastrointestinal AA amyloidosis diminished, but serum creatinine levels did not improve as a result of the treatment. In another study, long-term TNF blockade treatment with infliximab, etanercept or adalimumab of 36 patients with AA amyloidosis as a complication of rheumatic diseases reduced the median levels of proteinuria by 59.7% during the first 24 months (Fernandez-Nebro et al., 2010), while both mean serum creatinine levels and creatinine clearance remained stable. Finally, anti-TNF treatment was also shown to be effective for clinical improvement in AA amyloidosis associated with Crohn's disease (Pettersson et al., 2008) or TRAPS (Drewe et al., 2000). Putting these various findings together indicates that the treatment of AA amyloidosis with TNF inhibitors is promising but that its efficacy appears variable. Anakinra has also been found to control the clinical symptoms or progression of renal amyloid disease in autoinflammatory syndromes such as TRAPS, familial cold autoinflammatory syndrome and cryopyrin-associated periodic syndrome (Pettersson et al., 2008).

On the basis of the findings of the central role of IL-6 in the SAA1 gene activation and the powerful suppressive activity of tocilizumab on SAA, it is anticipated that tocilizumab may serve as an innovative drug for the treatment of AA amyloidosis. In a murine AA amyloidosis model, anti-IL-6 receptor ab (MR16-1) produced marked suppression of amyloid deposition in various organs when administered either preventively or therapeutically (Mihara et al., 2004). While reports regarding the efficacy of tocilizumab on AA amyloidosis are limited, Okuda & Takasugi were the first to report an excellent clinical response to treatment with tocilizumab in a patient with AA amyloidosis complicating juvenile idiopathic arthritis (Okuda & Takasugi, 2006). Tocilizumab immediately normalized the SAA level, followed by the disappearance of gastrointestinal symptoms such as diarrhea and abdominal pain after 1 month and resolution of proteinuria after 2 months of the treatment. Moreover, serial gastrointestinal biopsy specimens showed marked and lasting regression of AA protein deposits. We also reported that in an RA patient with AA amyloidosis who had been refractory to treatment with prednisolone, disease modifying anti-rheumatic drugs or TNF inhibitors including etanercept and infliximab, tocilizumab administration promptly stopped the diarrhea and diminished the disease activity of RA (Nishida et al., 2009). Surprisingly, three months after the tocilizumab treatment amyloid A protein deposits had completely disappeared. Subsequently, two other cases of AA amyloidosis associated with RA also showed the ameliorative clinical effect of tocilizumab on gastrointestinal symptoms due to intestinal amyloidosis (Sato et al., 2009; Inoue et al., 2010) and in one of the two cases amyloid A fibril deposits were found to have disappeared after three courses of tocilizumab treatment. Moreover, Kishida et al. reported observing the clinical ameliorative effect of tocilizumab on a patient with adult-onset Still's disease complicated by AA amyloidosis as well as marked regression of amyloid A protein in duodenal mucosa and submucosa after tocilizumab treatment (Kishida et al., 2010). These dramatic effects of tocilizumab on AA amyloidosis raise the possibility that tocilizumab may become an innovative drug for the treatment of AA amyloidosis, although further clinical studies are required to evaluate its efficacy and safety.

5. Conclusion

Recent analyses of molecular mechanisms regulating SAA production have revealed that proinflammatory cytokines such as IL-1β, TNFα and IL-6 are key players in this process. Biological modifiers including IL-1 receptor antagonist, TNF inhibitors and IL-6 receptor ab, on the other hand, have been demonstrated to be effective for the suppression of serum levels of SAA and for clinical improvement associated with AA amyloidosis. Our findings showed that among proinflammatory cytokines IL-6 appears to play a major role in the induction of the SAA1 gene, so that it is anticipated that IL-6 blockade may constitute the most powerful strategy for the treatment of AA amyloidosis. Indeed, the treatment of chronic inflammatory diseases with tocilizumab could markedly reduce serum concentrations of SAA and several recent case reports described how tocilizumab treatment led to the disappearance or marked regression of amyloid fibril. Tocilizumab may therefore be suitable as a first-line drug for patients who are complicated with, or at high risk of developing AA amyloidosis, although further clinical evaluation will be needed.

6. Acknowledgement

This work was supported by the Program for Promotion of Fundamental Studies in Health Sciences of the National Institute of Biomedical Innovation.

7. References

Akira, S. (1997). IL-6-regulated transcription factors. *The International Journal of Biochemistry & Cell Biology*, Vol.29, No.12, (December 1997), pp. 1401-1418.

Betts, J.C.; Cheshire, J.K.; Akira, S.; Kishimoto, T. & Woo, P. (1993). The role of NF-kB and NF-IL6 transactivating factors in the synergistic activation of human serum amyloid A gene expression by interleukin-1 and interleukin-6. *The Journal of Biological Chemistry,* Vol.268, No.34, (December 1993), pp. 25624-25631.

Charles, P.; Elliott, M.J.; Davis, D.; Potter, A.; Kalden, J.R.; Antoni, C.; Breedveld, F.C.; Smolen, J.S.; Eberl, G.; deWoody, K.; Feldmann, M. & Maini, R.N. (1999). Regulation of cytokines, cytokine inhibitors, and acute-phase proteins following anti-TNF-alpha therapy in rheumatoid arthritis. *The Journal of Immunology* Vol.163, No.3, (August 1999), pp. 1521-1528.

De Vries, M.K.; Van Eijk, I.C.; Van Der Horst-Bruinsma, I.E.; Peters, M.J.; Nurmohamed, M.T.; Dijkmans, B.A.; Hazenberg, B.P. & Wolbink, G.J. (2009). Erythrocyte sedimentation rate, C-reactive protein level, and serum amyloid a protein for patient selection and monitoring of anti-tumor necrosis factor treatment in ankylosing spondylitis. *Arthritis & Rheumatism,* Vol.61, No.11, (November 2009), pp. 1484-1490.

Drewe, E.; McDermott, E.M. & Powell, R.J. (2000). Treatment of the nephritic syndrome with etanercept in patients with the tumor necrosis factor receptor-associated periodic syndrome. *The New England Journal of Medicine,* Vol.343, No.14, (October 2000), pp. 1044-1045.

Elkayam, O.; Hawkins, P.N.; Lachmann, H.; Yaron, M. & Caspi, D. (2002). Rapid and complete resolution of proteinuria due to renal amyloidosis in a patient with rheumatoid arthritis treated with infliximab. *Arthritis & Rheumatism,* Vol.46, No.10, (October 2002), pp. 2571-2573.

Elliott, M.L.; Maini, R.N.; Feldmann, M.; Long-Fox, A.; Charles, P.; Katsikis, P.; Brennan, F.M.; Walker, J.; Bijl, H.; Ghrayeb, J. & Woody, J.M. (1993). Treatment of rheumatoid arthritis with chimeric monoclonal antibodies to tumor necrosis factor alpha. *Arthritis & Rheumatism,* Vol.36, No.12, (December 1993), pp. 1681-1690.

Emery, P. & Luqmani, R. (1993). The validity of surrogate markers in rheumatic diseases. *British Journal of Rheumatology,* Vol.32, Suppl.3, pp. 3-8.

Fernandes-Nebro, A.; Olive, A.; Castro, M.C.; Varela, A.H.; Riera, E.; Irigoyen, M.V.; De Yebenes, M.J.G. & Garcia-Vicuna, R. (2010). Long-term TNF-alpha blockade in patients with amyloid A amyloidosis complicating rheumatic diseases. *The American Journal of Medicine,* Vol.123, No.5, (May 2010), pp. 454-461.

Gattorno, M.; Pelagatti, M.A.; Meini, A.; Obici, L.; Barcellona, R.; Federici, S.; Buoncompagni, A.; Plebani, A.; Merlini, G. & Martini, A. (2008). Persistent efficacy of anakinra in patients with tumor necrosis factor receptor-associated with periodic syndrome. *Arthritis & Rheumatism,* Vol.58, No.5, (May 2008), pp. 1516-1520.

Gillmore. J.D.; Lovat, L.B.; Persey M.R.; Pepys, M.B. & Hawkins, P.N. (2001). Amyloid load and clinical outcome in AA amyloidosis in relation to circulating concentration of serum amyloid A protein. *Lancet,* Vol.358, No.9275, (July 2001), pp. 24-29.

Goldbach-Mansky, R.; Dailey, N.J.; Canna, S.W.; Gelabert, A.; Jones, J.; Rubin, B.I.; Kim, H.J.; Brewski, C.; Wiggs, W.; Hill, S.; Turner, M.L.; Karp, B.I.; Aksentijevich, I.; Pucino, F.; Penzak, S.R.; Haverkamp, M.H.; Stein, L.; Adams, B.S.; Moore, T.L.; Fuhlbrigge, R.C.; Shaham, B.; Jarvis, J.N.; O'Neil, K.; Vehe, R.K.; Beitz, L.O.; Gardner, G.; Hannan, W.P.; Warren, R.W.; Horn, W.; Cole, J.L.; Paul, S.M.; Hawkins, P.N.; Pham, T.H.; Snyder, C.; Weasley, R.A.; Hoffamann, S.C.; Holland, S.M.; Butman, J.A. & Kastner, D.L. (2006). Neonatal-onset multisystem inflammatory disease responsive to interleukin-1 beta inhibition. *The New England Journal of Medicine,* Vol.355, No.6, (Aug 2006), pp. 581-592.

Gottenberg, J-E.; Merle-Vincent, F.; Bentaberry, F.; Allanore, Y.; Berenbaum, F.; Fautrel, B.; Combe, B.; Durbach, A.; Sibilia, J.; Dougados, M. & Mariette, X. (2003). Anti-tumor necrosis factor alpha therapy in fifteen patients with AA amyloidosis secondary to inflammatory arthritides: a followup report of tolerability and efficacy. *Arthritis & Rheumatism,* Vol.48, No.7, (July 2003), pp. 2019-2024.

Hagihara, K.; Nishikawa, T.; Isobe, T.; Song, J.; Sugamata, Y. & Yoshizaki, K. (2004). IL-6 plays a critical role in the synergistic induction of human serum amyloid A (SAA) gene when stimulated with proinflammatory cytokines as analyzed with an SAA isoform real-time quantitative RT-PCR assay system. *Biochemical Biophysical Research Communications*, Vol.314, No.2, (February 2004), pp. 363-369.

Hagihara, K.; Nishikawa, T.; Sugamata, Y.; Song, J.; Isobe, T.; Taga, T. & Yoshizaki, K. (2005). Essential role of STAT3 in cytokine-driven NF-kappaB-mediated serum amyloid A gene expression. *Genes to Cells,* Vol.10, No.11, (November 2005), pp. 1051-1063.

Hawkins, P.N.; Lachmann, H.J.; Aganna, E. & McDermott, M.F. (2004). Spectrum of clinical features in Muckle-Wells syndrome and response to anakinra. *Arthritis & Rheumatism,* Vol.50, No.2, (February 2004), pp. 607-612.

Inoue, D.; Arima, H.; Kawanami, C.; Takiuchi, Y.; Nagano, S.; Shimoji, S.; Mori, M.; Tabata, S.; Yanagita, S.; Matsushita, A.; Nagai, K.; Imai, Y. & Takahashi T. (2010). Excellent therapeutic effect of tocilizumab on intestinal amyloid a deposition secondary to active rheumatoid arthritis. *Clinical Rheumatology,* Vol.29, No.10, (October 2010), pp. 1195-1197.

Kishida, D.; Okuda, Y.; Onishi, M.; Takebayashi, M.; Matoba, K.; Jouyama, K.; Yamada, A.; Sawada, N.; Mokuda, S. & Takasugi, K. (2010). Successful tocilizumab treatment in a patient with adult-onset Still's disease complicated by chronic active hepatitis B and amyloid A amyloidosis. *Modern Rheumatology,* Oct 8 [Epub ahead of print]

Kuroda, T.; Wada, Y.; Kobayashi, D.; Murakami, S.; Sakai, T.; Hirose, S.; Tanabe, N.; Saeki, T.; Nakano, M. & Narita, I. (2009). Effective anti-TNF-alpha therapy can induce rapid resolution and sustained decrease of gastroduodenal mucosal amyloid deposits in reactive amyloidosis associated with rheumatoid arthritis. *The Journal of Rheumatology,* Vol.36, No.11, (November 2009), pp. 2409-2415.

Lachmann, H.J.; Goodman, H.J.; Gilbertson, J.A.; Gallimore, J.R.; Sabin, C.A.; Gillmore, J.D. & Hawkins, P.N. (2007). Natural history and outcome in systemic AA amyloidosis. *The New England Journal of Medicine,* Vol.356, No.23, (June 2007), pp. 2361-2371.

Leslie K.S.; Lachmann, H.J.; Bruning, E.; McGrath, J.A.; Bybee, A.; Gallimore, J.R.; Roberts, P.F.; Woo, P.; Grattan, C.E. & Hawkins, P.N. (2006). Phenotype, genotype, and sustained response to anakinra in 22 patients with autoinflammatory disease associated with CIAS-1/NALP3 mutations. *Archives of Dermatology,* Vol.142, No.12, (December 2006), pp 1591-1597.

Li, Q. & Verma, I.M. (2002). NF-kB regulation in the immune system. *Nature Review of Immunology* , Vol.10, (October 2002), pp. 725-734.

Mihara, M.; Shiina, M.; Nishimoto, N.; Yoshizaki, K.; Kishimoto, T. & Akamatsu, K. (2004). Anti-interleukin 6 receptor antibody inhibits murine AA-amyloidosis. *The Journal of Rheumatology,* Vol.31, No.6, (June 2004), pp 1132-1138.

Merlini, G. & Bellotti, V. (2003). Molecular mechanisms of amyloidosis. *The New England Journal of Medicine,* Vol.349, No.6, (August 2003), pp. 583-596.

Nakamura, T.; Higashi, S.; Tomoda, K.; Tsukano, M. & Shono, M. (2010). Etanercept can induce resolution of renal deterioration in patients with amyloid a amyloidosis secondary to rheumatoid arthritis. *Clinical Rheumatology*, Vol.29, No.12, (December 2010), pp. 1395-1401.

Nakashima, K.; Yanagisawa, M.; Arakawa, H.; Kimura, N.; Hisatsune, T.; Kawabata, M.; Miyazono, K. & Taga, T. (1999). Synergic signaling in fetal brain by STAT3-Smad1 complex bridged by p300. *Science*, Vol.284, No.5413, (April 1999), pp. 479-482.

Nishida, S.; Hagihara, K.; Shima, Y.; Kawai, M.; Kuwahara, Y.; Arimitsu, J.; Hirano, T.; Narazaki, M.; Ogata, A.; Yoshizaki, K.; Kawase, I.; Kishimoto, T. & Tanaka T. (2009). Rapid improvement of AA amyloidosis with humanised anti-interleukin 6 receptor antibody treatment. *Annals of The Rheumatic Diseases*, Vol.68, No.7, (July 2009), pp. 1235-1236.

Nishikawa, T.; Hagihara, K.; Serada, S.; Isobe, T.; Matsumura, A.; Song, J.; Tanaka, T.; Kawase, I.; Naka, T. & Yoshizaki, K. (2008). Transcriptional complex formation of c-Fos, STAT3, and hepatocyte NF-1 alpha is essential for cytokine-driven C-reactive protein gene expression. *The Journal of Immunology*, Vol.180, No.5, (March 2008), pp. 3492-3501, 2008.

Nishimoto, N.; Sasai, M.; Shima, Y.; Nakagawa, M.; Matsumoto, T.; Shirai, T.; Kishimoto, T. & Yoshizaki, K. (2000). Improvement of Castleman's disease by humanized anti-interleukin-6 receptor antibody therapy. *Blood*, Vol.95, No.1, (January 2000), pp. 56-61.

Nishimoto, N.; Yoshizaki, K.; Maeda, K.; Kuritani, T.; Deguchi, H.; Sato, B.; Imai, N.; Suemura, M.; Kakehi, T.; Takagi, N. & Kishimoto, T. (2003). Toxicity, pharmacokinetics, and dose-finding study of repetitive treatment with the humanized anti-interleukin 6 receptor antibody MRA in rheumatoid arthritis. Phase I/II clinical study. *The Journal of Rheumatology*, Vol.30, No.7, (July 2003), pp. 1426-1435.

Nishimoto, N.; Yoshizaki, K.; Miyasaka, N.; Yamamoto, K.; Kawai, S.; Takeuchi, T.; Hashimoto, J.; Azuma, J. & Kishimoto, T. (2004). Treatment of rheumatoid arthritis with humanized anti-interleukin-6 receptor antibody: a multicenter, double-blind, placebo-controlled trial. *Arthritis & Rheumatism*, Vol.50, No.6, (June 2004), pp. 1761-1769.

Nishimoto, N.; Kanakura, Y.; Aozasa, K.; Johkoh, T.; Nakamura, M.; Nakano, S.; Nakano, N.; Ikeda, Y.; Sasaki, T.; Nishioka, K.; Hara, M.; Taguchi, H.; Kimura, Y.; Katao, Y.; Asaoku, H.; Kumagai, S.; Kodama, F.; Nakahara, H.; Hagihara, K.; Yoshizaki, K. & Kishimoto, T. (2005). Humanized anti-interleukin-6 receptor antibody treatment of multicentric Castleman disease. *Blood*, Vol.106, No.8, (October 2005), pp. 2627-2632.

Nishimoto, N.; Terao, K.; Mima, T.; Nakahara, H.; Takagi, N. & Kakehi, T. (2008). Mechanisms and pathologic significances in increase in serum interleukin-6 (IL-6) and soluble IL-6 receptor after administration of an anti-IL-6 receptor antibody, tocilizumab, in patients with rheumatoid arthritis and Castleman disease. *Blood*, Vol.112, No.10, (November 2008), pp. 3959-3964.

Obici, L.; Raimondi, S.; Lavatelli, F.; Bellotti, V. & Merlini, G. (2009). Susceptibility to AA amyloidosis in rheumatic diseases: a critical overview. *Arthritis & Rheumatism*, Vol.61, No.10, (October 2009), pp. 1435-1440.

Okuda, Y. & Takasugi, K. (2006) Successful use of a humanized anti-interleukin-6 receptor antibody, tocilizumab, to treat amyloid A amyloidosis complicating juvenile idiopathic arthritis. *Arthritis & Rheumatism*, Vol.54, No.9, (September 2006), pp. 2997-3000.

Ortiz-Santamaria, V.; Valls-Roc, M.; Sanmarti, M. & Olive, A. (2003). Anti-TNF treatment in secondary amyloidosis. *Rheumatology (Oxford)*, Vol.42, No.11, (November 2003), pp. 1425-1426.

Perfetto, F.; Moggi-Pignone, A.; Livi, R.; Tempestini, A.; Bergesio, F. & Matucci-Cerinic, M. (2010). Systemic amyloidosis: a challenge for the rheumatologist. *Nature Review of Rheumatology*, Vol.6, (July 2010), pp. 417-429.

Perry, M.E.; Stirling, A. & Hunter, J.A. (2008). Effect of etanercept on serum amyloid A protein (SAA) levels in patients with AA amyloidosis complicating inflammatory arthritis. *Clinical Rheumatology*, Vol.27, No.7, (July 2008), pp. 923-925.

Pettersson, T.; Konttinen, Y.T. & Maury, C.P.J. Treatment strategies for amyloid A amyloidosis. *Expert Opinion on Pharmacotherapy*, Vol.9, No.12, (August 2008), pp. 2117-2128.

Ravindran, J.; Shenker, N.; Bhalla, A.K.; Lachmann, H. & Hawkins, P. (2004). Case report: response in proteinuria due to AA amyloidosis but not Felty's syndrome in a patient with rheumatoid arthritis treated with TNF-alpha blockade. *Rheumatology (Oxford)*, Vol.43, No.2, (February 2004), pp. 669-672.

Sato, H.; Sakai, T.; Sugaya, T.; Otaki, Y.; Aoki, K.; Ishii, K.; Horizono, H.; Otani, H.; Abe, A.; Yamada, N.; Ishikawa, H.; Nakazono, K.; Murasawa, A. & Gejyo, F. (2009). Tocilizumab dramatically ameliorated life-threatening diarrhea due to secondary amyloidosis associated with rheumatoid arthritis. *Clinical Rheumatology*, Vol.28, No.9, (September 2009), pp. 1113-1116.

Smolen, J.S.; Beaulieu, A.; Rubbert-Roth, A.; Ramos-Remus, C.; Rovensky, J.; Alecock, E.; Woodworth, T.; Alten, R. & OPTION Investigators. (2008). Effect of interleukin-6 receptor inhibition with tocilizumab in patients with rheumatoid arthritis (OPTION study): a double-blind, placebo-controlled, randomized trial. *Lancet*, Vol.371, No.9617, (March 2008), pp. 987-997.

Tanaka, T.; Narazaki, M. & Ogata, A. (2010). Tocilizumab for the treatment of rheumatoid arthritis. *Expert Review of Clinical Immunology*, Vol.6, No.6, (November 2010), pp. 843-854.

Tanaka, T.; Narazaki, M. & Kishimoto, T (2011). Anti-interleukin-6 receptor antibody, tocilizumab for the treatment of autoimmune diseases. *FEBS Letters*, March 17. [Epub ahead of print]

Thornton, B.D.; Hoffman, H.M.; Bhat, A. & Don, B.R. (2007). Successful treatment of renal amyloidosis due to familial cold autoinflammatory syndrome using an interleukin 1 receptor antagonist. *American Journal of Kidney Diseases*, Vol.49, No.3, (March 2007), pp 477-481.

Uhlar, C.M. & Whitehead, A.S. (1999). Serum amyloid A, the major vertebrate acute-phase reactant. *European Journal of Biochemistry*, Vol.265, No.2, (October 1999), pp. 501-523.

Van Eijk, I.C.; De Vries, M.K.; Levels, J.H.; Peters, M.J.; Huizer, E.E.; Dijkmans, B.A.; Van Der Horst-Bruinsma, I.E.; Hazenberg, B.P.; Van De Stadt, R.J.; Wolbink, G.J. & Nurmohamed, M.T. (2009). Improvement of lipid profile is accompanied by atheroprotective alterations in high-density lipoprotein composition upon tumor necrosis factor blockade: a prospective cohort study in ankylosing spondylitis. *Arthritis & Rheumatism*, Vol.60, No.5, (May 2009), pp. 1324-1330.

Verschueren, P.; Lensen, F.; Lerut, E.; Claes, K.; De Vos, R.; Van Damme, B. & Westhovens, R. (2003). Benefit of anti-TNFalpha treatment for nephrotic syndrome in a patient with juvenile inflammatory bowel disease associated spondyloarthropathy complicated with amyloidosis and glomerulonephritis. *Annals of the Rheumatic Diseases*, Vol.62, No.4, (April 2003), pp. 368-369.

Yamada, T.; Wada, A.; Itoh, Y. & Itoh, K. (1999). Serum amyloid A1 alleles and plasma concentrations of serum amyloid A. *Amyloid*, Vol.6, pp. 199-204.

Zhang, D.; Sun, M.; Samols, D. & Kushner, I. (1996). STAT3 participates in transcriptional activation of the C-reactive protein gene by interleukin-6. *The Journal of Biological Chemistry*, Vol.271, No.16, (April 1996), pp. 9503-9509.

Zhang. Z. & Fuller, G.M. (2000). Interleukin 1beta inhibits interleukin 6-mediated rat gamma fibrinogen gene expression. *Blood*, Vol.96, No.10, (November 2005), pp. 3466-3472.

12

Cardiac and Multi-Organ Transplantation in Patients with Amyloidosis

Eugenia Raichlin[1] and Sudhir S. Kushwaha[2]
[1]*University of Nebraska Medical Center, Division of Cardiology, Omaha, NE,*
[2]*Mayo Clinic, Rochester, MN,*
USA

1. Introduction

1.1 AL amyloidosis

Background

Amyloidosis is a group of diseases characterized by the extracellular deposition of a proteinaceous material in various organs and tissues, leading to progressive multiple organ failure and death. The presence of cardiac involvement and its relative predominance varies with the type of amyloidosis, tends to progress rapidly and has a very poor prognosis.
AL amyloidosis is the most common form of the disease. The heart in AL amyloidosis is affected in close to 50% of cases and amyloid deposition can be very rapidly progressive with increased untreated myocardial wall thickening at rates of up to 1.45–2.16 mm/month (Kristen *et al.*, 2007). Heart failure (HF) is the presenting clinical manifestation in about half of these patients (Dubrey *et al.*, 1998). Even among patients in whom another organ system dysfunction predominates, the presence of cardiac amyloidosis is frequently the worst prognostic factor (Kyle *et al.*, 1995). Once HF occurs, the median survival is less then six months in untreated patients (Dubrey *et al.*, 1998; Kyle *et al.*, 1995). Although the overall survival of AL amyloidosis patients can be improved by the use of high dose chemotherapy and autologous stem-cell transplantation (ASCT) (Dey *et al.*, 2010), the advanced cardiac disease at the time of diagnosis place these patients at a risk of 30% peri-treatment mortality (Falk *et al.*, 1998). Marked wall thickening, elevated brain natriuretic peptide or elevated troponin predict poor outcomes and an ejection fraction < 40% is considered an absolute contraindication to high-dose chemotherapy and ASCT (Dispenzieri *et al.*, 2003; Dispenzieri *et al.*, 2004; Falk *et al.*, 2005). However, it has been suggested that cardiac transplantation can restore health and permit subsequent administration of intensive chemotherapy.

1.2 Cardiac transplantation for AL amyloidosis

Cardiac transplantation for AL amyloidosis was first described in 1994 (Hall *et al.*, 1994). Early experience came from individual case reports and small series, which demonstrated that short and medium term mortality, did not differ from that in other disorders (Dubrey *et al.*, 2001; Hosenpud *et al.*, 1991). However reports generated from a survey of heart transplantation (HTx) centers in the USA, Canada and Europe showed outcomes significantly inferior to those seen in cardiac transplantation for primary cardiomyopathy

(Hosenpud *et al.*, 1990; Hosenpud *et al.*, 1991). Survival at four years was 39% and systemic progression was seen in the majority of patients. The Heart Transplant Centers in the European consortium reported a five-year survival of 38% in recipients with AL amyloidosis compared with 67% in recipients with HF due to non-amyloid cases (Dubrey *et al.*, 2004). Amyloid deposition occurred in the graft in every case in which it was sought histologically, and progressive systemic amyloidosis contributed to mortality in 70% of patients (Dubrey *et al.*, 2001). United Network for Organ Sharing data (Kpodonu *et al.*, 2005) are the largest published series of patients undergoing cardiac transplantation for AL amyloidosis which included 69 cardiac transplantations performed at 24 different centers in the USA, found a five-year survival of 54%. However, survival was not analyzed according to amyloid type in this study. Based on these discouraging outcomes amyloid heart disease has been considered a contraindication for HTx. Moreover, the need for adjunctive chemotherapy to suppress production of monoclonal light chains became obvious from the findings of several series that confirmed that relatively rapid development of cardiac allograft amyloid (Dubrey *et al.*, 1995; Valantine *et al.*, 1989;).

In 2004, Skinner *et al.* reported a complete hematologic response, defined as no evidence of an underlying plasma cell dyscrasia one year after treatment, in 40% of patients with primary AL amyloidosis who received high-dose melphalan followed by autologous stem cell transplantation (Dey *et al.*, 2010; Skinner *et al.*, 2004). Recently cardiac transplantation followed by high-dose chemotherapy and ASCT has been shown to be feasible in carefully selected patients with AL amyloidosis and severe HF (Dey *et al.*, 2010; Gillmore *et al.*, 2006; Kristen *et al.*, 2009; Lacy *et al.*, 2008; Maurer *et al.*, 2007; Mignot *et al.*, 2008; Sattianayagam *et*

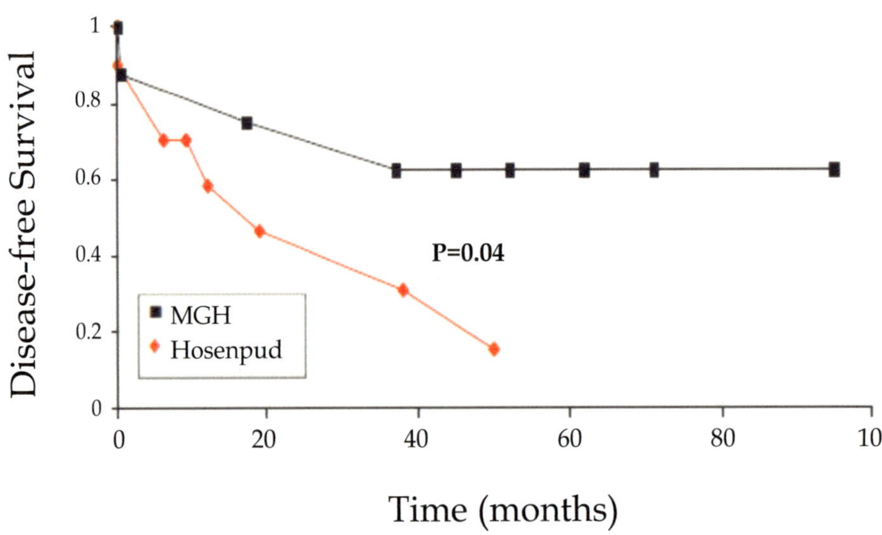

Reproduced from Dey *et al.*, 2010

Fig. 1. Kaplan-Meier disease free survival estimates, according to treatment MGH, orthotopic heart transplant followed by hematopoietic stem-cell transplant for cardiac amyloidosis; Hosenpud, orthotopic heart transplant alone for cardiac amyloidosis. Comparisons of survival between two groups of patients were made using the log-rank and Wilcoxon tests

al., 2010). This treatment is aimed at preventing recurrence of amyloid in the cardiac allograft or progression of extra cardiac amyloidosis, thus long-term remission and apparent improvement in long term survival in carefully selected patients can been achieved. (Fig. 1)
Gillmore et al., reported five patients with AL amyloidosis and predominant cardiomyopathy undergoing sequential HTx followed by ASCT: three patients survived for more than nine years without evidence of recurrence and two patients died of progressive amyloidosis at 33 and 90 months after HTx (Gillmore et al., 2006). This study also showed that relapse of the plasma cell dyscrasia after ASCT was associated with characteristic echocardiographic evidence of cardiac amyloidosis and rise in serum NT-pro-BNP. Maurer *et al.*, reported on 10 patients who underwent HTx for AL amyloidosis (Maurer *et al.*, 2007). In this study among eight patients who received subsequent ASCT, two died from sepsis and lymphoma. The median survival from cardiac transplantation of 9.7 years in this series is comparable to US all-cause cardiac transplant survival (Sattianayagam *et al.*, 2010).
The largest case scenarios came from Mayo Clinic and Massachusetts General Hospital (Dey *et al.*, 2010; Lacy *et al.*, 2008). In report of Dey *et al.*, five of eight patients who underwent sequential HTx / ASCT were alive with a good functional status at a median follow-up of 56 months (range, 7–101 months). None have evidence of recurrent amyloidosis, with four

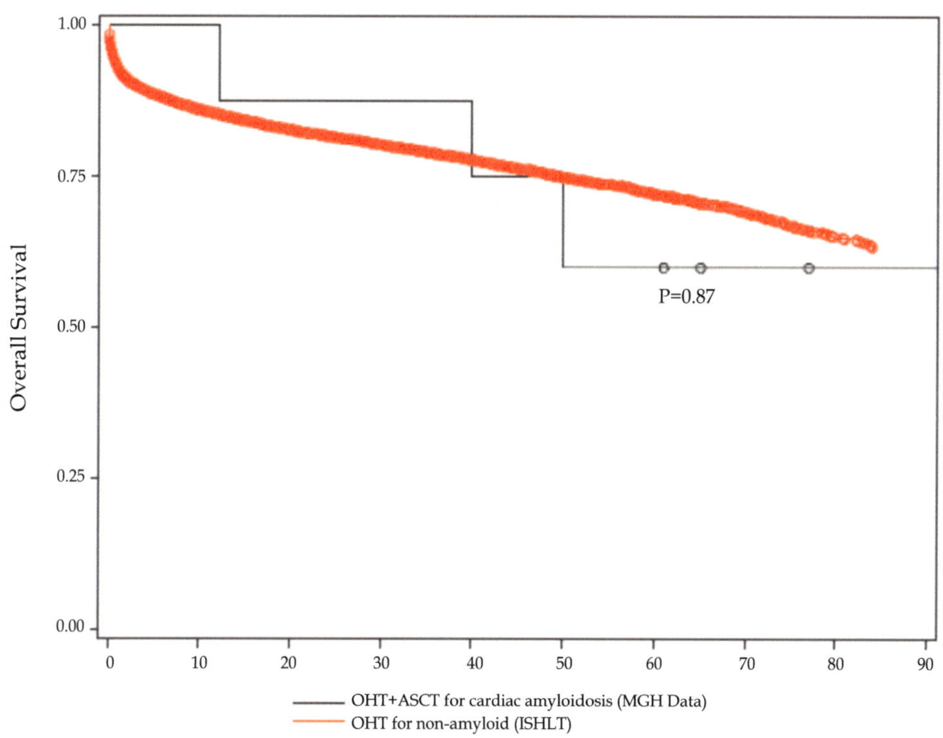

OHT, orthotopic heart transplant; ASCT, autologous hematopoietic stem-cell transplant; MGH – Massachusetts General Hospital; ISHLT, International Society for Heart and Lung Transplantation. Reproduced from Dey *et al.*, 2010

Fig. 2. Kaplan-Meier overall survival estimates, according to treatment. Comparisons of survival between OHT and OHT+ASCT groups of patients (p=0.87, log-rank and Wilcoxon tests)

remaining in complete hematologic remission. The survival of these patients (Figure 2) was 60% at seven years, which is not significantly different from the outcomes of 17,389 patients collected in the database of the International Society for Heart and Lung Transplantation who underwent HTx for non-amyloid heart disease during the same time. Lacy *et al.*, from the Mayo Clinic have published a series of 11 carefully selected patients undergoing sequential HTx /ASCT. They reported a one and five-year survival of 82% and 65%, respectively (Lacy *et al.*, 2008). Although two patients died from transplant-related toxicity and three patients died from progressive amyloidosis, the survival was comparable to patients undergoing HTx for non-amyloid disease.

Thus, the data indicates that reasonable outcomes are achievable in patients with severe cardiac AL amyloidosis after HTx if underlying dyscrasia plasma cell is successfully treated afterward.

1.3 Selection criteria

In the early experience of cardiac transplantation for AL amyloidosis, patients were not screened to exclude extensive systemic involvement and a significant degree of systemic involvement may have accounted for the particularly poor prognosis. Careful patient selection may have contributed at least partially to improved outcomes in more recent studies.

The baseline evaluation of all patients being considered for transplantation includes bone marrow aspirate and biopsy, echocardiogram, serum and 24-hour urine monoclonal protein studies, immunoglobulin-free light-chain assay, a chemistry panel including creatinine, liver function tests and renal clearance estimates (Gertz *et al.*, 2005).

In the Mayo Clinic series, selection criteria for cardiac transplantation included advanced cardiomyopathy, age under 60 years, and absence of myeloma or extensive extra-cardiac amyloidosis (Lacy *et al.*, 2008). (Table 1)

In the MGH data, however, in addition to advanced cardiac disease extra cardiac solid organ involvement by amyloidosis was present in all patients at the time of evaluation: all but one of the patients had evidence of amyloid deposition in the gastrointestinal tract, significant proteinuria was present in two and peripheral neuropathy in three HTx patients. Monoclonal plasma cells comprised 5% to 10% of marrow cellularity (Dey *et al.*, 2010).

1.4 Waiting period

Unfortunately, patients with AL amyloidosis and severe HF have an extraordinarily poor prognosis on completing their cardiac transplant evaluation. Of 26 patients evaluated in the MGH series, 18 patients were selected and listed for HTx/ASCT, but only half survived to HTx (Dey *et al.*, 2010). In the Mayo Clinic experience, of 54 patients evaluated, 27 patients were selected and listed for HTx but nine died while on the waiting list and six were removed from the list due to progressive disease. Only 11 patients (20%) underwent cardiac transplantation. In the study of Sattianayagam *et al.*, less than 2% of all patients with systemic AL amyloidosis assessed at the United Kingdom National Amyloidosis Center underwent cardiac transplantation (Sattianayagam *et al.*, 2010).

Despite the significant risk of death associated with the use of vigorous chemotherapy in patients with AL cardiac amyloidosis, it should be considered in selected patients: a clinical improvement in HF despite an unchanged echocardiographic appearance has been reported (Dubrey *et al.*, 1996). This improvement may result from the abolition of the production of freshly produced light chains, which have been shown to be toxic to myocardial cells,

Routine cardiac transplantation evaluation with the following additional studies:	• Serum protein electrophoresis • Urine protein electrophoresis (24-hour urine) • Factor X and thrombin time (special coagulation studies) • Bone marrow biopsy with aspirate, labeling index and smear • Labeling index in peripheral blood with number of circulating plasma cells • Serum carotene • β_2-microglobulin • C-reactive protein • 24-hour urine creatinine clearance • 48-hour stool collection for fat • Subcutaneous fat aspirate • Metastatic bone survey with single views of humeri and femurs
Pulmonary assessment will proceed as follows:	Recurrent pleural effusions, refractory to treatment will necessitate: • Chest CT • Possible lung biopsy dependent on CT findings
Liver assessment will proceed as follows:	• If alkaline phosphatase <1.5-fold upper limit of normal (350), then proceed with transplant evaluation • If alkaline phosphatase 1.5- to 3-fold upper limit of normal, then proceed to liver biopsy: 1. If there is portal tract amyloid deposition, then there is an absolute contraindication 2. If vascular amyloid only, then proceed with transplant evaluation • If alkaline phosphatase is ≥3.0-fold upper limit of normal (750), absolute then there is an contraindication to HT
Renal assessment will proceed as follows:	Lothalamate clearance should exceed 50 ml/min/1.73 m^2 • If urinary albumin is <250 mg/24 hours, then proceed with transplant evaluation • If urinary albumin is 250 to 1,000 mg/24 hours, then proceed to renal biopsy 1. If vascular amyloid only, is present then proceed with transplant evaluation 2. If interstitial or glomerular amyloid is present, then there is an absolute contraindication to cardiac transplant
Blood/marrow plasma cell labeling index assessment will proceed as follows:	Plasma cell labeling index • If plasma cell labeling index is ≥2%, then exclude from consideration for transplant evaluation • If plasma cell labeling index is ≥1%, then proceed to metastatic bone survey to exclude myeloma-associated bony lesions • If plasma cell labeling index is <1%, then proceed with transplant evaluation Peripheral blood labeling index • If peripheral blood plasma cell labeling index is >1%, then absolute contraindication to cardiac transplant Plasmacytosis • If plasma cell differential on marrow aspirate is <10%, then proceed with transplant evaluation • If plasma cell differential on marrow aspirate is 10% to 20%, then do metastatic bone survey to exclude myeloma-associated bony lesions • If plasma cell differential on marrow aspirate, marrow biopsy or cytoplasmic immunoglobulin–positive plasma cells are ≥20%, then contraindication to there is an absolute cardiac transplant
Intestinal assessment will proceed as follows:	• 48-hour stool collection for fecal fat to rule out malabsorption • Serum carotene if low level could indicate malabsorption • Endoscopic and flexible sigmoidoscopic evaluation with biopsy 1. If vascular amyloid deposition only, then proceed with transplant evaluation 2. If mucosal amyloid deposition, then there is an absolute contraindication to cardiac transplantation

Adapted from Lacy *et al.*, 2008

Table 1. Cardiac Transplantation: pre-transplant evaluation of AL amyloid patients

suggesting that AL amyloidosis is not simply an infiltrative cardiomyopathy but rather a toxic infiltrative disorder (Brenner *et al.*, 2004; Falk *et al.*, 2005; Liao *et al.*, 2001; Nakamura *et al.*, 2002). Despite the risk and delayed clinical benefits (Skinner *et al.*, 1996), successful outcomes have been reported in small numbers of patients treated with chemotherapy followed by cardiac transplantation (Mignot *et al.*, 2008). At the United Kingdom National Amyloidosis Center five patients were fit enough to receive chemotherapy and achieved a partial hematologic response before cardiac transplantation. Similarly, one patient at Mayo Clinic and two patients at MGH received systemic therapy consisting of melphalan and prednisone before cardiac transplantation. In cases when a substantial delay before the cardiac transplant is likely, the earlier application of plasma-cell-targeted therapeutic approaches with newer agents, such as bortezomib and lenalidomide (Kastritis *et al.*, 2007; Sanchorawala *et al.*, 2007) which are effective and better tolerated than conventional chemotherapeutic agents, beginning at the time of the evaluation process may be beneficial, and improve patients' chances for receiving an HTx. A similar approach may also be considered for patients who are not ready for ASCT after cardiac transplantation since a prolonged time without treatment may allow progression of the amyloidosis and therefore both impair the candidacy of these patients for ASCT and increase their transplant related mortality (Dey *et al.*, 2010; Lacy *et al.*, 2008).

1.5 Timing of ASCT after the HTx

During the last several years, ASCT has undergone further refinement, including changes in supportive care and a better understanding of the complications of ASCT that are unique to amyloid patients. The optimal timing of ASCT after the HTx is debatable. Pursuing ASCT too soon may be problematic if the patient continues to require intensive immunosuppression to prevent organ rejection. Waiting too long may result in the amyloidosis progressing in other organs. Therefore, at the present time, it is recommended that ASCT be pursued approximately six to seven months after HTx (Dey *et al.*, 2010; Lacy *et al.*, 2008).

1.6 Recurrence of cardiac amyloidosis

Although in the United Kingdom study the patients were followed for two to six years with serial endomyocardial biopsies with no evidence of recurrent amyloid deposition during this time (Dubrey *et al.*, 2004), five of the 11 patients reported by Lacy *et al.*, demonstrated biopsy-proven recurrence in the cardiac allograft. Interestingly, none of these patients had symptoms, echocardiographic evidence, or biochemical evidence of cardiac amyloidosis. A similar observation was reported by Dey *et al.*, demonstrating that amyloid deposition in their heart transplant patients has had little clinical consequence, with no echocardiographic evidence of amyloid cardiomyopathy. By contrast, Gilmore showed that relapse of the plasma cell dyscrasia after ASCT was associated with characteristic echocardiographic evidence of cardiac amyloidosis and rise in serum NT-pro-BNP. The varying results may be secondary to multiple factors, including the type of chemotherapy used, the timing of ASCT following heart transplant, the type of underlying plasma cell dyscrasia as well as individual patient factors (Luk *et al.*, 2009). Nevertheless, the recurrent disease despite aggressive multimodality therapy is a reminder that it may be difficult to prevent recurrent protein deposition in patients with AL amyloidosis. Although conclusions are limited by the small sample size, it is likely that ASCT following cardiac transplantation results in a lack of clinically significant recurrent amyloidosis despite the presence of recurrent amyloid deposition and prolongs the interval of disease recurrence in the cardiac allograft. However, it is possible that future survival of patients with disease recurrence in the cardiac allograft beyond the time described may be limited (Dey *et al.*, 2010).

1.7 Conclusions

Although a multidisciplinary approach dedicated to early diagnosis, appropriate and timely screening for HTx and a multimodality plasma cell dyscrasia specific strategy may offer long-term remission for carefully selected patients with cardiac amyloidosis, HTx for amyloid cardiomyopathy continues to generate controversy because of the donor shortage and concerns about recurrence either in the transplanted heart or other vital organs. Clinical trials are still required to clarify which patients are most likely to achieve durable remissions after HTx and which chemotherapy strategy is most effective to eradicate the plasma cell clone.

1.8 Combined heart and kidney transplantation in patients with AL amyloidosis

AL amyloidosis is a multi-organ disease and the proportion of patients with cardiac AL amyloidosis and minimal systemic disease at the time of diagnosis is less than 5% (Dubrey *et al.*, 1998). Cardiac amyloidosis frequently coexists with renal involvement which is characterized by nephrotic proteinuria and progressive worsening of renal function. However there are only two published cases of combined organ transplantation in patients with AL amyloidosis. Because of significant renal impairment, one patient received a combined heart and kidney transplantation (CHKTx) followed by ASCT at MGH and is reported to be alive up to 65 months with no evidence of recurrence. In case of partial hematologic remission induced by two courses of oral melphalan plus prednisone, followed by CHKTx, without ASCT, resulting in excellent renal and cardiac allograft function at three years has been reported (Audard *et al.*, 2009).

2. Familial amyloidosis (ATTR)

2.1 Introduction

Familial amyloidosis (ATTR) is a fatal autosomal-dominant multisystem disorder induced by deposition in several organs of abnormal serum ATTR (prealbumin) protein which is mainly produced in the liver. Amongst the over 40 mutations described, the Portuguese variant (ATTR Met30) is the most frequent and not associated with cardiomyopathy. Orthotopic liver transplantation is established as the treatment of choice for ATTR Met30 with stabilization or remission of symptoms. In patients with a non-ATTR Met30 mutation and cardiomyopathy, after isolated liver transplantation (ILTx), the amyloid fibril deposition in the heart is increased suggesting that wild-type ATTR probably constitutes amyloid in the heart similar to the phenomenon observed in senile systemic amyloidosis (Stangou *et al.*, 1998; Westermark *et al.*, 1990; Yazaki *et al.*, 2000). This leads to progression of cardiomyopathy following ILTx in patients carrying a non-ATTR Met30 mutation and suggests that CHLTx is the procedure of choice (Pomfret *et al.*, 1998). The first case of CHLTx in familial amyloidosis patients was reported by (Rela *et al.*, 1995), however, the world-wide experience of this is small, and less than 25 cases of CHLTx have been reported in the medical literature.

2.2 Survival after CHLTx in ATTR amyloidosis

CHLTx experience has been analyzed for ATTR disease in the United Kingdom and the five-year survival has been shown to be comparable with survival after transplantation for other diseases suggesting that this procedure should be indicated for several non-ATTR Met30 variants with recognized risk for progressive amyloid cardiomyopathy (Dubrey *et al.*, 2004). A relatively large series from Mayo Clinic demonstrates the feasibility and excellent short and long term success that can be achieved with CHLTx for selected high-risk patients with familial amyloidosis. Indeed, patient survival after CHLTx was shown to be equivalent to those with IHTx. (Figure 3)

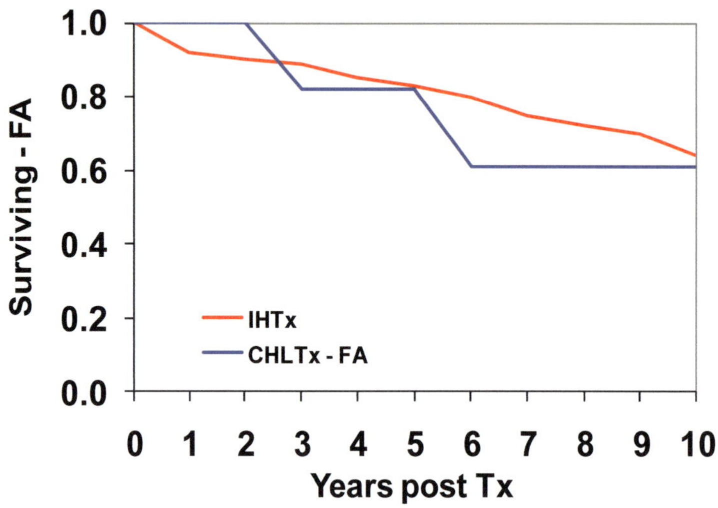

IHTx - isolated heart transplantation. CHLTx - combined heart and liver transplantation.
Reproduced from Raichlin *et al.*, 2009

Fig. 3. Survival rates for FA patients at 1 month, 1 year, 5 and 10 years were 100%, 100%, 75%, and 60% and did not differ from IHTx (97%, 93%, 83% and 65%, p=0.39, Log-Rank test)

In the Mayo Clinic study, among 11 patients with ATTR the most frequent mutations were ALA 60 (4), and TYR 77 (3), followed by PRO 24 (1), SER (1) and ASP 18 GLU (1). One patient had an undefined mutation. This study showed that specific ATTR mutations do not affect the therapeutic success of CHLTx. Indeed, ALA 60 ATTR has been reported as a mutation of particularly poor prognosis and five of eight patients with ALA60 mutation described in the literature have died after ILTx (Kotani *et al.*, 2002; Sharma *et al.*, 2003). Moreover, the Tyr 77 ATTR (German variant) mutation is also typically associated with prominent and progressive cardiac involvement after ILTx (Garcia-Herola, 1999). In the Mayo Clinic report three of the four patients with ALA 60 ATTR mutation remain alive and one died of progressive renal failure; three patients with the TYR 77 ATTR variant remain alive and had no amyloid deposition on the last endomyocardial biopsy.

Autonomic disturbances, modified body mass index, duration of symptoms, polyneuropathy, disability score, orthostatic hypotension, gastrointestinal and urinary tract dysfunction are important factors in the preoperative evaluation (Grazi *et al.*, 2003; Sharma *et al.*, 2003; Pilato *et al.*, 2007) and optimizing the timing for CHLTx appears to be crucial.

2.3 Surgical approaches for CHLTx

Several different surgical approaches have been described for CHLTx:

1. Transplantation of the heart but maintaining the patient on cardio-pulmonary bypass during the liver transplant was described. Subsequent concerns about substantial

coagulopathy and increased bleeding changed the strategy to performing liver implantation following separation from cardiopulmonary bypass (Befeler *et al.*, 1999; Grazi *et al.*, 2003; Shaw *et al.*, 1985; Detry *et al.*, 1997; Nardo *et al.*, 2004). Improved surgical and anesthetic techniques during liver transplant, and the potential benefits to the transplanted heart to remain on cardio-pulmonary bypass during liver implantation led to revising this strategy for CHLTx. In the case study by Hennessey and colleagues, this technique was suggested to provide a considerably shortened liver ischemia time and decreased blood transfusion compared to the sequential approach (Hennessey *et al.*, 2010).

2. Transplantation of the heart with discontinuation of cardio-pulmonary bypass, leaving the chest opened. The liver transplantation was performed as a second step through a bilateral sub-costal incision with extension in the midline to the sternotomy (Couetil *et al.*, 1995) and was accomplished by a caval sparing hepatectomy with an anastomosis between the donor supra-hepatic cava and the recipient left/middle hepatic vein trunk. Biliary tubes were inserted through the donor cystic duct stumps whenever possible, and the abdomen was closed over drains after achieving hemostasis. (Raichlin *et al.*, 2009) One of the major advantages of this procedure is that CHLTx can be performed with minimal deviation from the standard procedures of IHTx and ILTx.
3. Staged heart and liver transplantation was first reported by Figuera (Figuera *et al.*, 1986) for patients who underwent HTx and were hemodynamically unstable after cardiac reperfusion. Subsequent liver transplantation was deferred, and the patients underwent deceased donor liver transplantation from a second donor.(Barreiros *et al.*, 2010; Pilato *et al.*, 2007)

In the Mayo Clinic study simultaneous CHLTx was feasible in 87% (13 of 15) of patients and appears favorable if cardiac function and hemodynamics are satisfactory (Raichlin *et al.*, 2009).

Based on the experience of several centers (Befeler *et al.*, 1999; Raichlin *et al.*, 2007a) it seems that renal failure secondary to hypo-perfusion from cardiopulmonary and veno-venous bypass, blood loss and the nephrotoxic effects of peri-operative medications (including inotropic agents and immunosuppressive drugs) complicate the early post-operative course of many patients following CHLTx. As demonstrated in the study from Mayo Clinic, none of the preoperative evaluations were able to predict such postoperative complications. Within one month following transplantation renal function improved in the CHLTx patients and was comparable with the isolated heart transplantation (IHTx) group. However, three patients (30%) developed late end-stage renal failure presumably as a result of calcineurin inhibitor toxicity (clinical picture was not consistent with amyloid glomerulopathy) and required hemodialysis. Therefore, renal function was significantly worse in the CHLTx patients at the late follow-up. It was previously demonstrated that the risk of chronic renal failure after transplantation of a non-renal organ depends on the type of organ transplanted and at five years the cumulative incidence of chronic renal failure was lower after IHTx (10.9±0.2) compared to ILTx (18.1±0.20) (Gonwa *et al.*, 2001; Ojo *et al.*, 2003). Calcineurin inhibitor sparing (Sirolimus based) immunosuppression probably should be considered in CHLTx patients to prevent progressive calcineurin inhibitor - induced renal damage (Raichlin *et al.*, 2007a; Raichlin *et al.*, 2007b).

2.4 Acute cellular rejection

Acute cellular rejection of the liver is infrequent in CHLTx (Raichlin et al., 2009). The more aggressive immunosuppression regimen employed for CHLTx compared with that used for

ILTx may make rejection of liver allografts a relatively infrequent event. Interestingly, heart rejection was less frequent in CHLTx than in those receiving IHTx. (Figure 4) To explain the favorable low rejection rate an induction of partial tolerance has been proposed as a mechanism. The liver has been demonstrated to permit acceptance of other simultaneously transplanted organs operating via shedding soluble HLA antigens (Davies *et al.*, 1989; McMillan *et al.*, 1997). It has been hypothesized that maintaining a concentration of soluble HLA in the circulation would lead to tolerance to the allotype of the soluble HLA. This concept may help explain the protection of a simultaneous heart transplant by a successful human liver transplant (Vogel *et al.*, 1988). Therefore, less intensive immunosuppression therapy for these patients after CHLTx than for IHTx may be justified.

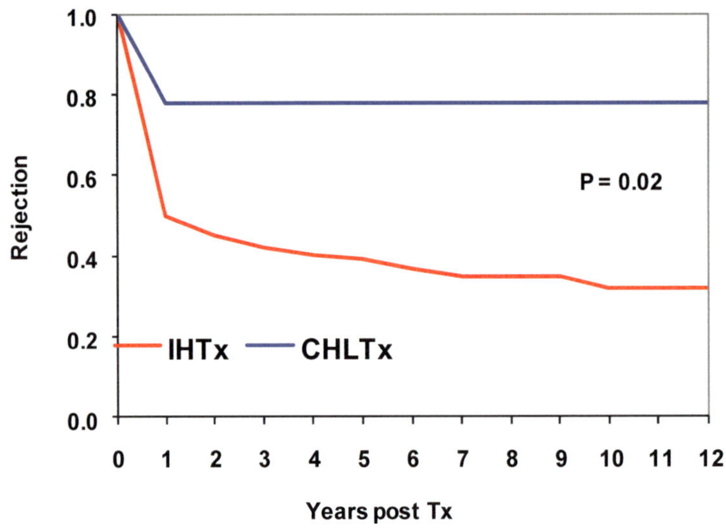

IHTx - isolated heart transplantation. CHLTx - combined heart and liver transplantation.
Reproduced from Raichlin *et al.*, 2009

Fig. 4. Freedom from cardiac allograft rejection (International Society for Heart and Lung Transplantation ≥ Grade 2) for at 1 month was 83% and did not change further. For IHTx freedom from rejection at 1 month, 1 year, 3 years and 10 years was 80%, 48%, 42% and 32% respectively (p=0.02, Log-Rank test)

2.5 Postoperative course and complications

In the Mayo Clinic report for recipients of CHLTx the mean intensive care unit stay did not differ (p=0.23) and the mean hospital stay was not significantly longer than for IHTx (p=0.09).

2.6 Pulmonary embolism

Pulmonary embolism is a rare complication in early period post IHTx (Berroeta *et al.*, 2006). In Mayo Clinic study two patients developed pulmonary embolism and were treated with anticoagulation. This high incidence of pulmonary embolism in recipients of CHLTx probably reflects the prolonged immobilization period and delayed recovery of anticoagulant proteins in this group of patients (Stahl *et al.*, 1990).

2.7 Cardiac allograft function

In the Mayo Clinic study, during a mean 65 month follow up, all heart allografts displayed normal systolic function on echocardiography with mean left ventricular ejection fraction 65% ± 7% and no signs of left ventricular heart. Congo red stain and/or sulfated alcian blue stain was negative for amyloid in all patients. There has been no significant cardiac allograft vasculopathy in any of these.

2.8 Use of amyloidotic livers for domino liver transplantation

Since livers explanted from patients with FA contain only microscopic amyloid deposits and are otherwise essentially normal, and it typically takes approximately 50 years for TTR deposition to progress to clinically apparent disease, the FA liver can be used as a domino donor liver for selected older patients awaiting liver transplantation. CHLTx does not preclude domino donation of FA recipients' liver. In contrast to caval sparing hepatectomy with an anastomosis between the donor supra-hepatic cava and the recipient left/middle hepatic vein trunk caval excision with veno-venous and portal-venous bypass was employed for FA patients serving as domino liver donors. None of the domino donors experienced any technical problems related to donation or veno-venous and porto-venous bypass. (Azoulay *et al.*, 1999; Raichlin *et al.*, 2009)

3. Conclusion

CHLTx for ATTR is a successful therapy for this disease and can be performed safely, with a acceptable level of morbidity. Given the 10-year survival of 60% with an associated freedom of rejection of 83%, the procedure is consistently curative in patients with ATTR and cardiac involvement. Specific ATTR mutations do not affect outcome. Cardiac allograft rejection after CHLTx is significantly less frequent than with IHTx and may justify less intensive immunosuppression therapy for these patients. In addition calcineurin sparing (sirolimus based) immunosuppression to prevent progressive calcineurin-induced renal damage should be considered in CHLTx recipients.

4. References

Audard V, Matignon M, Weiss L, *et al.* Successful long-term outcome of the first combined heart and kidney transplant in a patient with systemic Al amyloidosis. *Am J Transplant.* 2009;9:236-40

Azoulay D, Samuel D, Castaing D, *et al.* Domino liver transplants for metabolic disorders: experience with familial amyloidotic polyneuropathy. *J Am Coll Surg.* 1999;189:584-93

Barreiros AP, Post F, Hoppe-Lotichius M, *et al.* Liver transplantation and combined liver-heart transplantation in patients with familial amyloid polyneuropathy: a single-center experience. *Liver* Transpl, 2010; 16:314-23

Befeler AS, Schiano TD, Lissoos TW, *et al.* Successful combined liver-heart transplantation in adults: report of three patients and review of the literature. Transplantation. 1999;68:1423-7

Berroeta C, Flament F, Lathyris D, *et al.* Pulmonary embolism: an uncommon cause of dyspnea after heart transplantation. *J Cardiothorac Vasc Anesth.* 2006;20:236-8. Epub 2005 Dec 1

Brenner DA, Jain M, Pimentel DR, *et al.* Human amyloidogenic light chains directly impair cardiomyocyte function through an increase in cellular oxidant stress. *Circ Res.* 2004;94:1008-10. Epub 2004 Mar 25

Couetil JP, Houssin DP, Soubrane O, *et al.* Combined lung and liver transplantation in patients with cystic fibrosis. A 4 1/2-year experience. *J Thorac Cardiovasc Surg.* 1995;110:1415-22; discussion 1422-3

Davies HS, Pollard SG, Calne RY. Soluble HLA antigens in the circulation of liver graft recipients. *Transplantation* 1989;47:524-7

Detry O, Honore P, Meurisse M, *et al.* Advantages of inferior vena caval flow preservation in combined transplantation of the liver and heart. *Transpl Int.* 1997;10:150-1

Dey BR, Chung SS, Spitzer TR, *et al.* Cardiac transplantation followed by dose-intensive melphalan and autologous stem-cell transplantation for light chain amyloidosis and heart failure. *Transplantation* 2010 Oct 27;90(8):905-11

Dispenzieri A, Kyle RA, Gertz MA, *et al.* Survival in patients with primary systemic amyloidosis and raised serum cardiac troponins. *Lancet* 2003;361:1787-9

Dispenzieri A, Gertz MA, Kyle RA, *et al.* Serum cardiac troponins and N-terminal pro-brain natriuretic peptide: a staging system for primary systemic amyloidosis. *J Clin Oncol.* 2004;22:3751-7

Dubrey S, Simms RW, Skinner M, Falk RH. Recurrence of primary (AL) amyloidosis in a transplanted heart with four-year survival. *Am J Cardiol.* 1995;76:739-41

Dubrey S, Mendes L, Skinner M, Falk RH. Resolution of heart failure in patients with AL amyloidosis. *Ann Intern Med.* 1996;125:481-4

Dubrey SW, Cha K, Anderson J, *et al.* The clinical features of immunoglobulin light-chain (AL) amyloidosis with heart involvement. *Qjm.* 1998;91:141-57

Dubrey SW, Burke MM, Khaghani A, Hawkins PN, Yacoub MH, Banner NR. Long term results of heart transplantation in patients with amyloid heart disease. *Heart.* 2001;85:202-7

Dubrey SW, Burke MM, Hawkins PN, Banner NR. Cardiac transplantation for amyloid heart disease: the United Kingdom experience. *J Heart Lung Transplant.* 2004;23:1142-53

Falk RH RJ, Dubrey SW, Mendes LA, Sanchorawala V, Ekery, D CR, Vosburgh E, Skinner M. . The effect of cardiac involvement on the outcome of intravenous melphalan therapy and autologous stem cell rescue for AL amyloidosis. In: Kyle RA GM, eds., ed. *Amyloid and the Amyloidoses: VIIIth International Symposiumon Amyloidosis.* Rochester, MN: Parthenon 1998:181–183

Falk RH. Diagnosis and management of the cardiac amyloidoses. *Circulation.* 2005;112:2047-60.

Figuera D, Ardaiz J, Martin-Judez V, *et al.* Combined transplantation of heart and liver from two different donors in a patient with familial type IIa hypercholesterolemia. *J Heart Transplant.* 1986;5:327-9

Garcia-Herola A, Prieto M, Pascual S, *et al.* Progression of cardiomyopathy and neuropathy after liver transplantation in a patient with familial amyloidotic polyneuropathy caused by tyrosine-77 transthyretin variant. *Liver Transpl Surg* 1999;5:246-8

Gertz MA, Comenzo R, Falk RH, *et al.* Definition of organ involvement and treatment response in immunoglobulin light chain amyloidosis (AL): a consensus opinion from the 10th International Symposium on Amyloid and Amyloidosis, Tours, France, 18-22 April 2004. *Am J Hematol.* 2005;79:319-28

Gillmore JD, Goodman HJ, Lachmann HJ, *et al.* Sequential heart and autologous stem cell transplantation for systemic AL amyloidosis. *Blood.* 2006;107:1227-9. Epub 2005 Oct 6

Gonwa TA, Mai ML, Melton LB, *et al.* End-stage renal disease (ESRD) after orthotopic liver transplantation (OLTX) using calcineurin-based immunotherapy: risk of development and treatment. *Transplantation* 2001;72:1934-9

Grazi GL, Cescon M, Salvi F, *et al.* Combined heart and liver transplantation for familial amyloidotic neuropathy: considerations from the hepatic point of view. *Liver Transpl.* 2003;9:986-92

Hall R, Hawkins PN. Cardiac transplantation for AL amyloidosis. *Bmj.* 1994;309:1135-7

Hennessey T, Backman SB, Cecere R, *et al.* Combined heart and liver transplantation on cardiopulmonary bypass: report of four cases. 2010; *Can*;57:355-60

Hosenpud JD, Uretsky BF, Griffith BP, O'Connell JB, Olivari MT, Valantine HA. Successful intermediate-term outcome for patients with cardiac amyloidosis undergoing heart transplantation: results of a multicenter survey. *J Heart Transplant.* 1990;9:346-50

Hosenpud JD, DeMarco T, Frazier OH, *et al.* Progression of systemic disease and reduced long-term survival in patients with cardiac amyloidosis undergoing heart transplantation. Follow-up results of a multicenter survey. *Circulation.* 1991;84:III338-43

Kotani N, Hattori T, Yamagata S, *et al.* Transthyretin Thr60Ala Appalachian-type mutation in a Japanese family with familial amyloidotic polyneuropathy. *Amyloid* 2002;9:31-4

Kpodonu J, Massad MG, Caines A, Geha AS. Outcome of heart transplantation in patients with amyloid cardiomyopathy. *J Heart Lung Transplant.* 2005;24:1763-5

Kristen AV, Sack FU, Schonland SO, *et al.* Staged heart transplantation and chemotherapy as a treatment option in patients with severe cardiac light-chain amyloidosis. *Eur J Heart Fail.* 2009;11:1014-20

Kyle RA, Gertz MA. Primary systemic amyloidosis: clinical and laboratory features in 474 cases. *Semin Hematol.* 1995;32:45-59

Kristen AV, Perz JB, Schonland SO, *et al.* Non-invasive predictors of survival in cardiac amyloidosis. *Eur J Heart Fail.* 2007;9:617-24

Lacy MQ, Dispenzieri A, Hayman SR, *et al.* Autologous stem cell transplant after heart transplant for light chain (Al) amyloid cardiomyopathy. *J Heart Lung Transplant.* 2008;27:823-9

Liao R, Jain M, Teller P, *et al.* Infusion of light chains from patients with cardiac amyloidosis causes diastolic dysfunction in isolated mouse hearts. *Circulation.* 2001;104:1594-7

Luk A, Ahn E, Lee A, Ross HJ, Butany J. Recurrent cardiac amyloidosis following previous heart transplantation. *Cardiovasc Pathol* 2009;19:9

Maurer MS, Raina A, Hesdorffer C, *et al.* Cardiac transplantation using extended-donor criteria organs for systemic amyloidosis complicated by heart failure. *Transplantation.* 2007;83:539-45

McMillan RW, Gelder FB, Zibari GB, Aultman DF, Adamashvili I, McDonald JC. Soluble fraction of class I human histocompatibility leukocyte antigens in the serum of liver transplant recipients. *Clin Transplant* 1997;11:98-103

Mignot A, Bridoux F, Thierry A, *et al.* Successful heart transplantation following melphalan plus dexamethasone therapy in systemic AL amyloidosis. *Haematologica.* 2008;93:e32-5

Nakamura M, Satoh M, Kowada S, *et al.* Reversible restrictive cardiomyopathy due to light-chain deposition disease. *Mayo Clin Proc.* 2002;77:193-6

Nardo B, Beltempo P, Bertelli R, *et al.* Combined heart and liver transplantation in four adults with familial amyloidosis: experience of a single center. *Transplant Proc* 2004;36:645-7

Ojo AO, Held PJ, Port FK, *et al.* Chronic renal failure after transplantation of a nonrenal organ. N Engl J Med 2003;349:931-40

Pilato E, Dell'Amore A, Botta L, Arpesella G. Combined heart and liver transplantation for familial amyloidotic neuropathy. *Eur J Cardiothorac Surg.* 2007;32:180-2Raichlin E, Khalpey Z, Kremers W, *et al.* Replacement of calcineurin-inhibitors with sirolimus as primary immunosuppression in stable cardiac transplant recipients. Transplantation. 2007;84:467-74

Raichlin E, Bae JH, Khalpey Z, *et al.* Conversion to sirolimus as primary immunosuppression attenuates the progression of allograft vasculopathy after cardiac transplantation. *Circulation.* 2007;116:2726-33

Raichlin E, Daly RC, Rosen CB, *et al.* Combined heart and liver transplantation: a single-center experience. *Transplantation* 2009;88:219-25

Sanchorawala V, Skinner M, Quillen K, Finn KT, Doros G, Seldin DC. Long-term outcome of patients with AL amyloidosis treated with high-dose melphalan and stem-cell transplantation. *Blood* 2007;110:3561-3

Sattianayagam PT, Gibbs SD, Pinney JH, *et al.* Solid organ transplantation in AL amyloidosis Outcomes of heart transplantation for cardiac amyloidosis: subanalysis of the Spanish registry for heart transplantation. *Am J Transplatn.* 2010;10(9):2124-31

Sharma P, Perri RE, Sirven JE, *et al.* Outcome of liver transplantation for familial amyloidotic polyneuropathy. *Liver Transpl* 2003;9:1273-80

Shaw BW, Jr., Bahnson HT, Hardesty RL, Griffith BP, Starzl TE. Combined transplantation of the heart and liver. *Ann Surg* 1985;202:667-72

Skinner M, Anderson J, Simms R, *et al.* Treatment of 100 patients with primary amyloidosis: a randomized trial of melphalan, prednisone, and colchicine versus colchicine only. *Am J Med.* 1996;100:290-8

Skinner M, Sanchorawala V, Seldin DC, *et al.* High-dose melphalan and autologous stem-cell transplantation in patients with AL amyloidosis: an 8-year study. *Ann Intern Med.* 2004;140:85-93

Stahl RL, Duncan A, Hooks MA, Henderson JM, Millikan WJ, Warren WD. A hypercoagulable state follows orthotopic liver transplantation. *Hepatology* 1990;12:553-8

Stangou AJ, Hawkins PN, Heaton ND, *et al.* Progressive cardiac amyloidosis following liver transplantation for familial amyloid polyneuropathy: implications for amyloid fibrillogenesis. *Transplantation* 1998;66:229-33

Valantine HA, Billingham ME. Recurrence of amyloid in a cardiac allograft four months after transplantation. J Heart Transplant. 1989;8:337-41

Vogel W, Steiner E, Kornberger R, *et al.* Preliminary results with combined hepatorenal allografting. Transplantation 1988;45:491-3

Westermark P, Sletten K, Johansson B, Cornwell GG, 3rd. Fibril in senile systemic amyloidosis is derived from normal transthyretin. Proc Natl Acad Sci U S A 1990;87:2843-5

Yazaki M, Tokuda T, Nakamura A, *et al.* Cardiac amyloid in patients with familial amyloid polyneuropathy consists of abundant wild-type transthyretin. Biochem Biophys Res Commun 2000;274:702-6

13

Autologous Stem Cell Transplantation in the Treatment of Amyloidosis – Can Manipulation of the Autograft Reduce Treatment-Related Toxicity?

Çiğdem Akalın Akkök and Øystein Bruserud
Department of Immunology & Transfusion Medicine, Oslo University Hospital, Ullevaal, Oslo
Department of Medicine, Haukeland University Hospital and Institute of Internal Medicine, Section of Hematology, University of Bergen
Norway

1. Introduction

Autologous stem cell transplantation (ASCT) is used for disease stabilization and improvement of performance status in patients with immunoglobulin light chain amyloidosis. This therapeutic strategy has a relatively high treatment-related mortality. Therefore the limited treatment efficiency (cure is not possible) versus the risk of severe toxicity must be considered in each individual patient. The treatment-related mortality (TRM) has been up to 24% (Jaccard et al., 2007) and even 70% in certain studies (Moreau et al., 1998), but mostly lower mortality is reported (Vesole et al., 2006). These differences are probably due to patient selection criteria because TRM seems, among the other factors, to be associated mainly with cardiac amyloidosis. However, two main questions need to be answered with regard to efficiency versus toxicity of ASCT in amyloidosis. Firstly, one would appraise ASCT to be an effective treatment also in patients with cardiac amyloidosis, and ASCT could be considered also for these patients if the risk of severe toxicity could be reduced. Secondly, it can be difficult to select patients without cardiac amyloidosis for ASCT due to some uncertainity in assessment of cardiac involvement.

Determination of cardiac involvement is routinely performed by echocardiography despite the fact that the sensitivity of echocardiography is limited. Endomyocardial biopsy provides more reliable diagnosis but is associated with 1-2% complications (Cooper et al., 2007; Yilmaz et al., 2010). Thus, increased safety for patients with cardiac involvement may also reduce the risk of severe toxicity for patients without detectable cardiac involvement.

Dimethyl sulfoxide (DMSO) is used for cryopreservation of the stem cell autografts and the amount of DMSO infused together with the transplant may probably contribute to the early TRM in patients with amyloidosis. Several reports have described fatal outcome of autograft infusion, especially in patients with cardiac amyloidosis (Saba et al., 1999; Zenhäusern et al., 2000). By reducing the amount of infused DMSO, it may be possible to reduce the risk of ASCT-associated mortality and thereby make this treatment available for additional patients. In this chapter we will review various strategies that can be used to reduce the amount of DMSO infused together with autologous stem cell grafts.

2. Autologous stem cell transplantation in primary systemic amyloidosis

Primary systemic amyloidosis (AL) is a serious disease with a short survival (12-18 months) when conventional treatment with melphalan and prednisone is given (Dispenzeri et al., 2001). Patients with manifest cardiac involvement, being the worst prognostic indicator (Dubrey et al., 1998), have even poorer prognosis and a shorter survival; 4-6 months. Cardiac involvement is seen approximately in 50% of patients and half of them have congestive heart failure (Eshaghian et al., 2007). Arrhythmias and/or heart failure are the most frequent reasons of death in these patients.

Autologous stem cell transplantation is performed for disease stabilization and improvement of performance status in eligible AL patients. However, this therapeutic strategy has a high TRM; 15% to 70%, depending mostly on the patient selection criteria; meaning multiorgan involvement and especially advanced cardiac amyloidosis (Skinner et al., 2004; Moreau et al., 1998). Considering that TRM is less than 4% for patients with multiple myeloma (Segeren et al., 2003), even the lowest reported 15% TRM is unacceptably high for AL pateints. Therefore, patient selection for transplantation is a key issue (Tichelli et al., 2008). Underdiagnosed cardiac involvement may also be assumed to be an underlying factor in the high early TRM. DMSO used for cryopreservation of the stem cell autografts, is a cardiotoxic agent, and when infused together with the transplant DMSO may contribute to the treatment-related toxicity in AL patients. Several case reports have described fatal outcome of autograft infusion, especially in patients with cardiac amyloidosis (Saba et al., 1999; Zenhäusern et al., 2000). Severe arrhythmias including atrial fibrillation are reported in the early stage of transplantation. Reduction of complications related to stem cell infusion may be achieved by different strategies for decreasing the amount of DMSO in the infused autologous stem cell grafts, since DMSO reduction may in turn promote/endorse improvement of early phase survival in AL patients.

3. Cardiac involvement in primary amyloidosis

Cardiac involvement is quite often in AL amyloidosis, occurring in up to 63 percent of the patients (Merlini et al., 2008). Symptoms are related to the localization and the degree of the amyloid accumulation in the heart. Since cardiac involvement that may result in congestive heart failure is rapidly fatal, it is important to realize the condition and choose the right treatment option as soon as possible.

Assessment of heart involvement is mostly made by evaluation of the clinical symptoms, electrocardiography (ECG), detection of biomarkers N terminal Pro brain natriuretic peptide (NT-proBNP) and troponins, scintigraphy, echocardiography, magnetic resonance imaging (MRI) and/or endomyocardial biopsy. Except for the latter method all the assessments are non-invasive. Low voltage, arrhythmias and conduction abnormalities may be found in ECG (Eshaghian et al., 2007). The biomarkers are sensitive markers of heart damage, but they are not specific for damage caused by amyloid light chains. NT-proBNP was reported to be very valuable in diagnosis of ventricular dysfunction (Krishnaswamy et al., 2001), in assessing prognosis of heart failure and after myocardial infarction (Palladini et al., 2003). In one study, NT-proBNP appeared to be more sensitive than conventional echocardiographic parameters in detecting clinical improvement or worsening of amyloid cardiomyopathy during follow-up, meaning that NT-proBNP is a powerful prognostic determinant in AL amyloidosis (Palladini et al., 2003) and not necessarily diagnostic. However, as mentioned above high values of NT-ProBNP and cardiac troponins are seen also in other cardiac diseases like coronary artery disease and atrial fibrillation. NT-ProBNP is elevated as a

result of left ventricular dysfunction in congestive heart failure. On the other hand, a normal NT-ProBNP can be used to eliminate myocardial amyloidosis.
Scintigraphy with various tracers has some value in diagnosis; either with technetium 99 m-pyrophosphate to differentiate AL amyloidosis from other transthyretin-associated amyloidosis or with I^{123}-labeled serum amyloid P (Hazenberg et al., 2006). Increased interventricular septum thickness and "granular sparkling" of the myocardium at echocardiography is helpful but not specific and sensitive enough. Increased myocardial echogenity and valve-thickening are also frequent findings by echocardiography (Dubrey et al., 1998). Late gadolinium enhancement-cardiac MRI may detect early cardiac abnormalities in patients with amyloidosis with normal left ventricular thickness (Syed et al., 2010).
Finally, demonstration of amyloidosis by endomyocardial biopsy confirms the diagnosis in a patient whose echocardiography shows a mean left ventricular wall thickness more than 12 mm, when no other cardiac cause can be identified (Gertz et al., 2004). Tissue biopsies from other organs than the heart, showing amyloid deposits are not diagnostic for cardiac amyloidosis (Eshaghian et al., 2007). On the other hand, the endomyocardial biopsy being a diagnostic, yet invasive method may be associated with complications like bleeding, arrhythmias, thrombosis, infection, injury to the recurrent laryngeal nerve, heart block, injury to the vein/artery of the catheterization, pneumothorax and tricuspid regurgitation due to damage to the valve. Another seldom complication can be the rupture of the heart with pericardial tamponade (Cooper et al., 2007; Yilmaz et al., 2010). Complication rates vary between 0.6 and 6 percent (Cooper et al., 2007; Yilmaz et al.; 2010), and the frequency of the complications depends on various factors including the experience of the operator, clinical status of the patient, and presence or absence of left bundle-branch block (Cooper et al.; 2007).

4. Adverse effects related to stem cell infusion

In allogeneic stem cell transplantation setting, allografts harvested from healthy donors are usually infused to patients freshly. Autologous stem cell grafts, however, must be cryopreserved because of the time needed for in vitro quality controls (e.g. aerobic and anaerobic bacterial cultures, CD34+ cell enumeration and/or colony-forming unit assays) of the grafts and administration of high-dose chemotherapy before stem cell infusion. Autografts are commonly stored in nitrogen tanks at minus 160-180°C after controlled-rate freezing either on the harvesting day or the day after. Various controlled-rate freezers provide gentle cooling by -1 to -2°C/min to about -40 to -50°C, thereafter -5 to -10°C/min to about -80 to -90°C/min. At this point some centres transfer the bags to nitrogen tanks for storage, others continue the controlled-rate freezing until the temperature is equivalent to the nitrogen containers'. Despite the fact that liquid phase of nitrogen provides more stable temperature for storage, higher risk of contamination from other bags is documented and vapor phase appears consequently to be safer (Fountain et al.; Tedder et al., 1995). Cryoprotectants prevent intracellular formation of ice crystals that can damage cellular structures, and are therefore added to autografts before freezing (Szmant, 1975). The most commonly used cryoprotectant is DMSO, which is associated with well-known adverse effects during and shortly after autograft infusion, corresponding to the early transplantation stage. Besides DMSO itself, the adverse effects can also be due to DMSO-induced histamine release, and cell debris/lysis products released by graft white blood cells (WBCs) (Calmels et al., 2007; Milone et al., 2007; Saur-Heilborn et al., 2004). The frequency and severity of the adverse effects seems to increase with the amount of infused DMSO (Halle et al. 2001; Stroncek et al., 1991; Zambelli et al. 1998), a high number of granulocytes in the autograft (Cordoba et al., 2007), and a high patient age (Milone et al., 2007). Mild adverse reactions like transient nausea, vomiting, headache, flushing, chest tightness, hypotension, bradycardia, and abdominal cramps are common (Alessandrino et al., 1999; Donmez et al., 2007; Zambelli et al. 1998), whereas serious reactions like hypertension, arrhythmias, cardiac arrest, anaphylaxis, respiratory arrest, multiorgan failure, and neurologic complications are rare (Bauwens et al., 2005; Chen-Plotkin et al., 2007; Nishihara et al., 1996; Hentschke et al., 2006). The risk of DMSO-associated fatal complications, however, is increased for certain diseases, for example, primary amyloidosis (Benekli et al., 2000; Saba et al., 1999; Zenhäusern et al., 2000).

5. Reduction of infused DMSO

Infusion of lesser DMSO may improve the treatment-related mortality in primary amyloidosis patients, especially in the early transplantation period. There are several methods of reducing the amount of infused DMSO and consequently decreasing the risk of adverse effects in association with stem cell infusion:

5.1 Reduction of the autograft volume and increasing the cell concentration

Increasing the cell concentration in the autograft and thereby reducing both the autograft volume and the amount of DMSO needed for cryopreservation is a simple strategy (Cabezudo et al., 2000; Martin-Henao et al., 2005; Rowley et al., 1994). The final mononuclear cell concentration in the autografts varies between transplantation centers; the most common concentration being 2×10^8/mL (Windrum et al., 2005). Some centres use higher and some use lower concentrations (for example 1×10^8/mL), whilst others do not have any limits (Windrum et al., 2005). Several reports describe cryopreservation with high cell concentrations not resulting in additional loss of hematopoietic progenitor cell function, and not impairing the hematopoietic reconstitution (Cabezudo et al., 2000; Rowley et al., 1994), despite lower viability in samples with high concentration; 0.9 (range: 0.6-1) versus 2.9 (range: 2.2-4.7) $\times 10^8$/mL (Cabezudo et al., 2000).

Reduction of the autograft volume by centrifugation prior to cryopreservation of the stem cells, as we performed, results in lower autograft volumes that will consequently require reduced amounts of DMSO for cryopreservation (Akkok et al., 2009). Cell concentration before freezing was kept at minimum 2×10^8/mL in our study. We could therefore report low frequencies of side effects in our patients who also received DMSO-depleted autografts, since we followed a combination strategy with both volume reduction and DMSO-depletion procedure (the latter method will be explained detailed in 5.4) (Akkok et al., 2009).

5.2 Infusion of autografts over longer time

Infusion of autografts over longer time, if necessary several days (Martino et al., 1996), will reduce the daily DMSO exposure and limit the toxicity. The necessity is due to large volumes of the autografts to be returned to the patients. Patients in whom stem cell harvesting has to be performed in several subsequent days or patients who have to be re-mobilized usually have larger autograft volumes. Approximately 60% (57 out of 97 centres) of the European Group for Blood and Marrow Transplantation (EBMT) transplantation centres that replied a questionnaire, which was performed to assess current practice in the use of DMSO, had an upper limit in the amount of DMSO given per day varying between 20 to 80g (Windrum et al., 2005). Among the other centres the most frequently used limit was 1g/kg/day (33 out of 97 centres) or the centres did not have an upper limit of DMSO given per day.

Approximately one third of the centres preferred to return cells in split doses (Windrum et al., 2005). This study reveals the fact that there are no guidelines or agreement on the daily maximum dose of DMSO expected to be tolerated rather safely of the patients. In our study, when the total autograft volume exceeded 500 mL (i.e., total DMSO amount >50 mL for unmanipulated grafts), the stem cell infusion was divided into two separate sessions with at least a 2-hour interval or two subsequent days (Akkok et al., 2009).

5.3 Using DMSO concentrations lower than 10 percent

Using DMSO concentrations lower than 10 percent reduces complication rate (Akkok et al., 2009; Curcoy et al., 2002; Galmes et al., 2007; Windrum et al., 2005). There are only a few clinical studies where DMSO is used as the sole cryoprotectant at a 5 percent or lesser concentration (Akkok et al., 2009; Curcoy et al., 2002; Galmes et al. 1996, 2007). One other group used 3.5% DMSO, which is the lowest reported DMSO concentration in a clinical study but it was used in combination with 2.5% hydroxyethyl starch and followed by storage at -80°C (Halle et al., 2001). Galmés and colleagues, on the other hand, reported cryopreservation using only 5% DMSO and promptly hematopoietic engraftment as expected after short-time storage but slower hematopoietic recovery following long-time storage at -80°C (Galmes et al., 1996, 1999, 2007). Nevertheless, hematopoietic reconstitution was similar in both groups, when the patients were transplanted with more than 1.5×10^6/kg CD34+ cells (Galmes et al., 2007). In addition, they showed reduced infusion-related toxicity (19% versus 6.8%) compared to 10 % DMSO. However, the authors do not recommend storage of grafts at -80°C for longer than 6 months due to progressively diminishing viability of mononuclear cells (MNC) and recovery rates of colony-forming units; granulocyte-macrophage (CFU-GM) and burst-forming unit erythroid (BFU-E) reaching zero after 24 months, when grafts are cryopreserved with 5% DMSO (Galmes et al., 2007).

In a pediatric setting, Curcoy and colleagues reported successful engraftment after short time storage at -80°C by using only 5% DMSO (Curcoy et al., 2002). It was also illustrated by in vitro studies that the numbers of both total and viable CD34+ cells were higher, CD34+ cells were less apoptotic and necrotic plus early hematopoietic progenitor cells were better preserved with 5 compared to 10% DMSO (Abrahamsen et al., 2002, 2004). As we reported from our clinical study, autografts stored in nitrogen gave similar hematopoietic recovery with hematopoietic stem cells cryopreserved either using 5 or 10% DMSO (Akkok et al., 2008). These findings strongly suggest that cryopreservation of autologous stem cell grafts with 5 instead of 10% DMSO reduces the complication rate during stem cell infusion, without any adverse effect on time until hematopoietic reconstitution (Akkok et al., 2008; Games et al, 2007).

5.4 Washing autografts to remove DMSO

Washing autografts in order to remove as much DMSO as possible will also expectedly reduce the side effects associated with stem cell autograft infusion. However, there have been some conserns for this procedure based on the risk of CD34+ cell loss. Keeping this risk in mind, DMSO-depletion should be avoided when the CD34+ cell yield is barely 2×10^6/kg. Some of the studies where DMSO depletion was utilized, included a large group of patients without bone marrow disease and may not be representative for the present use of autologous peripheral blood stem cell transplantation for hematological malignancies with diffuse infiltration of malignant cells throughout the bone marrow (Calmels et al., 2003; Rodriguez et al., 2005). These preclinical studies investigated grafts of highly selected patients who relapsed or died before autotransplantation could be done (Calmels et al.,

2003; Rodriguez et al., 2005). Furthermore, Foïs et al. cryopreserved autografts with voluven + DMSO 10% and not DMSO alone, and they did not include detailed analyses of engraftment and transfusion. This makes it difficult to evaluate the impact of DMSO-depletion and compare with other studies (Foïs et al., 2007). Lemarie and colleagues used comprehensive automated washing to reach more than 20-fold reduction of DMSO-levels, whereas Syme and coworkers investigated patients with solid tumors and used a relatively extensive manual DMSO depletion (Lemarie et al., 2005; Syme et al., 2004).

In the preclinical studies mentioned above (Calmels et al., 2003; Rodriguez et al., 2005), the researhers used a device; CytoMate™, to perform the washing procedure with phosphate buffered saline (PBS) plus 5% Dextran-40, 5% ACD-A and 1-5% human serum albumin (HSA). While Calmels et al. achieved more than 96% elimination of DMSO and a mean recovery of viable total cells, CD34+ cells and lymphocyte subsets above 60%, Rodriguez et al. reported 98% DMSO elimination and 103% CD34+ cell recovery. Foïs and co-authors used an automatic cell washer (COBE 2991) and diluted thawed autografts with a saline and acid citrate dextrose anticoagulant (ACD) solution. Washing procedure was repeated twice or three times before suspension in a glucose 5% solution (Foïs et al., 2007). Manual washing repeated three times was the method utilized by Syme and colleagues (Syme et al., 2004). They prepared a washing solution also with saline and citrate dextrose solution USP Formula A, and resuspended the final product again in the washing solution before infusion.

Rowley et al. initiated a post-thaw DMSO-reduction study, where autografts cryopreserved with only 10% DMSO were thawed and diluted with 10% dextran-40 and 5% HSA (Rowley et al., 1999). Stem cell components were thereafter centrifuged to remove DMSO and resuspended in dextran and HSA before infusion. However, they had to stop the study for safety reasons due to severe infusion-related toxicity. Even though acute renal failure is a seldom complication associated with dextran use, dextran should probably not be the first choice in AL amyloidosis patients (Boldt, 2010), in whom dextran side effects like anaphylaxis may also bring additional risk. One of our studies described elsewhere, analysed a simple, one-step manual method for DMSO-depletion (Akkok et al., 2009). We diluted thawed autografts with a washing solution prepared by adding acid citrate dextrose (ACD) in saline. Following centrifugation the supernatant was removed and the autograft was resuspended with ACD-saline solution before infusion. By this means we achieved at least 6-fold reduction in the amount of infused DMSO, and the recovery data were comparable to the previous studies with regard to recovery of MNC and CD34+ cells (81.9 and 77 percent, respectively) (Akkok et al., 2009).

In the above mentioned study, we demonstrated that time until neutrophil engraftment was not affected by the DMSO-depletion (Akkok et al., 2009). Only three other earlier studies have investigated effects of DMSO-depletion on hematopoietic reconstitution, (Fois et al., 2007; Lemarie et al., 2005; Syme et al., 2004) and two of them described comparable neutrophil engraftment following DMSO-removal (Lemarie et al., 2005; Syme et al., 2004). Syme and colleagues described 1 day shorter time until neutrophil engraftment for patients receiving DMSO-depleted grafts, but this difference reached only borderline significance (Syme et al., 2004). Thus, DMSO-depletion of stem cell grafts seems to have minimal effects on neutrophil engraftment.

The significantly prolonged time until platelet engraftment for our patients receiving DMSO-depleted grafts was associated with a predictable increase in the number of platelet transfusions (Akkok et al., 2009). Lemarie et al. also described a slightly increased time until platelet engraftment for their patients, but the difference did not reach statistical significance (Lemarie et al. Transfusion 2005). In contrast, Syme et al. could not detect any effect of

DMSO-depletion on platelet engraftment time or platelet transfusion requirements (Syme et al., 2004). Taken together these results suggest that DMSO-depletion has relatively minor effects on platelet reconstitution.
Finally, both our group and others have shown that washing out DMSO, either manually or with an automated device, is associated with fewer adverse effects (Akkok et al., 2009; Fois et al., 2007; Lemarie et al. Transfusion 2005). However, DMSO is probably not the only reason of adverse effects; factors like patient's age (i.e. the higher the age the higher the frequency of adverse effects) and the content of infused non-mononuclear cells >0.5 x 10(8)/kg have been reported, yet for non-cardiovascular adverse effects (Milone et al., 2007). Despite a significant reduction, both Lemarie et al. and Foïs et al. reported adverse effects in approximately 20 percent of patients after automated DMSO-depletion, which is very similar to our result (Akkok et al., 2009; Fois et al., 2007; Lemarie et al. Transfusion 2005). However, since the washing procedure will also reduce the number of neutrophils and the levels of a wide range of platelet- and leukocyte-derived soluble mediators (e.g. cytokines, soluble adhesion molecules, intracellular mediators), this reduction may also influence the frequencies of adverse events. It is important that DMSO-depletion procedures are effective; i.e. a meaningful DMSO-removal can be achieved, the procedure is not very time-consuming and will not result in critical CD34+ cell loss.

6. Conclusion

Autologous stem cell transplantation has an important place in the management of primary amyloidosis patients. However, treatment-related mortality is very high especially in patients with cardiac amyloidosis compared with other hematologic disorders. Therefore, this therapeutic option can only be offered to one fourth of the patients. It may be assumed that underdiagnosed cardiac involvement may bring an additional risk for this patient group. The role of DMSO (used for cryopreservation of the autografts) in early treatment-related mortality is undecided. Nevertheless, it is shown that reduction of DMSO before stem cell infusion reduces adverse effects without essential disturbance of hematopoietic reconstitution, we therefore recommend cryopreservation with 5% DMSO in addition to removal of DMSO before stem cell infusion, whenever patients with primary amyloidosis have adequate yield of CD34+ cells in their autografts.

7. References

Abrahamsen, J.F.; Bakken, A.M. & Bruserud, O. (2002). Cryopreserving human peripheral blood progenitor cells with 5-percent rather than 10-percent DMSO results in less apoptosis and necrosis in CD34+ cells. *Transfusion,* Dec;42(12):1573-80

Abrahamsen, J.F.; Rusten, L.; Bakken, A.M. & Bruserud, O. (2004). Better preservation of early hematopoietic progenitor cells when human peripheral blood progenitor cells are cryopreserved with 5 percent dimethylsulfoxide instead of 10 percent dimethylsulfoxide. *Transfusion,* May;44(5):785-9

Akkök, Ç.A.; Liseth, K.; Nesthus, I.; Løkeland, T.; Tefre, K., Bruserud, Ø. & Abrahamsen, J.F. (2008). Autologous peripheral blood progenitor cells cryopreserved with 5 and 10% DMSO alone give comparable hematopoietic reconstitution after transplantation. *Transfusion,* May;48(5):877-83

Akkök, C.A., Holte, M.R., Tangen, J.M., Ostenstad, B., Bruserud, O. (2009). Hematopoietic engraftment of dimethyl sulfoxide-depleted autologous peripheral blood progenitor cells. (2009). *Transfusion,* Feb;49(2):354-61

Benekli, M.; Anderson, B.; Wentling, D.; Bernstein, S.; Czuczman, M. & McCarthy, P. (2000). Severe respiratory depression after dimethylsulphoxide-containing autologous stem cell infusion in a patient with AL amyloidosis. *Bone Marrow Transplant,* 25:1299-301

Boldt, J. (2010). Safety of nonblood plasma substitutes: less frequently discussed issues. *Eur J Anaesthesiol,* Jun;27(6):495-500

Cabezudo, E.; Dalmases, C.; Ruz, M.; Sanchez, J.A.; Torrico, C.; Sola, C.; Querol, S. & García, J. (2000). Leukapheresis components may be cryopreserved at high cell concentrations without additional loss of HPC function. *Transfusion,* 40:1223-7

Calmels, B.; Houze, P.; Hengesse, J.C.; Ducrot, T.; Malenfant, C. & Chabannon C. (2003). Preclinical evaluation of an automated closed fluid management device: Cytomate, for washing out DMSO from hematopoietic stem cell grafts after thawing. *Bone Marrow Transplant,* May;31(9):823-8

Cooper, L.T.; Baughman, K.L.; Feldman, A.M.; Frustaci, A.; Jessup, M.; Kuhl, U.; Levine, G.N.; Narula, J.; Starling, R.C.; Towbin, J. & Virmani, R. (2007). American Heart Association, American College of Cardiology, European Society of Cardiology. The role of endomyocardial biopsy in the management of cardiovascular disease: a scientific statement from the American Heart Association, the American College of Cardiology, and the European Society of Cardiology. *Circulation,* 116(19):2216-33

Curcoy, A.I.; Alcorta, I.; Estella, J.; Rives, S.; Toll, T. & Tuset, E. (2002). Cryopreservation of HPCs with high cell concentration in 5-percent DMSO for transplantation to children. *Transfusion,* Jul 42(7):962

Dispenzieri, A.; Lacy, M.Q.; Kyle, R.A.; Therneau, T.M.; Larson, D.R.; Rajkumar, S.V.; Fonseca, R.; Greipp, P.R.; Witzig, T.E.; Lust, J.A. & Gertz, M.A. (2001). Eligibility for hematopoietic stem-cell transplantation for primary systemic amyloidosis is a favorable prognostic factor for survival. *J Clinical Oncology,* 19:3350-56

Dubrey, S.W.; Cha, K.; Anderson, J.; Chamarthi, B.; Reisinger, J.; Skinner, M. & Falk R.H. (1998). The clinical features of immunoglobulin light-chain (AL) amyloidosis with heart involvement. *QJM,* Feb;91(2):141-57

Eshaghian, S.; Kaul, S. & Shah, P.K. (2007). Cardiac amyloidosis: new insights into diagnosis and management. *Rev Cardiovasc Med,* Fall;8(4):189-99

Fois, E.; Desmartin, M.; Benhamida, S.; Xavier, F.; Vanneaux, V.; Rea, D.; Fermand, J.P.; Arnulf, B.; Mounier, N.; Ertault, M.; Lotz, J.P.; Galicier, L.; Raffoux, L.; Benbunan, M.; Marolleau, J.P.; Larghero, J. (2007). Recovery, viability and clinical toxicity of thawed and washed haematopoietic progenitor cells: analysis of 952 autologous peripheral blood stem cell transplantations. *Bone Marrow Transplant,* 40:831–835

Fountain, D.; Ralston, M.; Higgins, N.; Gorlin, J.B.; Uhl, L.; Wheeler, C.; Antin, J.H.; Churchill, W.H. & Benjamin, R.J. (1997). Liquid nitrogen freezers: a potential source of microbial contamination of hematopoietic stem cell components. *Transfusion,* 37:585-91

Galmes, A.; Besalduch, J.; Bargay, J.; Matamoros. N.; Duran, M.A.; Morey, M.; Alvarez, F. & Mascaro, M. (1996). Cryopreservation of hematopoietic progenitor cells with 5-percent dimethyl sulfoxide at -80 degrees C without rate-controlled freezing. *Transfusion,* Sep;36(9):794-7

Galmes, A.; Besalduch, J.; Bargay, J.; Novo, A.; Morey, M.; Guerra, J.M. & Duran, M.A. (1999). Long-term storage at -80 degrees C of hematopoietic progenitor cells with 5-percent dimethyl sulfoxide as the sole cryoprotectant. *Transfusion,* Jan;39(1):70-3

Galmes, A.; Gutierrez, A.; Sampol, A.; Canaro, M.; Morey, M.; Iglesias, J.; Matamoros, N.; Duran, M.A.; Novo, A.; Bea, M.D.; et al. (2007). Long-term hematological reconstitution and clinical evaluation of autologous peripheral blood stem cell transplantation after cryopreservation of cells with 5% and 10% dimethylsulfoxide at -80 degrees C in a mechanical freezer. *Haematologica*, Jul;92(7):986-9

Gertz, M.A. & Zeldenrust, S.R. (2009). Treatment of Immunoglobulin Light Chain Amyloidosis. *Curr Hematol Malig Rep*, 4:91–8

Halle, P.; Tournilhac, O.; Knopinska-Posluszny, W.; Kanold, J.; Gembara, P.; Boiret, N.; Rapatel, C; Berger, M.; Travade, P.; Angielski, S.; Bonhomme, J. & Deméocq, F. (2001). Uncontrolled-rate freezing and storage at -80 degrees C, with only 3.5-percent DMSO in cryoprotective solution for 109 autologous peripheral blood progenitor cell transplantations. *Transfusion*, May;41(5):667-73

Hazenberg, B.P.; van Rijswijk, M.H.; Piers, D.A.; Lub-de Hooge, M.N.; Vellenga, E.; Haagsma, E.B.; Hawkins, P.N. & Jager, P.L. (2006). Diagnostic performance of 123I-labeled serum amyloid P component scintigraphy in patients with amyloidosis. *Am J Med*, Apr;119(4):355.e15-24

Jaccard, A.; Moreau, P.; Leblond, V.; Leleu, X.; Benboubker, L.; Hermine, O.; Recher, C.; Asli, B.; Lioure, B.; Royer, B.; Jardin, F.; Bridoux, F.; Grosbois, B.; Jaubert, J.; Piette, J.C.; Ronco, P.; Quet, F.; Cogne, M.; Fermand, J.P.; Myélome Autogreffe (MAG) and Intergroupe Francophone du Myélome (IFM) Intergroup. (2007). High-dose melphalan versus melphalan plus dexamethasone for AL amyloidosis. *N Engl J Med*, 357: 1083–93

Lemarie, C.; Calmels, B.; Malenfant, C.; Arneodo, V.; Blaise, D.; Viret, F.; Bouabdallah, R.; Ladaique, P.; Viens, P. & Chabannon C. (2005). Clinical experience with the delivery of thawed and washed autologous blood cells, with an automated closed fluid management device: CytoMate. *Transfusion*, May;45(5):737-42

Martin-Henao, G.A.; Torrico, C.; Azqueta, C.; Amill, B.; Querol, S. & Garcia, J. (2005). Cryopreservation of hematopoietic progenitor cells from apheresis at high cell concentrations does not impair the hematopoietic recovery after transplantation. *Transfusion*, 45:1917-24

Martino, M.; Morabito, F.; Messina, G.; Irrera, G.; Pucci, G. & Iacopino P. (1996). Fractionated infusions of cryopreserved stem cells may prevent DMSO-induced major cardiac complications in graft recipients. *Haematologica*, 81:59-61

Merlini, G. & Palladini, G. (2008). Amyloidosis: is a cure possible? *Annals of Oncology*, Jun;19 Suppl 4:iv63-6

Milone, G.; Mercurio, S.; Strano, A.; Leotta, S.; Pinto, V.; Battiato, K.; Coppoletta, S.; Murgano, P.; Farsaci, B.; Privitera, A. & Giustolisi, R. (2007). Adverse events after infusions of cryopreserved hematopoietic stem cells depend on non-mononuclear cells in the infused suspension and patient age. *Cytotherapy*, 9:348-55

Moreau, P.; Leblond, V.; Bourquelot, P.; Facon, T.; Huynh, A.; Caillot, D.; Hermine, O.; Attal, M.; Hamidou, M.; Nedellec, G.; Ferrant, A.; Audhuy, B.; Bataille, R.; Milpied ,N. & Harousseau, J.L. (1998). Prognostic factors for survival and response after high-dose therapy and autologous stem cell transplantation in systemic AL amyloidosis: a report on 21 patients. *Br J Haematol*, 101: 766–769

Palladini, G. & Merlini, G. (2009). Current treatment of AL amyloidosis. *Haematologica*, Aug; 94(8):1044-8

Rodriguez, L.; Velasco, B.; Garcia, J. & Martin-Henao, G.A. (2005). Evaluation of an automated cell processing device to reduce the dimethyl sulfoxide from hematopoietic grafts after thawing. *Transfusion*, Aug;45(8):1391-7

Rowley, S.D.; Bensinger, W.I.; Gooley, T.A. & Buckner, D. (1994). Effect of cell concentration on bone marrow and peripheral blood stem cell cryopreservation. *Blood*, 83:2731-6

Rowley, S.D.; Feng, Z.; Yadock, D.; Holmberg, L.; Macleod, B. & Heimfeld, S. (1999). Post-thaw removal of DMSO does not completely abrogate infusional toxicity or the need for pre-infusion histamine blockade. *Cytotherapy,* 1(6):439-46

Saba, N.; Sutton, D.M.; Ross, H.J.; Siu, S.; Crump, R.M.; Keating, A. & Stewart, A.K. (1999). High treatment-related mortality in cardiac amyloid patients undergoing autologous stem cell transplant. *Bone Marrow Transplant,* 24:853-5

Skinner, M.; Sanchorawala, V.; Seldin, D.C.; Dember, L.M.; Falk, R.H.; Berk, J.L.; Anderson, J.J.; O'Hara, C.; Finn, K.T.; Libbey, C.A.; Wiesman, J.; Quillen, K.; Swan, N. & Wright, D.G. (2004) High-dose melphalan and autologous stem-cell transplantation in patients with AL amyloidosis: an 8-year study. *Annals of Internal Medicine,* 140, 85–93

Segeren, C.M.; Sonneveld, P.; van der Holt, B.; Vellenga, E.; Croockewit A.J.; Verhoef, G.E.G.; Cornelissen, J.J.; Schaafsma, M.R.; van Oers, M.H.J.; Wijermans, P.W.; Fibbe, W.E.; Wittebol, S.; Schouten, H.C.; van Marwijk Kooy, M.; Biesma, D.H.; Baars, J.W.; Slater, R.; Monique M. C. Steijaert, M.M.C.; Buijt I & Lokhorst H.M. (2003). Overall and event-free survival are not improved by the use of myeloablative therapy following intensified chemotherapy in previously untreated patients with multiple myeloma: a prospective randomized phase 3 study. *Blood,* 101:2144-51

Syed, I.S.; Glockner, J.F.; Feng, D.; Araoz, P.A.; Martinez, M.W.; Edwards, W.D.; Gertz, M.A.; Dispenzieri, A.; Oh, J.K.; Bellavia, D.; Tajik, A.J. & Grogan M. (2010). Role of cardiac magnetic resonance imaging in the detection of cardiac amyloidosis. *JACC Cardiovasc Imaging,* Feb;3(2):155-64

Syme, R.; Bewick, M.; Stewart, D.; Porter, K.; Chadderton, T. & Gluck, S. (2004). The role of depletion of dimethyl sulfoxide before autografting: on hematologic recovery, side effects, and toxicity. *Biol Blood Marrow Transplant,* Feb;10(2):135-41

Szmant, H.H. (1975). Physical properties of dimethyl sulfoxide and its function in biological systems. *Ann N Y Acad Sci,* 243:20-3

Tedder, R.S.; Zuckerman, M.A.; Goldstone, A.H.; Hawkins, A.E.; Fielding, A.; Briggs, E.M.; Irwin, D.; Blair, S.; Gorman, A.M.; Patterson, K.G. et al. (1995). Hepatitis B transmission from contaminated cryopreservation tank. *Lancet,* 346:137-40

Tichelli, A.; Bhatia, S. & Socie, G. (2008). Cardiac and cardiovascular consequences after haematopoietic stem cell transplantation. *British Journal of Haematology,* 142:11–26

Vesole, D.H.; Perez, W.S.; Akasheh, M.; Boudreau, C.; Reece, D.E. & Bredeson C.N. (2006) High-dose therapy and autologous hematopoietic stem cell transplantation for patients with primary systemic amyloidosis: a Center for International Blood and Marrow Transplant Research Study. *Mayo Clin Proc,* 81: 880–888

Windrum, P.; Morris, T.C.; Drake, M.B.; Niederwieser, D. & Ruutu, T. (2005). EBMT Chronic Leukaemia Working Party Complications Subcommittee. Variation in dimethyl sulfoxide use in stem cell transplantation: a survey of EBMT centres. *Bone Marrow Transplant,* 36:601-3

Yilmaz, A.; Kindermann, I.; Kindermann, M.; Mahfoud, F.; Ukena, C.; Athanasiadis, A.; Hill, S.; Mahrholdt, H.; Voehringer, M.; Schieber, M.; Klingel, K.; Kandolf, R.; Böhm, M. & Sechtem, U. (2010) Comparative evaluation of left and right ventricular endomyocardial biopsy: differences in complication rate and diagnostic performance. *Circulation,* 122(9):900-9

Zenhäusern, R.; Tobler, A.; Leoncini, L.; Hess, O.M. & Ferrari, P. (2000). Fatal cardiac arrhythmia after infusion of dimethyl sulfoxide-cryopreserved hematopoietic stem cells in a patient with severe primary cardiac amyloidosis and endstage renal failure. *Ann Hematol,* 79:523-6